MEDICINE IN THE CRUSADES

This is the first book to be published on any aspect of medicine in the crusades. It will be of interest not only to scholars of the crusades specifically, but also to scholars of medieval Europe, the Byzantine world and the Islamic world. Focusing on injuries and their surgical treatment, Piers Mitchell considers medical practitioners, hospitals on battlefields and in towns, torture and mutilation, emergency and planned surgical procedures, bloodletting, analgesia and anaesthesia. He provides an assessment of the exchange of medical knowledge that took place between East and West in the crusades, and of the medical negligence legislation for which the kingdom of Jerusalem was famous. The book presents a radical reassessment of many outdated misconceptions concerning medicine in the crusades and the Frankish states of the Latin East.

PIERS MITCHELL is Research Fellow at the Wellcome Trust Centre for the History of Medicine at University College London and Honorary Lecturer at Imperial College London. He is the author of numerous articles on disease in the crusades.

MEDICINE IN THE CRUSADES

Warfare, Wounds and the Medieval Surgeon

PIERS D. MITCHELL

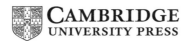

PUBLISHED BY THE PRESS SYNDICATE OF THE UNIVERSITY OF CAMBRIDGE
The Pitt Building, Trumpington Street, Cambridge, United Kingdom

CAMBRIDGE UNIVERSITY PRESS
The Edinburgh Building, Cambridge, CB2 2RU, UK
40 West 20th Street, New York, NY 10011–4211, USA
477 Williamstown Road, Port Melbourne, VIC 3207, Australia
Ruiz de Alarcón 13, 28014 Madrid, Spain
Dock House, The Waterfront, Cape Town 8001, South Africa

http://www.cambridge.org

First published 2004

Printed in the United Kingdom at the University Press, Cambridge

Typeface Adobe Garamond 11/12.5 pt.   *System* LATEX 2$_\varepsilon$ [TB]

A catalogue record for this book is available from the British Library

ISBN 0 521 84455 x hardback

Contents

Illustrations

Tables

Preface

It is rather unusual for someone normally labelled as an osteoarchaeologist to write on medical history. However, this multiskilling became necessary as a consequence of my palaeopathological research on crusader period excavations from the eastern Mediterranean. I was both surprised and frustrated to find that there was very little relevant historical work with which to compare my findings. In order to properly interpret the signs of a weapon injury or disease on a crusader skeleton a sound knowledge of contemporary history and medical practice is immensely helpful. As no one has yet undertaken the kind of historical work I was hoping to find, I ended up having to do it myself. This required exchanging my academic second home of Jerusalem for the Wellcome Centre for the History of Medicine at UCL in the University of London. In my time as a research fellow there I have benefited greatly from the expertise to be found within its walls. Over the years the evidence that accumulated became so large that instead of publishing just the one book covering all my findings, the work has had to be divided into several more manageable sections. A proportion of this has also formed my University of London doctoral thesis. I would like to thank those friends and colleagues who gave opinions on sections of this work or helped with certain translations, especially Vivian Nutton whose translation of Frankish medical legislation forms an invaluable section of the book.

The topics discussed here focus on weapon injuries and surgery, the fundamentals of military medicine. This is not only of interest to me as I am a practising trauma and orthopaedic surgeon, but also because for many people the crusades are synonymous with medieval warfare. I hope that these core topics, together with the range of complementary chapters, will give the reader a view of Frankish life that will both interest and provoke a change in the conventional opinion that many historians hold on the crusades and the Latin East.

Introduction

The crusades could be said to be the most fascinating events of the medieval world. The mass migration in sequential waves of tens of thousands of people from Europe to the eastern Mediterranean for such a disparate number of reasons created a complex and unique society. The armies were not just composed of trained soldiers but ranged from the nobility to paupers, clergy to criminals, businessmen to con artists.[1] For the many crusaders who might never even have ventured beyond the next village prior to their expedition the journey itself was a major challenge.[2] The overland and sea journeys could lead to malnutrition, frostbite, drowning and the potential for the spread of communicable conditions from fleas to tuberculosis. An individual with a culture and an immune system developed for cooler northern Europe might have been at considerable risk migrating to the Middle East. First, he would encounter new diseases to which he might have little immunity, such as the parasites dracunculiasis and schistosomiasis.[3] Moreover, a culture developed for a different region would have increased a crusader's risk of succumbing to conditions resulting from the different climate, such as heat stroke or food poisoning.

Soldiers involved in a long siege would have faced yet more dangers. While we would expect the risk of death or wounding from weapon injuries, the mere fact that siege conditions necessitated staying in the same place for so long significantly increased the risk of ill health from other causes. Dysentery was well described in the chronicles[4] and we would expect such gastrointestinal diseases to have resulted from contamination of drinking water supplies with human latrine waste. Fevers and epidemics were often mentioned by those recounting life in army encampments.[5] In many cases we will never know exactly which infections occurred in any particular

---

[1] Setton 1955–89; Mayer 1988; Riley-Smith 1991; Riley-Smith 1999a.   [2] Hamilton 1999.
[3] Adamson 1976; Adamson 1988.   [4] John of Joinville 1874 p. 6; John of Joinville 1955 p. 24.
[5] John of Joinville 1874 p. 164; John of Joinville 1955 p. 99; Richard de Templo 1864 p. 124; Richard de Templo 1997 p. 126.

epidemic, but there a number of possibilities. Malarial parasites have been found in Egyptian mummies[6] and this confirms their presence in the region well before the time of the crusades. Some Frankish written sources mention whether a fever was periodic in nature[7] and the time period at which the fever returns in malaria (quartan/tertian) is a classic sign of the disease. If an army was encamped close to marshes for a long period of time, we might expect a significant proportion of the troops to have been bitten by mosquitoes and run the risk of contracting malaria. Trachoma, also known in the past as ophthalmia, is an infection of the eyes which is spread by flies. It may have a protracted and chronic course which can end in blindness. Trachoma is also believed to have been present in the eastern Mediterranean well before the crusades and was probably endemic in ancient Egyptian times.[8] This disease was still debilitating in more recent military expeditions to the Levant in the nineteenth and twentieth centuries.[9] It is yet another condition that we would expect to have become endemic both in the soldiers who made up the crusading armies and also the settlers who decided to stay in the east after the military campaign came to a close. Scurvy is the nutritional deficiency that results from insufficient intake of vitamin C in the diet. While the loss of teeth is perhaps the best-known consequence in severe cases, an individual may die from spontaneous bleeding if the deficiency continues for long enough. Scurvy is clearly described in the troops of a number of Frankish sieges.[10] In a medieval army it must have been very difficult to maintain personal hygiene, eat an adequate diet or live a lifestyle that would have minimised the risk of contracting any one of the wide range of diseases that existed. In consequence thousands appear to have died from such diseases in the Latin East.

The First Crusade set out for Jerusalem in 1096 and the invaders established the kingdom of Jerusalem in the south, the county of Tripoli in the centre, with the principality of Antioch and county of Edessa in the north. The island of Cyprus was added to these Frankish states during the Third Crusade in 1189–92 (Figure 1). While the king was based in the city of Jerusalem in the twelfth century, after the loss of Frankish territory following the battle of Hattin in 1187 the monarchy moved to the coastal city of Acre. Nearly two hundred years after the initial conquest, the loss of Acre in 1291 effectively signalled the end of the mainland Frankish states, although Cyprus remained in Frankish hands. The scramble of individuals, military groups and religious organisations for land, power and royal

---

[6] Miller *et al.* 1994.   [7] *Assises de Jérusalem* 1843, 1, pp. 167–9.
[8] Feigenbaum 1957; Meyerhof 1936.   [9] Vetch 1807; MacCallan 1913 p. 2; Cornand 1979.
[10] Ambroise 1897 p. 114; Ambroise 1939 p. 65; John of Joinville 1874 p. 166; John of Joinville 1955 p. 100.

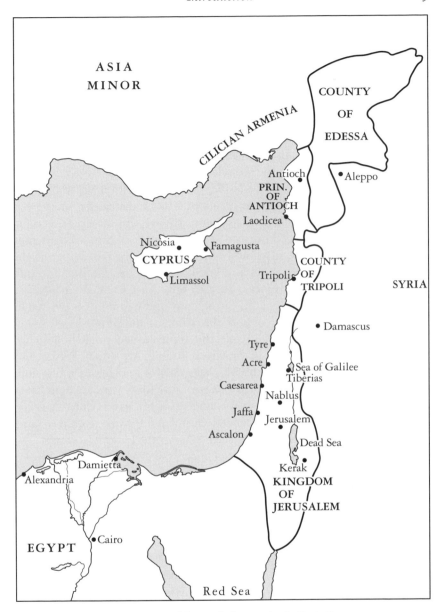

Figure 1. Map of the Frankish states in the Latin East
This map shows the important towns mentioned in the text. However, the borders
changed over time, so that the area covered by the Frankish states at any one instant would
not have been identical to that shown in this map.

favour with each conquest or defeat has made this period an intriguing one for the modern historian. The interaction between the crusaders and the local Christians, Jews and Muslims who lived under Frankish rule, and also relations with the neighbouring Christian territories of Armenia and Byzantium to the north and Muslim territory to the north-east, east and south of the Frankish states made the situation even more complex. Needless to say, this collision of cultures would be expected to have profound implications for diseases of all kinds as well as the efforts made by medical practitioners to treat their patients.

Medicine and disease in the crusades are topics that have interested historians for many years, as the number of articles written on the subject clearly demonstrates.[11] This interest appears to be increasing, as the last decade has seen more than twice as many articles published on this topic as the entire total produced prior to 1990. The work of Susan Edgington, Benjamin Kedar, Tony Luttrell and others has brought refreshing insight to particular aspects of crusader and Frankish medicine. Unlike the study of more recent medical advances, research into crusader medicine utilises archaeology and palaeopathology, cartography and manuscripts written in the many different languages of both the crusaders and those already living in the eastern Mediterranean. To do this topic justice would require an author proficient in medieval Latin, Greek, Arabic, Armenian, Persian and Syriac as well as the various vernacular languages of France, Italy, England, Germany and Spain. I have yet to meet an individual with such archaeological, medical and linguistic talents and probably never will. However, despite these limitations the evidence accumulated for this work is so large that only certain aspects of the medical history of the Latin East can be covered in this volume. I have chosen to concentrate on weapon injuries and their treatment since the battlefield is usually the first image that springs to mind when the crusades are considered. It was the *cyrurgicus*, the medieval surgeon, who would have treated such wounds. His practice included what in modern times is called military medicine. Associated topics that complement this core theme are also investigated, including injuries resulting from torture, the evidence for medical practitioners, hospitals, elective surgery, medical legislation and the exchange of medical knowledge between cultural groups thrown together by the crusades. Other equally fascinating areas such as malnutrition, epidemic disease, parasites, psychiatric illness, the crusaders' attitudes to disease, the role of religion and miracles in healing, the spread of disease with the crusades and the macabre methods

[11] Walsh 1919; Ell 1996; Ficarra 1996; Dolev 1996.

employed to transport the physical remains of the deceased back home are to be covered in a future work.

The subject area covered by the word 'surgery' in the medieval period is much larger than in modern times. With the exception of those suffering from a few notable diseases, it is usual for a modern surgeon to take on the care of a patient only when an operation is likely to be required. The medical treatment of a patient with drugs and other non-operative techniques is normally managed by physicians. At the time of the crusades, surgery covered all those diseases which might at some point need an operation as well as those conditions that were visible at the surface of the body.[12] That meant that the surgeon would still be required to be competent in the use of other treatments of the time such as dietary modification, drugs, blood-letting and bathing.[13] This explains the wide variety of conditions covered in the surgical texts of the twelfth to fourteenth centuries. From a modern surgical viewpoint we would expect to find sections on the treatment of weapon injuries, fractures, abscesses, bladder stones, haemorrhoids and anal fistulae. However, also included in the typical medieval *cyrurgia* would be a range of skin diseases such as leprosy, ascites (dropsy) and venereal diseases[14] which would normally be managed by modern physicians. For this study I have concentrated on the actual application of surgical techniques to illustrate the role of surgery in the crusades, rather than discussing all the evidence for the treatment of any disease found in the surgical texts of the time.

The sources that provide evidence for this project can broadly be divided into written texts and archaeological excavation. A large number of chronicles were written describing events during the crusades[15] and over forty have provided evidence for this study. Some were written by soldiers or clerics who participated in a particular crusade and recorded their journey, so that on their return they could tell those from their home town or monastery what the experience was really like. They often saw events from the perspective of their particular subgroup in the crusade, such as those from a particular region of Europe or those in the entourage of a certain noble. In consequence their version of events would tend to favour members of their own group and such accounts are prone to discrediting or gossiping about the activities of other sections of the army. This is especially the case when old rivalries already existed between the groups back in Europe. Many pilgrims travelling in peacetime also wrote of the route they took and

---

[12] Talbot 1967 pp. 88–124; McVaugh 1998b.   [13] Siraisi 1981 pp. 109–10; Hunt 1990.
[14] Theodorich Borgognoni 1498; Theodorich Borgognoni 1955–60.   [15] France and Zajac 1998.

noted the highlights along the way. While some were secular, a significant proportion of these accounts were written by clerics for the use of other clerics. However, despite being eye witnesses they were just as prone to memory lapses as any of us, and were sometimes fed incorrect information by ignorant guides.

Others who had never been to the Latin East used the oral testimony or written works of these eye witnesses to write works themselves, and these 'secondhand' chronicles have to be interpreted with appropriate caution. A number copied their battle scenes from classical works such as the *Aeneid* and consequently fabricated a great story – but one that is of limited use to the modern medical historian. There is evidence from Graeco-Roman times that such epics with a recreational as well as historical function often included fabricated examples of battle scenes to make the story more exciting[16] and it is possible that the same technique was used in the medieval period too. However, if such invented episodes were included then we would expect them to be at least plausible to the medieval listener and so still give some kind of a guide to contemporary medical practice where this is mentioned. Clearly the need to fabricate would have been much less likely in works by eye witnesses to events and in those accounts describing the experiences of well-known individuals to whom the author would have had access, in contrast to others who wrote of the crusades from a different place and time. However, cross-referencing with other chronicles may demonstrate that vivid and original descriptions in some chronicles written by those who stayed in Europe were probably based on the verbal eye witness accounts of others, and consequently are still a valuable source of information.[17] Even among the eye witness works there were plenty of sections copied from older sources.[18] Sometimes this was because certain areas were too unsafe for pilgrims to travel through to allow a firsthand report, while other sources were copied as they were regarded as infallible.[19]

Of course, the key elements of historiography, those of evidence and narrative structure, were approached by medieval readers and writers with rather different expectations from our own. A major purpose of recording history was to expose the divine will working through mankind, and the crusades were a classic example of this. Furthermore, many authors fail to provide us with evidence of a systematic or thorough effort on their part to find ways to detect mistaken or biased information. The concepts of trustworthiness and accuracy of information were not sufficiently

[16] Salazar 2000.   [17] Edgington 1998a; Gilo of Paris 1997 pp. xiii–xxiv.
[18] France 1998; Brefold 1994.   [19] Wilkinson, Hill and Ryan 1988 pp. 2–3.

distinguished, just as the difference between possibility and probability in the twelfth century was less marked than it is now. A number of issues recur in many medieval histories and chronicles. Where stories seem plausible to the author, but impossible or hard to corroborate, they were often included in the text. Authors were generally more tolerant of stories of miracles and wonders in foreign lands if they or their readers had never been there. Histories were often entertainment, and so needed to create imagery, not just record events. They were frequently written with a bias, such as for the cultural origins of the author, or to glorify a patron to whom a work was dedicated in order to advance the author's career. These texts may not have been written by someone with access to all the facts. A cleric acting as chaplain to a noble may have been ignorant of the activities of the foot-soldiers and other poor members of the crusade as he wrote, and perhaps have had to rely on court gossip. Many passages where the supposed words of individuals were written as a speech in these texts must be interpreted with great caution, as they were frequently made up by the author for literary effect. Those writing a history which covered many years, sometimes centuries, had to rely on the information in past texts. However, they nevertheless frequently embellished them with fabricated passages to improve readability, or allow reinterpretation of past history based on the issues of the day at the time of rewriting.[20] The medieval mindset was different from that of modern times, and we must view what was written then with this in mind.

Some Frankish settlers undertook histories of their own kingdom that often covered much longer time periods than the detailed, but short-term, coverage in the texts produced by the transient crusaders. The indigenous Christian communities that lived in areas covered by the Frankish states continued their own historical traditions and a few chronicles in Syriac and Armenian recorded life under the Latins. The Byzantines to the north were yet another source of texts, and they seemed to have a very complex relationship with the crusaders. They often intermarried and worked side by side with Frankish settlers in the early twelfth century, but at times fought against old enemies from Europe who also happened to have taken the cross. This animosity reached its peak with the Fourth Crusade that took Constantinople itself. The neighbouring Islamic states to the north, east and south of the Frankish states all contributed in the recording of historical events and some of this understandably addressed the interaction between themselves and these invaders from Europe, both when at war

---

[20] Partner 1977.

and in peacetime. However, Arabic sources are heavily underrepresented as publications available for the use of those interested in the crusades. This is partly because relatively few such texts have been edited and published at all (compared with Latin sources), and even fewer have been translated from Arabic into other languages which would further improve their accessibility.[21] Another possible reason is that the crusades were much less important to the Islamic world in the twelfth century than they were to Europe. The medieval Islamic world was so large that it seems that for most Muslim writers the crusades were no more than a remote frontier incident,[22] unworthy of much literary effort.

Medieval Arabic historiography has been divided by some into three groups in order to understand it more easily.[23] The first class of writing is chronography, and includes works and histories that follow events as they occurred over time. Examples of this kind that are used in this book are works by Ibn al-Furat and Ibn al-Athir. The second form of writing is biography, works that relate to the life of one person. Examples I have used here include those by Usama ibn Munqidh and Ibn Shaddad. Biographies and autobiographies were written for a range of reasons, just as today. Some were created to redress criticism of the author's life, others were narratives of conversion to Islam, some were entertainment, others spiritual guides, some were histories for the author's descendants and others still were just about a colourful character in history.[24] Many are not true biography as we would understand the concept today, but are really self-narratives, life representations or memoirs. In consequence, they may not be about the author's life as such, but rather concentrate on external events that took place around him. The third type of writing is prosography, and includes texts such as biographical dictionaries concentrating on specific social groups. One example used here is by Ibn Abi Usaybi'a. Arabic biographical dictionaries were first written about judges, jurists, mystics and Qur'an reciters.[25] However, by the tenth century AD most classes of people were covered by such dictionaries, even those whose contribution to Islam was more secular, as was the case for medical practitioners. Medieval Arabic historians were on the periphery of the academic establishment, as it was lawyers who were regarded as being of greatest importance. Most authors were historians part time, generating most of their wealth and social status from other professions. *Adab* literature was one style of writing that became popular as it required a combination of skills, attitudes and knowledge that

---

[21] Hillenbrand 1999 p. 9; Maalouf 1984; Atiya 1962 p. 2.   [22] Watt 1991 p. 81.
[23] Robinson 2003, pp. 55–79.   [24] Reynolds 2001 p. 89.   [25] Auchterlonie 1987 p. 2.

distinguished the author from a mere boorish ignoramus who chose to write. The function of the historian was to archive and entertain, but also to instruct and moralise. Historians attempted to teach rulers a lesson and to trigger their conscience, but they also legitimised ruling dynasties and reinforced traditional beliefs.[26] Consequently we must interpret medieval Arabic historical texts with this knowledge in mind.

One twelfth-century Islamic work has the potential to be extremely useful for its descriptions of medical practice in the Frankish kingdoms, but is also a classic example of the pitfalls of using any written source. Consequently it is worth briefly discussing this specific text. Usama ibn Munqidh claimed to have personally witnessed many battles and events in the era of the crusades, and he also claimed to be trained as a medical practitioner. His 'autobiography' is not an autobiography in the Western sense, where important or representative episodes are collected together to summarise the author's life. It instead belonged to the *adab* genre of Arabic literature, which aimed to instruct but also amuse and please its readers.[27] It was perfectly acceptable in this genre to stretch the truth to make a point and a number of the stories were probably stereotypes rather than actual incidents.[28] Consequently we are left in a dilemma. Do we take everything Usama wrote as truth, and know that we will be misled by some of his fictional stories? Do we discount everything he said and know that we are losing out on some fascinating events recorded by an eye witness? Do we try and differentiate the truth from the fiction, despite the fact that not even an *adab* expert would claim to get this right 100 per cent of the time? I am not an *adab* expert, nor an Islamic scholar. However, those who are do recognise the potential of using Usama, especially if we can see past the moral of each story and attempt to extract the more plausible information.[29]

This has left a wide range of very different chronicles, all written from different perspectives and with different hidden agendas. Some were written in the Latin East by eye witnesses but others were transcribed at a great distance from the events taking place, by those who could only base their work on the tales of others. While many were contemporary, a number were written decades after the event and some of the facts may have become blurred in the witnesses' minds or become modified with the hindsight of knowing how events would later unfold. Some were written in a factual manner, while others were created as a good story for the listener. This heterogeneity among the sources allows integration of the views from each perspective to perhaps enable a more balanced opinion to be constructed. However,

[26] Robinson 2003 pp. 187–8. [27] Conrad 1999. [28] Irwin 1998. [29] Hillenbrand 1999 p. 262.

the strengths and weaknesses of each source must also be considered before each sentence is accepted at face value.

As well as the chronicles, with their possibilities and pitfalls, there remains a wealth of other textual sources that contain relevant information. These include legal texts from the kingdom, letters written on campaign to relatives at home, the wills of those who were dying, the deeds of property sales in Frankish towns as well as the cartularies of military and religious orders. European sources include royal court records, papal bulls, academic medical texts and monastic histories of those countries that participated in the crusades. Clearly each of these has the potential to act as an indirect source of information with regard to crusader medical practice, although only a small proportion of each source will be relevant. The structured integration of information from such disparate sources is clearly fraught with difficulties but does greatly improve our knowledge of trauma and its medical treatment in the crusades.

Archaeological excavation has provided information both from the recovery of Frankish human skeletal remains and also of buildings and the bioarchaeological analysis of appropriate sites. Palaeopathological study of crusader cemeteries can provide clear proof for weapon injuries and many diseases that leave their mark on bone. The excavation of hospitals helps us to visualise the locations where written sources confirm that medical treatment took place. Study of pharmacy jars can show which medicines were in use, how they were traded around the Mediterranean and, if found in large numbers, may identify the location of an apothecary's shop. Medical equipment and surgical instruments also help us to visualise medical practice and confirm the use of particular medical treatments in the past. Bioarchaeological analysis of soil samples from Frankish sites provides evidence such as animal bone fragments, parasitic intestinal worm eggs, pollen and seeds. This kind of information can help us to understand what types of food were eaten, what medicines may have been used, and standards of hygiene. Frankish sites discussed include cities such as Acre, Caesarea, Jerusalem and Nablus, and also fortifications such as Belmont Castle, Le Petit Gérin, Jacob's Ford, Paphos and the Red Tower.

This integration of the textual and archaeological evidence is employed here as much as possible, to draw conclusions that each specialism alone could not substantiate. I hope that the subsequent discussions will improve our modern understanding of how effectively the crusaders and Frankish settlers coped with the considerable challenges associated with life in the time of the crusades.

CHAPTER I

Medical practitioners in the Frankish states

In the course of the 200-year history of the Frankish states it is likely that several hundred thousand people travelled from Europe to the eastern Mediterranean. Among them it would not be surprising if many hundreds, if not thousands, would have been medical practitioners. Even if we disregard those whose primary reason for the journey was a pilgrimage to Jerusalem rather than to practise their trade, we are still left with a significant number. Many had no choice but to go, since it was their duty to accompany their local nobility when they participated in a crusade. Others appear to have been under contract with their city authorities to attend the wounded from that town when the army was in action. Others still may have gone east for a fresh start or just to make money, as so many other Europeans did, whether they were soldiers, farmers or prostitutes.

While there are many references in contemporary chronicles to the activities of doctors in the Latin East, there has been very little work on named individuals other than Wickersheimer's preliminary work fifty years ago.[1] It seems that on the whole the records have mainly preserved details of the most prestigious individuals, which is not too surprising. This group was typically well educated, often having studied medicine at renowned centres of learning such as Salerno, Montpellier, Paris, Bologna or Padua.[2] Several years' study of the liberal arts (grammar, rhetoric, logic, arithmetic, astronomy, geometry and music) gained them the title master/*magister*, and a further period concentrating on the theory as well as the practical application of medicine completed their medical credentials. However, in the following discussion those masters should not be regarded as representative of the larger group of crusading medical practitioners as a whole. It is likely that many of these latter would be less well educated, often learning their trade by apprenticeship rather than at a university.[3]

---

[1] Wickersheimer 1951.   [2] Bayon 1953; Morris 1992; Siraisi 1994a.   [3] O'Boyle 1994.

Fortunately, terms used to describe practitioners in the medieval period often enable us to distinguish the various grades of competence in both the practice and theory of medicine, although the meanings did change over time.[4] The broad terms *medicus/miege/mire* were commonly used to designate doctors in the medieval period. They would take a history and examine the patient's pulse and urine[5] and then prescribe alterations to the diet, drugs and bloodletting as required. Many also practised surgery and treated wounds. Some of them held the title of master, having had an academic training at a centre of learning. In examples from the Frankish states a number of doctors referred to by the Latin term *medicus* were masters, but interestingly none of those referred to by the French terms *miege/mire* were. Sometimes the word *mire* took on a much broader meaning and was used for any medical practitioner, including a barber, apothecary or folk healer. *Physicus/fisicien*[6] designated a doctor with a high level of theoretical knowledge of natural science and medicine, together with study of the liberal arts at university. The majority of these *physici* at the time of the crusades seem to have been clergy.

The *cyrurgicus* was a surgeon, a term which only became common in the thirteenth century although it did exist before that. Surgeons are widely thought to have been less well educated than *physici* and were looked down on by some physicians, who saw surgery as a manual trade. While surgery was usually taught via the apprenticeship method in the twelfth and early thirteenth centuries,[7] by the end of the thirteenth century it was a subject studied at universities in southern Europe.[8] A number of surgeons who probably went on crusade, or who settled in the Latin East, had the title of master (see tables 1.1 and 1.2). Their job was more hands on than that of the *physicus* (so they were sometimes termed *practici*) since they would bandage or suture wounds, manipulate fractures and operate with a range of surgical instruments. The *barberus/rasorius* was poorly educated and tended to learn his trade as an apprenticeship. Barbers could perform bloodletting, some minor surgical procedures, wound care in battle and shaving. The *minutor/phlebotomus/sanguinator* was also poorly educated and only able to bloodlet. He could treat on the instructions of a doctor or be approached directly by a patient. Sometimes such practitioners were waged employees of a hospital. Both the barber and bloodletter became more common in the thirteenth century as there was a decline in the amount of bloodletting performed by doctors themselves. The *apothecarius/herbolarius/spicer*

---

[4] Jacquart 1981.   [5] McVaugh 1997; Wallis 2000.   [6] Bylebyl 1990.   [7] McVaugh 2000.
[8] Sigerist 1943; Bullough 1960; Siraisi 1973 pp. 165–71; Siraisi 1981 pp. 51–2 and pp. 108–10.

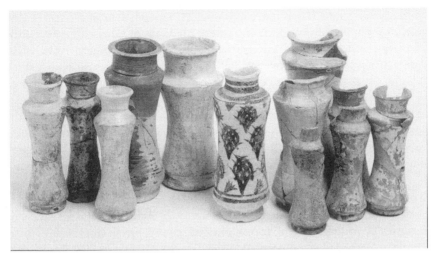

Figure 2. Pharmacy jars excavated from thirteenth-century Acre
Reproduced with the permission of the Israel Museum, Jerusalem.

would prepare drugs on the instruction of a doctor, but would also sell direct to patients who came to him for help. Again, the apothecary became more common in the thirteenth century as doctors prepared fewer and fewer drugs themselves.[9] While apothecaries are less likely to be mentioned in written sources than the better educated *medici* and *physici*, they certainly did exist throughout the Latin East. There are references to apothecary shops in the larger towns such as Antioch, Tyre and Famagusta.[10] A collection of Albarello jars of a shape typically used for the storage of drugs has also been excavated from a thirteenth-century building at Acre (Figure 2)[11] and such evidence confirms the presence of apothecaries. A good example of the different titles for medical practitioners can be seen in the infirmary of the Hospital of St John of Jerusalem in the 1180s. Statutes of the order dating from 1184–5 show that four *medici* and four *chirurgici* were employed there.[12] Other manuscripts from the same time refer to the four general doctors as *mieges* and state that a *fisicien* was employed to look after the weakest patients.[13] *Minutores* were also hired to bleed patients on the instructions of the doctors.

[9] Trease 1959; Matthews 1967.
[10] Marsilio Zorzi 1991 p. 140; *Le Cartulaire du Saint-Sépulchre* 1984 p. 177; Lamberto de Sambuceto 1883 pp. 67 and 78.
[11] Stern 1999. [12] *Cartulaire Général* 1894–1906, I, p. 458, cart. 690.
[13] Edgington 1998b; Kedar 1998.

Medieval Spain has often been seen as a parallel to the Latin East, since the populations of both areas were made up of Christians, Jews and Muslims, and both were intermittently in a state of religious war, with military confrontation between Christian states and neighbouring Muslim regions. The structure of medical practitioners in Spain may, therefore, be of interest when investigating the profession in the Frankish states. It seems that Jews and Muslims practised there alongside Christians[14] and that both Jews and Christians treated the Aragonese royal family in the early fourteenth century.[15] At the end of the thirteenth century, the king of Aragon employed a personal physician (*fisicus*), an apothecary, at least two barbers and also three surgeons who lived away from court and attended the king when summoned.[16] In times of crusade, when Christian states were at war with neighbouring Muslim kingdoms, there are also records of the medical facilities provided. A number of named surgeons, physicians, barbers and apothecaries have been identified at the siege of Almeria in Granada under King James II of Aragon in 1310. Arnold of Villanova also wrote a short medical work on advice on health in the king's army for this campaign and covered matters such as the healthiest place to site the army camp, how to check if water was safe to drink, the importance of burying the dead quickly in mass graves and how to treat those with weapon injuries.[17]

There has been much confusion in modern times as to the past attitudes of the church on the role of clergy in medicine. In the twelfth century the practice of medicine appears to have been permitted to everyone, but in the Council of Tours in 1163 it was forbidden for clergy in religious orders to leave their monasteries and abbeys to study medicine or law in a secular environment.[18] It was not medicine itself that was the problem but the period to be spent away from the religious environment that caused the objection. The secular clergy, who lived with the general population anyway, could still study medicine without controversy and the regular clergy could do so within the confines of an appropriate religious establishment. In 1215 canon 18 of the Fourth Lateran Council forbad certain clergy (subdeacons, deacons and priests) in religious orders from practising surgery involving incisions or cautery[19] as this was believed to preclude them from saying mass. This did not apply to those clergy in minor orders (such as porters, acolytes, exorcists and lectors) or the secular clergy and these two groups actually made up the majority of clerics. Similarly, there was no prohibition against anyone practising aspects of surgery where no tissue damage was

---

[14] Garcia-Ballester 1987; Garcia-Ballester 1994.   [15] McVaugh 1994.   [16] McVaugh 1993 pp. 6–7.
[17] McVaugh 1992.   [18] *Sacrorum Conciliorum* 1776, XXI, col. 1179, canon 8.
[19] *Disciplinary Decrees* 1937 p. 258, canon 18.

caused by the technique employed, such as setting broken bones or treating wounds with poultices. The old quote of *ecclesia abhorret a sanguine* (the church abhors the shedding of blood) appears never to have come from a medieval document,[20] despite its inclusion in almost all medical history books.

Medical practitioners' income in Europe varied greatly depending on their occupation, training, academic knowledge and employer.[21] The best paid were the physicians in royal courts who received a regular salary from the king. Often they would be given lucrative ecclesiastical appointments on their retirement from court.[22] Next came the royal court surgeons who earned a little less but still became very rich. Payment may have been in money of account, or the rights to the income from an estate or other source. Other benefits such as expensive clothing are commonly recorded in the manuscripts. Lesser educated practitioners such as barbers were also often salaried in royal courts, and these earned correspondingly less. Outside the system of patronage practitioners had to rely on fees for service, rather than a fixed retainer. Clergy who were qualified in medicine would have received regular income from their clerical duties and some accepted intermittent fees for treating the sick, although they were not supposed to do so.[23] Practitioners outside the clergy who worked with the general population, such as surgeons and barbers, typically worked just on a fee-for-service basis. It was often thought best to fix the fee when patients were at their most unwell as they would then agree to a higher price.[24]

While there does not appear to have been much specific regulation of doctors travelling on a crusade, once the fighting had stopped and peace returned the laws of the Frankish states came into force. A commentary on the laws of the kingdom of Jerusalem which specifically cover medical licensing, clinical practice and negligence was the *Assises de la Cour des Bourgeois*.[25] This is thought to have been collected together in its final form around 1240–4 in Acre, but some sections significantly predate this time.[26] These have been translated in the medical legislation chapter in this volume, where further discussion of the laws can be found. A further function of the surgeon is shown in another collection of thirteenth-century legal documents, the *Assises de la Haute-Cour*.[27] In the *Livre de Jean d'Ibelin* in this collection it is shown that those Franks in the Latin East who claimed to be too ill to attend court had to undergo medical examination

---

[20] Talbot 1967 p. 55.   [21] Hammond 1960; Rawcliffe 1988.   [22] Rawcliffe 2000.
[23] Getz 1998 pp. 6–7; Rawcliffe 1988.   [24] Jarcho 1944.
[25] *Assises de Jerusalem* 1839, I, docs. 231 and 233; Grandclaude 1923.
[26] Prawer 1951.   [27] *Assises de Jerusalem* 1841, I, pp. 338–40; Brittain 1966.

to confirm if this was true. This was to ensure that people did not fake illness to avoid their responsibilities. If the problem was a weapon injury or surgical problem then a *selorgien* was required to inspect it. A *fisicien* or *miege* was sent to assess pulse and urine if the complaint was medical. These doctors would then report back and confirm whether or not the excuse was reasonable.

A number of Latin practitioners were mentioned as witnesses in legal documents from the crusades. Some of these were written in the confusion of the army camp, where it might be expected that anyone academically trained would have been asked to witness documents. However, many documents were drawn up in optimal conditions, such as a major city in times of peace, and it has been proposed that it may have been normal for doctors to act in a legal capacity.[28] While a small proportion were described in the texts as a *notarius* (professional draughtsman of legal documents), most are not. The legal role of doctors in the Latin East is an interesting one. Many are noted just once in the records, which might suggest that they were just passing through on a crusade or pilgrimage to Jerusalem. Others are mentioned in documents dated a number of years apart which might suggest that a doctor had actually settled in the area.

Some medical practitioners are known to have definitely gone on crusade by references to their actual presence. They may have witnessed a charter drawn up in a Frankish city, been referred to in a document or included in a contemporary historical work describing the crusade in which they took part. Some doctors wrote medical works in their later life and actually described diseases or treatments which they mention encountering on crusade when they were younger. Others can be considered as very likely to have gone on crusade if there are records showing that they were in the service of a particular king or nobleman both before and after a crusade in which that noble is known to have taken part. Supportive evidence for these cases may sometimes be found in the form of records of papal indulgences or protection for the nobleman's estate while he was abroad. It is well accepted that the name of a noble on a list of those who took the cross did not guarantee his participation on a crusade, as some later changed their minds and bought their way out of their obligation with a donation to the church. However, doctors in the service of a noble would not have been in a position to do this, so that if their patron is known to have gone east then we can be reasonably certain that the doctor did too.

[28] Brundage 1993.

For others there may be less definite evidence for their involvement in the crusades, but sufficient circumstantial information to make it possible or even probable. A record from within a year or two of a crusade, which showed a doctor to be in the service of a noble who is known to have gone east makes such a case possible. Any noble with a doctor in his service would have been bound to include him in his crusading entourage and would not really have left the doctor any choice but to go. It is, of course, possible that the doctor mentioned may have died or retired from service just before the crusade or alternatively just started working for the noble after his return from crusade. In view of this, there will always be some element of doubt as to the participation of practitioners with this less definite, circumstantial evidence in the records and so the evidence must be used with a little caution.

The following individuals have been arranged according to their country of origin. Those who do appear to have worked in the Latin East are discussed in detail, while those possible cases are listed in table 1.1 to avoid the chapter becoming too unwieldy. Within each group they are discussed in chronological order to highlight the evolution of the medical profession over the 200-year period in which the mainland Frankish states existed.

FRENCH PRACTITIONERS

The most frequent country of origin for medical practitioners who went on crusade seems to have been France. This is not too surprising as France was the major crusading nation in the medieval period and French culture was dominant within the Frankish states themselves. While the evidence for named practitioners is fairly detailed from the 1180s onwards, there are frustratingly few examples for the early years. However, we do know that medical treatment was taking place at this time (see chapter 5). In consequence, it seems most likely that the paucity of named practitioners is merely a reflection of the nature of the early sources which have survived, and of the linguistic style of crusading authors in the early twelfth century. The earliest reference to a doctor yet encountered is for the *medicus* Geffroi, who came from Nantes. He was witness to the will of Count Herbert of Thouars drawn up on 28 May 1102 at Jaffa.[29] Count Herbert had heard that his brother had died (although this was not in fact the case), took the news rather badly and subsequently become seriously ill.

---

[29] *Cartulaires du Bas-Poitou* 1877 pp. xv and 7–8; Wickersheimer 1936 p. 177.

Eudes de Champagne (Odo Campanus) was a French astrologer who lived in the second half of the twelfth century. He made a journey to Jaffa at the end of the twelfth century and refers to this in his book *Libellus de Efficatia Artis Astrologice*, which he is believed to have written some time between 1192 and 1202. This text itself appears to have been lost but large sections of it are quoted in the work of another French astrologer named Helinand de Froidmont, who lived between c.1160 and c.1229. Helinand lived in a monastery near Beauvais and it was there he wrote his *Chronica*, also known as the *Disputatio Contra Mathematicos*, around 1210–16.[30] It has been suggested[31] that Eudes de Champagne travelled in the entourage of Count Henry of Champagne when he travelled east in 1190 to join the Third Crusade, later ruling the kingdom of Jerusalem between 1192 and 1197.[32] In the *Libellus* Eudes covers various aspects of astrology, including his beliefs regarding the effect of the planets on the development and birth of the foetus. He thought that each stage of pregnancy was governed by the planets and other heavenly bodies. Saturn governed the first month, Jupiter the second, Mars the third, the sun the fourth, Venus the fifth, Mercury the sixth and the moon the seventh. In the last two months the effects of Jupiter and Saturn were thought responsible for preparing both the foetus and the mother's uterus for the birth. In view of passages such as this it has been suggested that Eudes may have been a doctor as well as astrologer.[33] Many physicians of the twelfth century also studied astrology,[34] so this is quite a plausible hypothesis. It was widely believed that bloodletting should be avoided during certain phases of the moon[35] and some doctors used the location of the planets in determining the prognosis of a sick patient.[36] However, Eudes is never actually referred to as a *medicus* or *physicus* or given the title *magister*, so it is possible that he was primarily an astrologer who also happened to have studied some medicine.

Magister Bertrandus and *Magister* Petrus Maurinus were *physici* present in Acre in 1221. They were witnesses to the will of Count Henry I of Rodez (1214–27), dated 18 October, which was written as he lay sick in the house of the Hospitallers.[37] Master Bertrand was described as a *notarius* as well as a *physicus*. One possibility was that they were in the service of the count of

---

[30] Eudes de Champagne 1974.   [31] D'Alverny 1967.
[32] Continuation of William of Tyre 1982 pp. 143 and 193; Continuation of William of Tyre 1996 pp. 2, 47 and 168.
[33] Malewicz 1974.   [34] French 1994.   [35] Voigts and McVaugh 1984.
[36] *Aggregationes* 1991; Sigerist 1942.
[37] *Documents Historiques* 1900 p. 19; Wickersheimer 1936 p. 649.

Rodez and they had survived the disastrous Fifth Crusade. This set out in 1217 for Egypt and surrendered to the Egyptian sultan in 1221, after which most of the forces who were allowed to go free headed to Acre to recover from their ordeal.[38] Another option to consider is that they may have been *physici* already in Acre, perhaps employed in the Hospital of St John for sick poor or working on a fee-for-service basis in the town and called in for an opinion as such an important noble was in the hospital. Interestingly, a master Petrus was described in 1226 as *medicus* to Princess Isabelle, daughter of John of Brienne.[39] John had become king of Jerusalem in 1210 when he married Queen Mary and after she died in 1212 he continued as regent to his daughter Isabel until 1225. Since the two documents mentioning master Petrus are dated so close together, it is interesting to speculate as to whether they may be referring to the same individual.

Hersende was a female physician to King Louis IX who went with him on crusade to Egypt in 1248–50. She is referred to, along with her wages of 12 Parisian deniers per day, in a document drawn up at Acre, dated August 1250.[40] The army travelled from Damietta to Acre in the spring of 1250 after its release from captivity by the Egyptian commander, which explains Hersende's presence there at that time. An educated female physician was unusual in the thirteenth century[41] and it was especially extraordinary for her to be so well respected that she should become personal physician to one of the major kings in Europe. Her position and the title *magistre* Hersende, *physica* suggest she may have had a university education. In the 1250s she married an apothecary named Jacques and they set up house in Paris.[42] Her marriage shows that she did not belong to a religious order, as many male physicians did at that time.

Other physicians from the Seventh Crusade include Robert de Duaco.[43] He was a *physicus* who went east with Louis IX to Egypt in 1249. He was a cleric from Douai who was also canon of Saint-Quentin and Senlis in the 1240s alongside his royal duties. Initially he was physician to Louis's wife Marguerite de Provence,[44] but by 1245 he was also physician to the king. Queen Marguerite went on the crusade with Louis but stayed in the coastal city of Damietta once it had been taken by the crusaders. Louis

[38] Oliver of Paderborn 1894; Oliver of Paderborn 1948; Minstrel of Reims 1876; Minstrel of Reims 1939.
[39] *Regesta Regni* 1893, 1, p. 256, doc. 975.   [40] Daumet 1918; Wickersheimer 1936 pp. 294–5.
[41] Green 1994; Talbot and Hammond 1965; Wickersheimer 1936; Jacquart 1979.
[42] *Archives de L'Hotel Dieu* 1894 pp. 534–5.   [43] Wickersheimer 1936 pp. 709–10.
[44] Riolan 1651 p. 92; *Chartularum Universitatis* 1889, 1, pp. 372–5.

then moved inland with the troops and it appears that the royal medical staff split at that point. Master Robert stayed in Damietta with the queen[45] while other doctors travelled with the rest of the army to treat the sick and injured during the campaign. Robert de Duaco survived the crusade to die in France on 20 May 1258.[46]

Pierre de Soissons was surgeon to Louis IX and went with him on the crusade to Egypt in 1248. Pierre is referred to in a document written at Jaffa in August 1252,[47] where he was given an annual pension of 20 Parisian livres per year. Significantly, he was not given the title of 'master' as the king's physicians were, which might suggest that he was less educated than them. He is the first crusading doctor so far identified in the texts who was referred to specifically as a surgeon. Up until the middle of the thirteenth century it appears that many doctors would have performed all the tasks which were later to be divided between the physician and surgeon.

Two physicians known to have participated in the crusade of 1270 were master Dude de Laon and master Martin. Master Dude came from Laon in northern France and was *physicus* and cleric to the king. He accompanied Louis IX to Tunis in north Africa, on what was to be the king's last crusade.[48] Dude treated Louis when he became unwell with dysentery but despite his best efforts, the king died, along with large numbers of the army.[49] Master Martin (described as *domini regis phisicus*) was another physician who accompanied Louis to Tunis in the summer of 1270.[50] Martin is mentioned in a letter written at Tunis from Pierre de Condé to Mathieu de Vendôme, dated 21 August 1270.[51]

Pierre de la Broce was one of three surgeons working for King Louis around the time of the 1270 crusade. Pierre had been *cyrurgicus* to Louis from 1261, when he first arrived at court.[52] At this point he was paid a basic salary of 2 sous per day plus clothing allowance and other benefits, but this increased by 6 deniers when the king was at court.[53] Pierre was married with a family, so clearly was not a cleric. He was given the post of chamberlain in 1266[54] and then went on crusade with the king to Tunis in 1270. After Louis died there he worked for his son Philippe III 'le Hardi', who was also present on the crusade. Pierre is mentioned in a document of Philippe III in Tunis dated September 1270.[55]

---

[45] Berthaud 1907.   [46] *Obituaires* 1902 p. 744.
[47] *Layettes de Trésor* 1875, III, p. 166, doc. 4022; Wickersheimer 1936 p. 662.
[48] Richard 1992 p. 325.   [49] *De Vita et Actibus* 1840 p. 39; Wickersheimer 1936 pp. 123–4.
[50] Wickersheimer 1936 p. 539.   [51] Delisle 1890 p. 75; Brachet 1903 p. 402.
[52] Baudouin d'Avensnes 1855 pp. 180–1.   [53] Chereau 1862.
[54] Guillaume de Nangis 1840 pp. 494–5.   [55] Langlois 1887 p. 15.

A considerable number of English doctors also participated in the crusades. It is theoretically possible that some may have trained at Oxford and Cambridge universities, as they both appear to have started to teach medicine by the thirteenth century.[56] However, there is no firm evidence that any of the practitioners discussed below trained at either of these institutions. It is therefore more likely that most either went to European universities or spent a number of years as apprentices to established local practitioners.

Gilbertus Anglicus (de Aquila) was perhaps the most famous English doctor from the time of the crusades.[57] He was a cleric who had become physician to the king of England by 1207.[58] His best-known work is the *Compendium Medicine*, written about 1240,[59] but he also wrote a *Commentary* on the *De Urinis* by Giles de Corbeil.[60] The *Compendium Medicine* covers surgical topics such as the management of wounds, fractures and many operations along with medical topics such as fevers, venereal disease and dietetics.[61] It is very likely that Gilbertus Anglicus went to the Latin East at some stage as his *Compendium Medicine* includes mention of his treatment of Bertram, a son of Hugh of Jubail (Gibelet) in the county of Tripoli. Bertram suffered with an ophthalmic condition, and apparently Gilbertus healed his eyes using an ointment when local Muslim and Syrian Christian doctors had been unable to help him.[62] It could be argued that Bertram may actually have come to Europe for treatment rather than Gilbertus travelling to the Frankish states. If this was in fact the case, the treatment would have happened somewhere in southern Europe at a port such as Salerno or Montpellier. Unfortunately, it is not known for sure where Gilbertus spent most of his life or if he ever went to Salerno or Montpellier. However, if Gilbertus did in fact travel to the Latin East then perhaps the most likely time for him to have gone was with the large English contingent accompanying King Richard I on the Third Crusade in 1189–92.

It is quite possible that Gilbertus went east in the service of either Hubert Walter, who was bishop of Salisbury at the time, or Earl Robert III of Leicester. In 1205, once Hubert Walter had become the archbishop of Canterbury, records show that Gilbertus Anglicus was his physician,[63] so it is possible that Gilbertus was also in his service the decade before. Bishop

---

[56] Bullough 1961; Bullough 1962b; Getz 1995.   [57] Talbot and Hammond 1965 pp. 58–60.
[58] *Monasticon Anglicanum* 1830, VI, pt 2, p. 1026.   [59] Getz 1991.   [60] Russel 1936.
[61] Handerson 1918.   [62] Gilbertus Anglicus 1510 fol. 137a.   [63] *Index Britanniae* 1902 p. 91.

Hubert landed at Tyre in 1189, survived the heavy losses at the siege of Acre and stayed with the army until the truce with Saladin.[64] Hubert had soldiers under his command and there are records of their injuries which would have needed medical attention, such as when the right hand of a certain Everard was cut off near Acre in August 1191.[65] Earl Robert III of Leicester also went on the Third Crusade and was a close companion of King Richard I. A charter (witnessed by Hubert Walter) confirmed the receipt of 100 shillings by Gilbertus from Robert of Leicester for his homage and service[66] and *magister* Gilbertus was witness to some of the earl's charters too.[67] As Robert only became earl in 1189 and he died in 1204, the charter must date from this period. Although Bishop Hubert and Robert of Leicester are mentioned many times in the chronicles of the Third Crusade, no mention of a doctor or other specific members of their entourages is recorded. However, since we know he worked for both these crusaders shortly after their return, the evidence for Gilbertus Anglicus' involvement in the east with at least one is promising.

The mention of a specific father and son from the Latin East should in theory help with the dating of Gilbertus' crusade. However, it is unfortunate that both Hugh and Bertram were extremely common names in the noble family concerned, which makes a definitive identification of a specific Bertram difficult, and an attempted analysis rather complicated. The only Bertram of Jubail identified by Rey to have had a father named Hugh was Bertram II.[68] This Bertram took part in the Seventh Crusade to Egypt with King Louis IX and he eventually died in 1259. As Bertram II's grandfather (Bertram I) only married around 1186, Bertram II could not possibly have been alive at the time of the Third Crusade. In consequence we are left with two theories. The first is that Gilbertus Anglicus did not go on the Third Crusade at all, and therefore must have gone with the English contingent on the crusades of 1217 or 1227. This would be more compatible with the Bertram and Hugh evidence. However, the king of England did not participate in this crusade and by that time Gilbertus was in his entourage. It seems unlikely that he would have gone east in the circumstances. The second option is that Gilbertus just made a mistake when writing his book. He wrote this many years after the Third Crusade and his memory could easily have failed him. Perhaps he treated Hugh, son of Bertram (rather than Bertram son of Hugh as he wrote). If that was the case then this would be compatible with their meeting on the

---

[64] Richard de Templo 1864 p. 116; Richard de Templo 1997 p. 119.
[65] Richard de Templo 1864 p. 250; Richard de Templo 1997 p. 238.
[66] *Rotuli Chartarum* 1837, 1(1), p. 141.   [67] *Documents Illustrative* 1920 p. 243.   [68] Rey 1895.

Third Crusade after all. As Bertram I had married his wife Dolète in the mid-1180s it is quite possible that their son Hugh would have been born prior to the crusade. If Gilbertus mistakenly remembered the relationship between Hugh and Bertram as that of father and son when it was in fact that of grandfather and grandson or elder and younger brother, then Bertram I himself may have in fact been the patient. Both Bertram I's grandfather and his elder brother were called Hugh. Attempting to determine the timing of Gilbertus' trip to the east based on the reference to Hugh and Bertram is inconclusive and tantalising. However, the evidence as it stands may be most compatible with the participation of a young Gilbertus on the Third Crusade. Gilbertus Anglicus is thought to have died somewhere between 1240 and 1250.

Ralph Besace was a medical cleric in the service of Richard I (*phisicus regis Ricardi*) for whom there is independent evidence of his presence on the Third Crusade of 1189–92. Matthew Paris recounted how master Ralph was an eye witness to Saladin's execution of nobles by decapitation.[69] Apparently Ralph had been sent to Saladin's camp by King Richard as an embassy to bargain for their release. A large number of Frankish captives were beheaded by Saladin around this time as he was furious about the mass beheadings of the population of Acre ordered by King Richard after its capture by the armies the Third Crusade.[70] Master Ralph continued as the king's physician until Richard's death and later became canon of St Paul's cathedral in London.[71]

Master John of St Albans was the English *physicus* who treated King Philip Augustus of France while he was ill during the siege of Acre in 1191.[72] He is also known as Jean de Saint-Gilles and Johanne Anglicus.[73] The Continuation of William of Tyre mentions the treatment of Philip's illness during the siege. 'He fell seriously ill of a double tertian fever. The illness afflicted him so grievously that he nearly died . . . The doctors offered their advice and God gave him grace to recover from his illness.'[74] There has been much discussion as to exactly what the various forms of tertian fever were[75] and it thought likely that they were umbrella terms for a number of infectious diseases, including malaria. The reason that information on master John's crusade was mentioned in the *Historia Minor* of Matthew Paris (a history of England), despite his working for the French royal court,

---

[69] Matthew Paris [Madden] 1866, II, p. 37.   [70] Ibn Shaddad 2001 pp. 168–77.
[71] Matthew Paris [Luard] 1880, v, p. 220–1; Talbot and Hammond 1965 p. 263.
[72] Matthew Paris [Madden] 1866, II, p. 38.   [73] Talbot and Hammond 1965 p. 179.
[74] Continuation of William of Tyre 1982 p. 131; Continuation of William of Tyre 1996 pp. 108–9.
[75] Jarcho 1987.

was probably because that they were both clerics from the Abbey of St Albans.[76] It has been suggested that master John was on loan to Philip from King Richard, since John was English.[77] This seems very unlikely as the two kings Richard and Philip did not get on at all well. In fact, they only agreed to go on crusade on the condition that both went, since neither trusted the other to resist the temptation to invade if one of them headed east alone and left his country unprotected.[78] It seems that master John came into the service of King Philip by a more conventional route. There is no evidence for his study at Oxford,[79] as has been suggested,[80] but he did appear to have attended university at Paris and then Montpellier, where he studied medicine.[81] It was from there that he became royal physician and Montpellier would have been a logical place for the king of France to look for his medical staff, on account of its prestige. Master John was still in the service of King Philip in 1198, as he gave a house in Paris to the Jacobites for the use of pilgrims.[82]

Two English *medici* are known to have participated in the Fifth Crusade in 1218. Master Roger was not only a *medicus* but also parson of Kippax in Yorkshire.[83] He went on crusade to Egypt with John de Lascy, the constable of Chester, and witnessed a document of his at Damietta.[84] It is known that he returned home alive as he witnessed a number of other Pontefract charters, including one in 1239.[85] Thomas was a *medicus* who travelled with the entourage of William the earl of Arundel to Egypt in 1218–21.[86] The earl managed to survive the first two years of the ordeal, unlike much of the army, but then died in 1221. Thomas then succeeded in transporting William's corpse back home where it was buried, at Wymondham in Norfolk.[87] There is no record of quite how he managed this, as the body would have to have been preserved to avoid its decomposition in the heat. However, medical texts available at the time (such as that of al-Razi) did sometimes include passages on how to preserve bodies after death to allow just such a journey.[88] When King Baldwin I died during an expedition to Egypt in 1118 his abdominal organs were removed and he was salted and embalmed with balsam and spices.[89] However, by the time his body reached Jerusalem the corpse apparently smelt terrible. Likewise after Emperor Frederick of Germany drowned on crusade in Armenia in June 1190 he was embalmed so

[76] Matthew Paris [Madden] 1866, II, p. 38.   [77] Wickersheimer 1936 p. 476.
[78] Roger of Wendover 1886, I, pp. 173–4; Roger of Wendover 1994, II, pp. 87–8.
[79] Emden 1957, III, p. 1623.   [80] Berthaud 1907.   [81] Berthaud 1907.
[82] Matthew Paris [Madden] 1866, II, p. 66.   [83] Talbot and Hammond 1965 p. 307.
[84] *Chartulary of St John of Pontefract* 1899 pp. 36–7.
[85] *Chartulary of St John of Pontefract* 1899 p. 277.   [86] Talbot and Hammond 1965 p. 330.
[87] Matthew Paris [Luard] 1876, III, p. 67; *Gesta Abbatum* 1867, I, p. 275.
[88] Levey 1970.   [89] Albert of Aachen, in press, bk 12, ch. 28.

that the body could be taken to Antioch.[90] An alternative method popular in the thirteenth century was to boil the corpse so that the bones could be returned home while the soft tissues were buried at the place of death.[91] Thomas was clearly a cleric, as he was made prior of Wymondham in 1224.[92] This may have been a show of gratitude for his efforts to return the earl's remains. Thomas himself eventually died in 1248.[93]

A master John of Brideport is recorded as having gone on crusade with the army of Prince Edward of England in 1270. This master John is distinct from the physician of the same name who was in the service of King Richard I in 1190. Back in 1258 we first hear of John of Brideport as the physician of William of Valence, the earl of Pembroke and brother to King Henry III.[94] On 10 July 1270 master John is included in a list of English crusaders who were given protection for four years so that they could go to the eastern Mediterranean with Prince Edward.[95] As the earl of Pembroke is known to have gone on the crusade[96] it seems that master John was probably still in his service and therefore would have been attached to him. John de Brideport was clearly a cleric as he had become parson of the church of Axeminster by April 1277.[97] Master John died in February 1293.[98] Another doctor named master Robert de Murisien was also included in the list of crusaders with John of Brideport.[99] Robert was referred to as Prince Edward's physician in 1265 and also parson of South Kelsey church, near Lincoln.[100]

One English surgeon is of interest at the time of Prince Edward's crusade of 1270. Hugo Sauvage (*cyrurgicus*) is listed among crusaders heading east with Prince Edward.[101] He had been in the family service of King Henry III and Eleanor of Provençe and appears to have been seconded to Edward for the crusade.[102] Hugo is the only English doctor specifically referred to as a surgeon (as opposed to a *medicus*) to have been confidently identified so far as having gone on crusade. It is likely that he would have treated Edward for the stab wounds he received during the assassination attempt at Acre in 1272.[103]

ITALIAN PRACTITIONERS

The earliest example of an Italian involved with medicine in the Latin East was Stephen of Pisa. Stephen moved to Antioch in the early years of

---

[90] Continuation of William of Tyre 1982 p. 98; Continuation of William of Tyre 1996 p. 88.
[91] Brown 1981.   [92] *Monasticon Anglicanum* 1821, III, p. 326.
[93] Matthew Paris [Luard] 1882, VI, p. 278.   [94] *Calendar of Patent Rolls* 1908 p. 623.
[95] *Calendar of Patent Rolls* 1913 p. 480; Talbot and Hammond 1965 p. 126.
[96] Lloyd 1988 p. 140.   [97] *Calendar of Patent Rolls* 1901 p. 200.   [98] Emden 1957, I, p. 264.
[99] *Calendar of Patent Rolls* 1913 p. 480.   [100] Talbot and Hammond 1965 p. 289.
[101] Röhricht 1881.   [102] Lloyd 1988 app. 4.   [103] Templar of Tyre 2000 p. 140.

the Frankish states and became involved with the school of manuscript translation which developed there. Master Stephen described himself as a philosopher rather than a doctor, but clearly included medical knowledge as integral to the study of philosophy. It is thought that he was treasurer of the Benedictine monastery of St Paul in Antioch.[104] The most famous medical translation he made while at Antioch was the *Regalis Dispositio* (The Royal Arrangement) in 1127, which was a Latin translation of the tenth-century Arabic surgical text *kitab al-malaki* by al-Majusi. He also wrote a work on astronomy known as the *Liber Mamonis*.[105] These texts and the role of the translation centres in the Latin East in the spread of knowledge in the medieval world are discussed in more detail in a later chapter.

Among the Italian doctors who went on crusade, perhaps the most famous was master Hugo of Lucca. His fame results from the surgical text of Theodorich Borgognoni (c.1205–98), the bishop of Cervia.[106] Theodorich was one of Hugo's pupils and he repeatedly credits Hugo with the knowledge presented in the *Chirurgia*. In his introduction Theodorich mentioned that the text was written 'according to the system of medicine of the excellent Hugo of Lucca, a most expert man in the aforementioned science'.[107] Hugo was born around 1160 and between 1214 and 1219 is known to have been under contract with the city of Bologna to accompany the army in the field.[108] Hugo's contract of October 1214, paying him 600 Bolognese lire per year, appears to have been the earliest undisputed example in medieval Italy where a doctor was hired long term by a city to treat its population.[109] It is quite remarkable that a man of his age (about sixty) should remain in active military service at a time when he was well past the average life expectancy.[110] It is known that he went with the Bolognese troops on the Fifth Crusade, to Egypt, in 1218–21.[111] Hugo was witness to a document written at Damietta in 1220 where he is referred to as '*domino* Hugone Medico de Luca'.[112] It is likely that the practical tips on the surgical management of weapon injuries included in Theodorich's *Chirurgia* resulted at least in part from the experience Hugo gained when treating the injuries of the Bolognese soldiers. Hugo of Lucca is thought to have died in 1257,[113] aged well over ninety years old.

[104] Hunt 1950.   [105] Burnett 2000.   [106] Del Gaizo 1894.
[107] Theodorich Borgognoni 1498 p. 106r; Theodorich Borgognoni 1955, I, p. 3.
[108] *De Claris Archigymnasii* 1896, II, p. 14, doc. 3; Sistrunk 1993.
[109] Nutton 1979.   [110] Shahar 1993.
[111] See Oliver of Paderborn 1894; Oliver of Paderborn 1948; Minstrel of Reims 1876; Minstrel of Reims 1939.
[112] *De Claris Archigymnasii* 1896, II, p. 532.   [113] Vedrani 1921, I(2) pp. 312–20.

Master Roberto was another *medicus* attached to the Bolognese troops in Egypt. He is mentioned in many documents written at Damietta, especially in the summer of 1220.[114] He was to be paid 50 bezants (gold coins) in the first year of service and 100 bezants per year from then on. It is probable that he knew Hugo as they were both from Lucca, both contracted with the Bolognese troops at Damietta and sometimes both are mentioned in the same documents.[115]

Master Constantin was born at Labour near Scala, in the district of Salerno. He is known to have migrated to the Frankish states because he became *physicus* to Jean of Brienne, while he was king of Jerusalem. John had married Queen Mary of Jerusalem in 1210 and he ruled until 1225, the period from 1212 being as regent for his daughter Isabel since Mary had died. Constantin later moved north to join the service of the emperor of Byzantium. *Magister* Constantinus must have returned to France in his later life as he was buried at the church of Saint-Jean-en-Valée in France, following his death on 25 August 1250.[116]

OTHER EUROPEAN PRACTITIONERS

Other areas of Europe are not so well represented in the manuscripts with regards to evidence for crusading medical practitioners. The only Hungarian doctor so far identified is Alexander. He was a *physicus* mentioned in a Hungarian list of crusaders in the *Transilvaniae Praepositus*.[117] According to the *Historia Salonitana* of Thomas Spalatensis he arrived at Damietta in 1217,[118] but it is not clear if he survived the expedition.

Few Spanish doctors appear to have taken part in the crusades to the eastern Mediterranean as they were involved with their own holy war against the Muslims who held the southern part of the Iberian peninsula. However, one Catalan who did travel east was Ramon Lull. He was born in Palma, Majorca around 1232–5 and became a Franciscan monk. He spent much of his life preaching and writing on religious philosophy, producing over 300 works. There is no evidence that he ever treated a patient and he was never referred to as a *medicus* or *physicus*. However, he was sometimes given the title *magister* and he did spend time at the medical centre of Montpellier, subsequently writing texts on medicine, hygiene and physiology. His works include *Liber Principiorum Medicinae, Ars Compendiosa Medicinae, Liber de Regionibus Sanitatis et Infirmitatis, Liber Medicinae Magnae, Ars Operativa*

[114] *Annali Bolognesi* 1789, II(2), pp. 431–3, 442–3 and 447–8.
[115] *Studien* 1891 p. 70, no. 47.   [116] *Cartulaire de Notre-Dame* 1865, III, p. 160.
[117] *Studien* 1891 p. 80.   [118] *Testimonia Minora* 1882 p. 231.

Table 1.1 *Further medical practitioners who may possibly have participated in a crusade*

French practitioners

Master Pierre Lombard	Physician to King Louis VII of France in 1138. Louis went on 2nd Crusade 1147–8[a]
Caius Clodius Cervianus	Doctor to Queen Eleanor, the wife of Louis VII[b]
Master Gilles de Corbeil	Physician to King Philippe-Auguste of France from 1180 to 1223. Philippe went on 3rd Crusade, 1190–1[c]
Guillelmus de Migeio	A *miege* who took the cross in 1218, to join the 5th Crusade to Egypt[d]
Master Roger de Provins	*Physicus* to King Louis IX of France in 1256. Louis went on 7th Crusade and returned 1252[e]
Nicolas Germinet	*Physicus* in Louis IX's service in 1249, at the time when Louis was in Egypt[f]
Johannes barberus	Barber to Louis IX in 1261. Might have gone to Egypt in 1249–52, or Tunis in 1270[g]
Master Roger	Physician to King Philippe III 'le Hardi' of France in 1274. Philippe went on the 1270 crusade to Tunis[h]
Guillaume de Salu	Surgeon to Louis IX in 1261, and Philippe III in 1274. Might have gone to Tunis in 1270[i]
Master Jean de Betisy	Surgeon to Louis IX and Philippe III until 1288. Might have gone to Tunis in 1270[j]

English practitioners

Master John of Brideport	*Medicus* to King Richard I of England in 1190–93. Might have gone on 3rd Crusade to the Holy Land[k]
Joseph medicus	In service with Richard I in 1171–2 and 1190. Might have gone on 3rd Crusade[l]
Master Malger	*Medicus* in service with Richard in 1190s. Might have gone on 3rd Crusade[m]
Master William Fiscamp	Physician to King Henry III of England from 1263, granted protection for one year in 1271. Might have gone on 1270 crusade with Edward[n]
Master Simon de Preston	Surgeon to Henry III 1268–75. Might have gone on 1270 crusade with Edward[o]

Italian practitioners

Galvano de Levanto	Genoese *medicus* in service of Pope Boniface VIII. Wrote a crusade proposal in 1295 for King Philippe 'le Bel' of France[p]
Guido de Vigevano	Wrote text in 1335 for King Philippe VI of France, on how to stay healthy on a crusade[q]

[a] *Glossarium* 1733, I, p. 643; *Cartulaire de Notre-Dame* 1865, III, p. 25.
[b] Anon. 1750 p. 193.
[c] D'Irsay 1925; Rath 1964; O'Boyle 1998.
[d] *Studien* 1891 p. 112; Powell 1986 p. 224.
[e] Johannis Saraceni 1855 p. 360; Chereau 1862.
[f] Brocard 1877; Wickersheimer 1936 p. 570.
[g] Chereau 1862; Wickersheimer 1936 p. 344.
[h] Jacquart 1981 p. 476.

Medica and *Liber de Modo Applicandi Novam Logicam ad Scientiam Iuris et Medicine.*[119] Although many treatises on alchemy were attributed to him to gain them credibility, he appears to have been rescued from these associations during the twentieth century.[120] He travelled extensively throughout Europe and when he heard the rumour that the Tartars had defeated the Muslims in battle and were allowing free access to pilgrims to visit the Holy Places, he went east. He stayed in Cyprus in 1300 while it was the last of the Frankish lands left in Christian hands, lodging with the Templars. We know that at the time of his visit the *medicus* of the Templars' house at Famagusta was a master Theodorus,[121] but no record of any meeting has survived. In Famagusta Lull learnt that the Tartars had not overrun the mainland, as he had hoped. However, he did travel to the Christian kingdom of Armenia in 1301 and may then have taken the overland pilgrimage route to the Holy Places. He was back in Majorca again by 1302. In total he made three famous trips to Bugia and Tunis in north Africa to preach, in an attempt to convert the Muslims there.[122] Initially he was just thrown out of these cities but on the third occasion, in 1315, one version has it that he was stoned to death.[123]

A number of other Latin doctors are known to have gone to the Latin East but I have been unable to identify their country of origin. For example, Emfred (Aufredus) de Novo Castro was the doctor to Robert of Artois, the brother of King Louis IX of France. Emfred is said to have accompanied Robert on the Seventh Crusade[124] where the nobleman died in the battle of Mansourah in Egypt. However, the original source for this assertion remains unidentified.[125] Others are known solely as witnesses to legal documents

---

i Chereau 1862; Jacquart 1981 p. 446.
j Le Confesseur 1840 p. 65; Berthaud 1907.
k *Great Roll of the Pipe* 1925 p. 3; Talbot and Hammond 1965 pp. 125–6; Gervase of Canterbury 1879, I, p. 518; *Cartulary of Oseney* 1929, I, pp. 246–7.
l *Great Roll of the Pipe* 1894 p. 86; *Great Roll of the Pipe* 1844 p. 18; Talbot and Hammond 1965 p. 199.
m Ralph de Diceto 1876, II, p. 168; Talbot and Hammond 1965 pp. 206–7.
n *Calendar of Patent Rolls 1258–1266* 1910 p. 276; *Calendar of Patent Rolls* 1913 p. 576; Talbot and Hammond 1965 pp. 393–4.
o *Calendar of Patent Rolls* 1913, p. 249; *Calendar of Close Rolls* 1900 p. 247; Talbot and Hammond 1965 pp. 324–5.
p Galvano de Levanto 1898; Leclerq 1965.
q Leopold 2000 pp. 42–3; Wickersheimer 1951; Samaran 1981.

[119] Anon. 1885; Delisle 1896 pp. 342–55. [120] Singer 1928; Pereira 1989.
[121] Lamberto de Sambuceto [Polonio], 1982, doc. 148, pp. 170–1.
[122] *Acta Aragonensia* 1908, II, pp. 879–901. [123] Hillgarth 1971; Peers 1929.
[124] Chereau 1862. [125] Wickersheimer 1951.

drawn up in the Frankish states. Often their country of origin is not obvious from the document and it seems unwise to speculate unless more evidence comes to light. Those that are only mentioned over a short time period and then no longer appear in later records may well have just been temporarily in the east, either as pilgrims or on military expeditions. They were often educated *magistri*, which was probably why they were used in such a legal capacity. In 1195 *magister* Bernardus *medicus* witnessed a document written in Cyprus on 29 September.[126] *Magister* Adjutus *medicus* was signatory to a document of 12 October 1200 written in Acre in the palazzo of the Benedictine monastery of St Mary of the Latins.[127] *Magister* Guillelmus *medicus* is recorded in a document from Acre dated 18 December 1207.[128] *Magister* Matthaeus *physicus* was signatory to a document from Acre drawn up on 30 April 1242,[129] while *magister* Johannes *medicus* witnessed a document written in the order of St John in Acre on 20 August 1244.[130] Later still, in 1279 a *magister* Rollandus *medicus* is the subject of a short document[131] written on 30 October at Laodicea (Latakiya) in the principality of Antioch.

FRANKISH SETTLERS

Certain information in the records suggest that many European practitioners settled in the east. Some may have accompanied a crusade and decided to stay in the east, while others may have emigrated in peacetime in an attempt to make a better living. Sometimes we can tell this by reference to their presence in documents dated many years apart. Robertus *medicus* was a Latin doctor who lived in the Frankish states. He is known from the records of his purchase of a house in Jerusalem for 80 bezants in 1137[132] and he was involved in further property dealings in 1167.[133] *Magister* Lambertus *medicus* was signatory to a document of 1200 written in Acre at the headquarters of the order of St Mary Latina[134] and is again mentioned in 1207.[135] This shows that he was most probably living in the Latin East long term, and not just passing through on a pilgrimage or military expedition. Other individuals can be identified as settlers by their activities in these documents, even if only mentioned once. Willelmus was a *medicus* who was recorded as dealing in property in Antioch in 1137.[136] Clearly someone

[126] *Regesta Regni* 1893, I, p. 193, doc. 723.   [127] *Regesta Regni* 1893, I, p. 206, doc. 775.
[128] *Regesta Regni* 1893, I, p. 221, doc. 824.   [129] *Regesta Regni* 1893, I, p. 288, doc. 1106.
[130] *Regesta Regni* 1893, I, p. 299, doc. 1122.   [131] *Regesta Regni* 1893, I, p. 374, doc. 1434.
[132] *Les Archives de Saint-Jean* 1883 pp. 73–4.   [133] *Regesta Regni* 1893, I, p. 112, doc. 430–1.
[134] *Regesta Regni* 1893, I, p. 206, doc. 775.   [135] *Regesta Regni* 1893, I, p. 221, doc. 824.
[136] *Le Cartulaire du Saint-Sépulchre* 1984, I, pp. 174–5.

passing through on a crusade would rent rather than buy property, so this suggests that Willelmus was a Frankish settler.

A significant number of medical practitioners are referred to in the documents collected together in the Genoese notarial registers of Lamberto di Sambuceto in Cyprus from 1289 to 1302.[137] It is very illuminating that many of his documents are either about, or are witnessed by, medical practitioners. Unlike the records of the royal court or military orders, many of the witnesses are from less prestigious groups such as barbers and apothecaries, and only a limited number were master *medici* and *physici*. The fact that nearly thirty barbers and apothecaries were mentioned in documents from just one part of Cyprus over a fifteen-year period suggests that probably a large number of them were present in the entire Latin East before that time. It is likely that our ignorance of them before this time merely stems from a lack of the kind of documents likely to mention them. Their names show that some were born in Europe (often they are Genoese, Pisan or Venetian), but interestingly after 1291 some were Frankish settlers who escaped from Acre. Almost all of them show evidence of living in Cyprus and they were not just temporary visitors passing through. Many are recorded as witnesses year after year, and may have acted in this way for a living. Indeed one, Petrus, was the unusual combination of barber and also *notarius*. Some apothecaries are mentioned in the documents as selling drugs to each other.[138] Many others were referred to as inhabitants of Famagusta. Interestingly, the only master barber I have so far come across, named Johanes, lived in Cyprus in 1289. The details of all the practitioners have been summarised in table 1.2.

NON-FRANKISH PRACTITIONERS

The majority of medical practitioners for whom we have evidence of their presence in the crusades were from Europe. However, there were also a considerable number of other doctors who were either indigenous to the Frankish states or emigrated there from Persia or the Mediterranean to work. Christian groups included the Melkites who followed the Greek Orthodox liturgical rite, Jacobites who followed their own Syriac rite, Maronites from the county of Tripoli, Copts from Egypt, Nestorians from Persia and Armenians from the principality of Antioch and county of Edessa.[139] However, the practice of medicine in the Latin East was not restricted to Christians and there is evidence for the activities of Jewish and Muslim practitioners.

---

[137] Lamberto de Sambuceto [Desimoni] 1883.
[138] Lamberto [Pavoni] 1987, doc. 197, pp. 236–7.   [139] Prawer 1976; Pahlitzsch 2001.

Table 1.2 *Medical practitioners in Frankish Cyprus, from Lamberto di Sambuceto*

Barbers
Enricus de Fossato (1289)[a]
Master Johanes (1289)[c]
Michael de Gênes (1289)[e]
Nicolaus de Sexto (1289)[g]
Thomas de Branducio (1289)[i]
Columbus (1290)[k]
Obertus de Clavaro (1290–1302)[m]
Bernardus Pisanus (1300)[o]
Dante (1300)[q]
Iohanninus de Accon (1300)[s]
Leo (1300)[u]
Maceotus (1300)[w]
Petrus notarius (1300)[y]
Polus (1300)[z]
Raimondinus de Torano (1300)[aa]
Thomas de Messana (1301)[bb]
Linardus (1302)[cc]

Apothecaries
Ansaldus (1290)[b]
Larius (1290)[d]
Pastura (1290)[f]
Bonensegnus (1299)[h]
Berthosius Florentinus (1300–2)[j]
Anthonius (1300)[l]
Beiaminus (1300)[n]
Marinus Veneticus (1301)[p]
Guiotus (1301)[r]
Guirardus de Garibaldo (1301)[t]
Iachetus (1301)[v]
Homodeus (1302)[x]

Medici
Master Jacobus de Mediolano (1289)[dd]
Guillelmus (1289–90)[ff]
Thodarus (1296)[hh]
Master Theodorus (1300)[jj]
Georgius (1302)[ll]

Surgeons
Master Jacobus de Terdana (1289–90)[ee]
Master Guillelmus (1289)[gg]
Master Jacobus de Fossano (1299–1304)[ii]
Master Enricus de Rezo (1301–2)[kk]
Master Recoverus de Pergamo (1301)[mm]
Master Rogerius (1301)[nn]
Recuperatus de Pergamo (1301)[oo]

Physicians
Master Bonaventura (1290)[pp]
Master Thomas (1301)[qq]
Master Albertus de Crema (1301–2)[rr]
Iohanus de Novaira (1302)[ss]
Master Bonifacius (1302)[tt]

---

[a] Lamberto [Balard] 1973 p. 73, doc. 32.
[b] Lamberto [Balard] 1973 p. 308, doc. 771.
[c] Lamberto [Balard] 1973 p. 122, doc. 293.
[d] Lamberto [Balard] 1973 p. 308, doc. 771.
[e] Lamberto [Balard] 1973 p. 82, doc. 82.
[f] Lamberto [Balard] 1973 p. 297, doc. 749.
[g] Lamberto [Balard] 1973 p. 91, doc. 126.
[h] Lamberto [Balard] 1983 pp. 138–9, doc. 116.
[i] Lamberto [Balard] 1973 p. 118, doc. 269.
[j] Lamberto [Desimoni] 1883 p. 78, doc. 150; p. 99, doc. 190; Lamberto [Polonio] 1982 pp. 64–5, doc. 56; pp. 497–8, doc. 417; and many more in between.
[k] Lamberto [Balard] 1973 p. 267, doc. 694.

While we might expect such practitioners to cater for the needs of their own religious communities, there appears to have been fairly fluid movement of practitioners between communities with differing cultural and religious backgrounds. Some of the newly arrived crusaders continued to use the Frankish doctors who came with them from Europe, but others seem to have been keen to make use of these new practitioners. William of Tyre describes this in his history of the kingdom, but also shows how suspicious he himself was of the local doctors.

> Our eastern princes, through the influence of their women, scorn the medicines and practice of our Latin physicians and believe only in the Jews, Samaritans, Syrians and Saracens. Most recklessly they put themselves under the care of such practitioners and trust their lives to people who are ignorant of the science of medicine.[140]

[l] Lamberto [Polonio] 1982 p. 168, doc. 146.

[m] Lamberto [Balard] 1973 p. 189, doc. 497; Lamberto [Pavoni] 1987 pp. 322–3, doc. 271.

[n] Lamberto [Polonio] 1982 pp. 12–14, doc. 12.

[o] Lamberto [Desimoni] 1883 pp. 34–5, doc. 67.

[p] Lamberto [Polonio] 1982 pp. 451–2, doc. 376.

[q] Lamberto [Desimoni] 1883 p. 78, doc. 149.

[r] Lamberto [Pavoni] 1982 pp. 54–5, doc. 42.

[s] Lamberto [Desimoni] 1883 p. 79, doc. 153.

[t] Lamberto [Pavoni] 1982 pp. 88–9, doc. 66.

[u] Lamberto [Desimoni] 1883 p. 26, doc. 47.

[v] Lamberto [Pavoni] 1982 pp. 28–30, doc. 23.

[w] Lamberto [Desimoni] 1883 p. 79, doc. 153.

[x] Lamberto [Pavoni] 1987 pp. 236–7, doc. 197.

[y] Lamberto [Polonio] 1982 pp. 123–5, doc. 110.

[z] Lamberto [Polonio] 1982 p. 90, doc. 176.

[aa] Lamberto [Polonio] 1982 pp. 138–9, doc. 124.

[bb] Lamberto [Pavoni] 1982 pp. 126–7, doc. 126.

[cc] Lamberto [Pavoni] 1987 pp. 209–10, doc. 177.

[dd] Lamberto [Balard] 1973 p. 75, doc. 45.

[ee] Lamberto [Balard] 1973 p. 141, doc. 94; pp. 243–4, doc. 646.

[ff] Lamberto [Balard] 1973 p. 93, doc. 137; p. 264, doc. 687.

[gg] Lamberto [Balard] 1973 p. 111, doc. 234.

[hh] Lamberto [Balard] 1983 pp. 17–9, doc. 13.

[ii] Lamberto [Balard] 1983 pp. 143–4, doc. 120; Lamberto [Pavoni] 1982 pp. 162–3, doc. 128a.

[jj] Lamberto [Polonio] 1982 pp. 170–1, doc. 148.

[kk] Lamberto [Polonio] 1982 pp. 292–3, doc. 247; Lamberto [Pavoni] 1987 p. 287, doc. 239a.

[ll] Lamberto [Pavoni] 1987 pp. 111–12, doc. 85.

[mm] Lamberto [Polonio] 1982 pp. 250–1, doc. 214; pp. 260–1, doc. 222; p. 262, doc. 223.

[nn] Lamberto [Polonio] 1982 pp. 107–8, doc. 92; p. 230, doc. 195.

[oo] Lamberto [Polonio] 1982 pp. 197–8, doc. 197.

[pp] Lamberto [Balard] 1973 p. 246, doc. 650.

[qq] Lamberto [Polonio] 1982 doc. 148; doc. 154; doc. 217; doc. 217a.

[rr] Lamberto [Pavoni] 1987 pp. 194–5, doc. 164.

[ss] Lamberto [Pavoni] 1987 pp. 208–9, doc. 208.

[tt] Lamberto [Pavoni] 1987 p. 107, doc. 81.

140 William of Tyre 1986, II, pp. 589–60; William of Tyre 1943, II, p. 292.

When King Amaury of Jerusalem became ill with dysentery in 1174, he asked first asked the advice of 'physicians from the Greek, Syrian and other nations' before turning to his own Frankish countrymen, and they were only consulted when the first group would not give him the purgative treatment he asked for.[141]

A commentary on the laws of the kingdom of Jerusalem dating from the 1240s, the *Assises de la Cour des Bourgeois*, included sections on the licensing of doctors prior to their practising in Frankish towns.[142] 'No foreign doctor, that is one coming from across the sea [Europe] or pagan lands should practise as a urine doctor until he has been examined by other doctors, the best in the land, in the presence of the bishop of the place.' The choice of words used show that doctors from different cultural backgrounds were allowed to practise in the Frankish states so long as they could demonstrate sound medical knowledge to the assessing board. Similarly, the regulations regarding the hiring of physicians and surgeons to work in the Hospital of St John in twelfth-century Jerusalem include two versions of an oath, presumably to allow doctors who were not Christian to work there.[143] Interestingly, a decree of the Frankish church of Nicosia in Cyprus was passed between 1252 and 1257 which forbad Christians there from employing the services of Muslim and Jewish physicians.[144] This strongly suggests that up to that time doctors from these groups were used by the Frankish population, or the law would not have needed to be introduced. The reasoning given for this ban was that non-Christians were not employing Christian doctors, so the church regarded this as contempt for Christianity by non-Christians. If this really was the case, then such a ruling was in effect a boycott of Jewish and Muslim practitioners by the Christian establishment, rather than a suggestion that Jewish and Muslim doctors were in any way substandard. While the outcome would have been surprisingly similar to that recommended by William of Tyre the century before (that Christians should avoid pagan doctors), the underlying reasoning was completely different. The ruling would not, obviously, have restricted access to Eastern Christian doctors by the Franks.

Practitioners indigenous to the eastern Mediterranean were paid in a similar manner to the newly arriving Europeans, discussed earlier. Many of these intermittently worked in the Frankish states and in neighbouring Muslim lands, depending on the circumstances. The best known were paid a regular fee for entering the service of the noble and wealthy and

---

[141] William of Tyre 1986, II, pp. 956–7; William of Tyre 1943, II, p. 395.
[142] *Assises de Jérusalem* 1839, I, docs. 231 and 233; see also Nutton's translation in this book.
[143] Edgington 1998b. [144] *Synodicum Nicosiense* 2001 p. 97, XIV.

some of these became immensely well off.[145] While some were only allowed to treat their sponsor, others, when not occupied with their contracted commitments, could take on private fee-for-service cases as well. Doctors who worked in a hospital were usually paid a regular salary.[146] However, the majority of practitioners took cases on an individual basis with a fee determined for each patient. Just as in Europe, it was thought honourable if a doctor treated the poor for free,[147] although quite what percentage of the total workload this might have comprised is not clear.

There were no universities as such in the Frankish states, in the way there were in Europe, although there were clearly centres of learning such as Antioch and Tripoli.[148] This may have been in part a result of the problem that few if any Frankish cities had a high enough population to sustain a European-style university.[149] Most of the non-European practitioners of whom we have any information appear to have learnt their skills from attachment to a particular scholar or trainer. This could have taken place in the Latin East or in neighbouring Islamic lands.[150] There is very little information on any Franks born in the country who wished to study medicine. Presumably the alternatives would have been to study in their home region under a respected practitioner via the apprenticeship method, or travel back to Europe for a university degree if they could afford it.

Eastern Christian groups were strongly represented among the local medical practitioners. The physician Abu Sa'id was with a Frankish army in 1138 in the county of Edessa. Barhebraeus wrote how the troops apparently set out from Samosata and were ambushed by Muslim forces under the lord of Mardin. A large part of the Frankish army was killed and many others captured and carried off as slaves. One of these captives was Abu Sa'id, whom Barhebraeus described as a minister, physician and philosopher.[151]

Abu Sulayman Dawud was an Eastern Christian who did well treating the Franks in the Latin East. He was a native of Jerusalem who emigrated to Fatmid Egypt and became well known for his ability in both medicine and astrology.[152] He returned to Jerusalem to work for King Amalric in the 1160s and treated his son Prince Baldwin, who had contracted leprosy.[153] One of Abu Sulayman's sons, al-Muhadhdhab Abu Sa'id, later took over from his father as Amalric's physician.[154] After the fall of Jerusalem to Saladin in 1187 Abu Sulayman returned to Egypt and stayed until his death.

[145] Jadon 1970a; Rosenthal 1978.   [146] Richards 1992.   [147] Biesterfeldt 1984.
[148] Usama ibn Munqidh 1929 pp. 237–8.   [149] Bullough 1962a.   [150] Leiser 1983.
[151] Barhebraeus 1932a p. 265.   [152] Cahen 1934.
[153] Mitchell 2000a.   [154] Hillenbrand 1999 p. 354.

Emperor Manuel I Comnenus of Byzantium (reigned 1143–80) was one of the more surprising practitioners to have been identified.[155] It was standard education for the Byzantine elite to study some medicine and apparently Manuel gained much satisfaction from practising his skill. This was despite the fact that following Byzantine etiquette it would have been inappropriate for him to lower himself to actually treat anyone. Emperor Manuel was also renowned for his sexual adventures at court as well as his fondness for Western customs. In 1148 he personally treated Conrad III, king of Germany, when he became ill on the Second Crusade and in 1159 he treated King Baldwin III of Jerusalem. This incident took place near Antioch when Baldwin fell from his horse while hunting and broke his arm. Even when the party had returned to Antioch and other doctors would certainly been present, 'he visited the king daily, himself renewing the poultices and healing ointments and then carefully replacing the bandages'.[156] Manuel died in September 1180, aged sixty-two.

Thabit was a doctor who is mentioned in the twelfth-century work of Usama ibn Munqidh [157] as treating some sick Franks at a castle. If we believe Usama's story as factual, then it seems that Thabit treated a knight with an abscess in his leg using a poultice, and a woman with mental illness by modification of her diet to improve the balance of her humours.

Barac was the physician to the count of Tripoli around 1161. William of Tyre recounts[158] how in the autumn of that year Barac was temporarily loaned to King Baldwin III of Jerusalem for a consultation.

The king was at Antioch. Desiring to take a physic before the approach of winter, as was his custom, he obtained certain pills from Barac, the physician of the count (of Tripoli), a part of which were to be taken at once and the rest after a short interval.

The physician Muwaffaq al-Din Ya'qub b. Siqlab worked in both Frankish Jerusalem and Muslim Damascus in the second half of the twelfth century.[159] His family were Melkites who came from Transjordan (to the east of the river) and they may well have been moved to Jerusalem in 1115 when King Baldwin I tried to increase the population of the city with local Christians. Ya'qub was born in 1165–6 and studied medicine in Jerusalem under another Eastern Christian known today only as 'the Antioch Philosopher' (died 1184–5). When in Frankish lands he would wear the medical

[155] Leven 1991; Lascaratos and Maletas 1996.
[156] William of Tyre 1986, II, p. 848; William of Tyre 1943, II, p. 280.
[157] Usama ibn Munqidh 1929 p. 162.
[158] William of Tyre 1986, II, p. 859; William of Tyre 1943, II, p. 292.   [159] Kohlberg and Kedar 1988.

dress of the Franks, namely a head shawl, a small turban and a collared upper coat. When working in Muslim areas he had to change this for a full sleeve silk robe and a turban, more typical Damascene dress.[160] Ya'qub's pupil Ibn Abi Usaybi'a wrote that he owned a number of medical books, including Galen, and would regularly quote long passages accurately. He tells us,

Ya'qub was an excellent and successful medical practitioner; he would first make a thorough study of the disease and would then commence treatment in accordance with the rules mentioned by Galen, while also making use of his own experience. He carefully studied the symptoms of a disease. Whenever he visited a patient he inquired about every single symptom and complaint and considered every symptom which might point to the nature of the disease. His treatment was therefore unsurpassable.[161]

Once Jerusalem had been lost to Saladin in 1187 he worked in a hospital in the city and then moved to Damascus. There he spent the rest of his career as physician to Sultan al-Mu'azzam until his death in 1228.[162]

Shaykh Abu Mansur was another Eastern Christian physician who practised in Jerusalem in the second half of the twelfth century, at the same time as Ya'qub b. Siqlab. Ibn Abi Usaybi'a tells us that they knew each other and practised medicine together.[163] This may have been the same Abu Mansur who was later one of Saladin's physicians.[164] Evidence for yet another Eastern Christian doctor from the same date is found in the records of the Holy Sepulchre of Jerusalem. A document dating from 1160–87 shows that a medicus named Bulfarage lived in a house on the *vicus* Sanctus Martinus in Jerusalem.[165] Bulfarage is likely to be a Frankish version of the Arabic name Abu'l-Faradj. Since he was allowed to live in Jerusalem at that time this suggests that he was probably Christian.

Theodore of Antioch was one of the best-known physicians to be born in the Frankish states. He was a Jacobite Christian thought to have been born in the 1190s and was brought up in Antioch, where he studied languages and philosophy.[166] His studies then took him to Mosul and then Baghdad, where he studied medicine until about 1220. After a time in the Lesser Armenian court he moved on to the court of Emperor Frederick II of Germany.[167] Master Theodore was active as a mathematician, philosopher, astrologer and also translated sections of Averroes and Aristotle into Latin.

[160] Ibn Abi Usaybi'a 1988.   [161] Ibn Abi Usaybi'a 1988.
[162] Ibn al-Qifti 1988.   [163] Ibn Abi Usaybi'a 1988.
[164] Jadon 1970b.   [165] *Le Cartulaire du Saint-Sepulchre* 1984 p. 321.
[166] Kedar and Kohlberg 1995.   [167] Barhebraeus 1663 p. 341.

His only medical work was the *Epistola Theodori Philosophi Imperatorem Fridericum*, a treatise on the rules for the preservation of health for his patron.[168] In February 1240 records show he was told to prepare syrups and violet sugar to be used by Emperor Frederick and others in the royal court.[169] Master Theodore had died by 1250 and there is evidence to suggest that he may have poisoned himself.[170]

Gregorius Barhebraeus (Ibn al-'Ibri, Grighor Abu'l-Faradj) was a Jacobite doctor who was born in 1225–6 at Malatya (Greek Melitene), on the Euphrates.[171] He was son of a doctor called Aaron, hence the name 'son of a Hebrew', and first learnt medicine from him. With the Mongol invasions his family moved west to Frankish Antioch around 1243 and at the age of seventeen Gregory became a monk. He went south to Frankish Tripoli and studied rhetoric and medicine under a Nestorian scholar named Ya'qub until 1246.[172] After these studies the Jacobite Patriarch Ignatius II appointed Gregory the bishop of Gubbash and by 1253 he had become the metropolitan of Aleppo. He wrote over thirty works on medicine, philosophy, astronomy, logic and religion and well as his historical epic *The Chronography*. He translated a medical treatise on simple remedies by al-Ghafiki from Arabic to Syriac, and his Syriac translation of the Qanun of Ibn Sina was incomplete at the time of his death. He died in 1286 and his tomb is in the church of the Mar Mattai monastery, near Mosul.

Saliba Barjacobi Vagii (Salibha Bar Ya'Kub Wagih) was also a Jacobite doctor who lived in the mid-thirteenth century. He was born in Edessa and studied medicine under Ya'qub in Frankish Tripoli, at the same time as Barhebraeus (1243–6).[173] When the Jacobite Patriarch Ignatius II sent Barhebraeus off to be bishop of Gubos, he appointed Saliba to be Jacobite bishop of Frankish Acre.[174] Despite various religious appointments in his life he was known to have continued to practise medicine. Ignatius was another Jacobite bishop who was a medical practitioner.[175] He was also bishop of Aleppo for a time and later retired to Tripoli to teach medicine there. These examples show a strong tradition for the study of medicine among the Jacobite religious community in the eastern Mediterranean at the time of the crusades. This has interesting parallels with the situation in Europe, where it was common for *physici* to be clerics as well. Despite high clerical office, some clearly continued to practise medicine and also to write medical works.

---

[168] Sudhoff 1915.   [169] *Historia Diplomatica* 1859, v(ii), pp. 750–1.   [170] Kedar and Kohlberg 1995.
[171] Barhebraeus 1932a pp. xv–xxxvi; *Geschichte der Christlichen* 1947, II, pp. 272–81; Segal 1971.
[172] Barhebraeus 1872, I–II, col. 668.   [173] Barhebraeus 1872, I–II, col. 668.
[174] Barhebraeus 1932a p. xvii.   [175] Barhebraeus 1872, I–II, cols. 728–30.

Benvenutus Grassus Hierosolimitanus (also known as Benvenutus Grapheus/Crassus) was a doctor specialising in diseases of the eye who is thought to have lived in the second half of the thirteenth century.[176] His only known work was the *Ars Probatissima Oculorum*[177] in which he provides clear descriptions of many of the ophthalmological diseases found around the Mediterranean at that time.[178] The text is thought to have been popular as it was translated from Latin into Provençal, Italian, French and English.[179] It was written in a very practical manner and was not particularly advanced with regard to medical theory. Benvenutus appears to have been a rather vain and self-confident man if the tone of his *Ars* was a true mirror of his character. Evidence in the text suggests that he was a Christian as it was written in Latin and includes many Christian terms, such as advising holding the cataract needle on the lens for as long as it takes to say four 'pater nosters'.[180] As many of his anecdotes and case studies are set in Italy he clearly spent a significant period of his career there. However, he also describes travelling widely, including to north Africa, and observing the local treatments for trachoma and other conditions. As well as the evidence for his Jerusalem origins from his name, he repeatedly used references to the east in the names of his treatments, such as the 'Jerusalemite collyrium' and 'Jerusalemite pills', while others are termed 'Alexandrine'. While it has been suggested that he might have used these terms as well as altering his name to gain credibility or prestige, a recent biography of Benvenutus thinks this rather unlikely.[181] For instance, Benvenutus recommended the use in his medicines of a high quality sugar termed *zucharum nabet*, a phrase used in the customs tariffs from Acre by the 1240s but apparently not in Europe until the fourteenth century.[182]

Maimonides (Abu 'Imran Musa Ibn Maimun) was the best-known Jewish physician to have spend time in the Frankish states, although it is unlikely that he ever practised there. He was born in 1139 and raised in Cordova in Spain, but left with his family in 1148 on account of religious persecution from a fanatical sect, the Almohades. The family eventually settled in Fez, Morocco, in 1158 but they left there in 1165 to move east. Maimonides arrived at Frankish Acre by ship before travelling south to Fustat in Egypt in the same year. Over the years he gradually became well known for his clinical acumen and medical knowledge, eventually

[176] Eldredge 1996 p. 4.
[177] Benvenutus Grassus 1474; Benvenutus Grassus 1929; Benvenutus Grassus 1996.
[178] Feigenbaum 1955a and 1955b.   [179] Eldredge 1996.
[180] Benvenutus Grassus 1474 p. 4v; Benvenutus Grassus 1929 p. 34.
[181] Kedar 1995.   [182] Kedar 1995.

becoming personal physician to Saladin.[183] His medical writings include *The Medical Aphorisms, A Commentary on the Aphorisms of Hippocrates, A Discourse on Asthma, The Extracts from Galen, Treatise on Haemorrhoids, Treatise on Sexual Intercourse, Treatise on Poisons and their Antidotes, Regimen of Health, Discourse on the Explanation of Fits* and *A Commentary on the Names of Drugs*.[184] These medical writings were firmly based on the works of Galen, whom he greatly admired.[185] It is now generally accepted that suggestions that King Richard I of England had asked Maimonides to be his personal physician while on the Third Crusade have no factual basis.[186] Besides his medical activities Maimonides was a rabbi and wrote many religious and philosophical works. He died on 13 December 1204, aged sixty-nine, and was buried at Tiberias in Galilee.

Other Jewish doctors who did live long term in the Latin East included R. Nehorai. He was mentioned in a pilgrim work of 1174–87.[187] Nehorai lived in Tiberius and was described as a *medicus* who also sold medicinal herbs. An interesting case is that of Samuel the *miege*. He is referred to in the chronicle of the Templar of Tyre as living in the Tyre in 1283. We know of him as he was responsible for carrying a copy of the Torah in a procession,[188] so clearly he was well respected within the Jewish community. A further example was Eli, a Jewish physician living in Frankish Cyprus. He was mentioned in a document of 1301 as a *medicus physicus* who lived in Famagusta.[189]

INTERPRETING THE EVIDENCE

In the course of this study around one hundred named medical practitioners and medical authors have been identified as having participated in the crusades, spent time in the Latin East or become settlers. Overall thirty-one are known to be definite members of crusading expeditions or pilgrims, while a further seventeen are possible crusading candidates (see table 1.1). Of those whose country of origin is known, the majority were from France (ten definite, ten possible), a significant number from England (eight definite, five possible) and Italy (four definite, two possible), while others came from Spain or Hungary (two definite). This means that the country of origin is known for twenty-four definite crusading practitioners, but unknown for

---

[183] Jadon 1970a.   [184] Bar-Sela, Hoff and Faris 1964; Rosner 1981; Rosner 1996.
[185] Lieber 1979.   [186] Lewis 1964.
[187] Petahyah of Regensburg 1746 col. MCCIV.   [188] Templar of Tyre 2000 p. 162.
[189] Lamberto de Sambuceto [Polonio] 1982, doc. 380, pp. 456–7.

the remaining seven. Of those crusading practitioners who did definitely spend time in the Latin East, thirteen were *physici*, eleven *medici/mieges*, three *cyrurgici*, two medical authors and one an astrologer, giving a total of thirty whose medical designation is known. Of this group, about half should theoretically have been able to treat trauma and weapon injuries, the rest being academics and *physici* who did not perform the necessary hands-on procedures.

Of those from France who definitely went on crusade, six out of ten (60 per cent) were masters. Among the English who definitely went east, six out of eight (75 per cent) were masters. From the Italian practitioners, all four definite participants were masters (100 per cent). At first glance this would suggest that English, French and Italian nobility appear to have had broadly similar access to medical staff who were highly qualified in the academic sense, although their skills in actually treating patients remain unknown. However, as most of the records refer to the medical staff of kings or nobles, we should not uncritically assume that the same pattern would have been seen in the much larger group of medical practitioners in the Latin East as a whole. There is little record of the less educated *miege*, *cyrurgicus* or *barberus* who worked freelance on crusades, unattached to a noble family. It is probable that there were far more of these than the highly educated masters who accompanied the nobles. Indeed, there are references to the activities of significant numbers of anonymous barbers in some of the later crusader chronicles.[190]

No practitioners termed surgeons or barbers lived earlier than the second half of the thirteenth century. The timing of the introduction of the words *cyrurgicus* and *barberus* closely parallels the findings of other studies in Europe.[191] While the majority of the named *physici* and many *medici* were clerics, there was no evidence that any of the surgeons or barbers were. Our understanding of the permitted role of clerics in the practice of surgery by the church, outlined previously, is completely compatible with the findings here. No clergy in major orders are seen to have been actively involved with operative surgery after 1215 and they were typically *physici*. Those clerics who were *medici*, and so may have practised some surgical techniques, appear to have come from the secular clergy, which was permitted. Interestingly none of the crusading surgeons were described as masters. This contrasts markedly with the pattern we see for the Italian surgeons settled on Cyprus from the 1290s, discussed below.

[190] John of Joinville 1874 p. 166; John of Joinville 1955 p. 100.
[191] Jacquart 1981 p. 235; Talbot and Hammond 1965 p. 375.

It is difficult to assess how the number of medical staff accompanying a king or noble may have varied over time or between countries. If we only consider definite crusaders whose noble has been identified then the resulting group is probably too small for such statistical analysis. While at first glance it would appear that King Louis IX had by far the largest number of practitioners, if it is remembered that he went on two crusades then the number per crusade is halved. Furthermore, the bias inherent in the sources makes such comparison open to criticism. Sources written by authors from the same country as a particular king or noble are much more likely to mention the medical staff in detail than those written by a foreigner who would not know the entourage so well. In consequence those crusades where our main evidence comes from sources from one country will tend to underestimate the number of practitioners brought by other countries. As a result it is probably not helpful to make statistical analyses until a much larger number of practitioners have been identified.

Some information has come to light on the incomes of a small proportion of practitioners discussed here. This may have been in part because many of the individuals identified were clergy and so should not in theory have been earning money from their practice of medicine.[192] The English *medicus* master Gilbertus Anglicus was paid 100 shillings (sous/soldi) per year by the earl of Leicester in the 1190s. The city of Bologna paid the *medicus* master Hugo of Lucca 600 Bolognese lire per year from 1214 and his colleague master Robertus of Lucca 100 gold bezants per year in the 1220s. King Louis IX paid the *physicus* Hersende 12 deniers per day in 1250, while the surgeon Pierre de Soissons was paid 20 Parisian livres per year in 1252. His *cyrurgici* Pierre de la Broce and Guillaume de Salu both received 2 sous per day in 1261, but Pierre received a further 6 deniers per day when the Louis was actually at court. Jean the *barbier* received just 6 deniers per day in 1261. It is often difficult to directly compare the earnings of doctors in the medieval period as the records may be for different currency from different areas at different times.[193] The common method of payment for more than trivial amounts would have been money of account, rather than a bag of coins.[194] This solved the problems of the physical shortage of coins, the difficulty in transporting large numbers of coins about and the different value of coins minted in different parts of Europe.[195] Each local region in Europe had its own system of money of account, and merchants would work out the relative value of units from different regions. Records for the

---

[192] Hammond 1960; Rawcliffe 1988.   [193] Spufford 1986.
[194] Spufford 1988 pp. 411–14; Pounds 1994 pp. 120–2.   [195] Metcalf 1995.

Table 1.3 *Salary given by King Louis IX to his crusading medical staff (1250–61)*

	Deniers/day
Jean the barber (1261)[a]	6
Magistre Hersende, *physica* (1250)	12
Pierre de Soissons, *cyrurgicus* (1252)	13
Guillaume de Salu, *cyrurgicus* (1261)[a]	24
Pierre de la Broce, *cyrurgicus* (1261)	24
extra when king at court	6

Note: [a] Probable participant, but not actually mentioned in documents from the Latin East.

practitioners discussed in table 1.3 were all in multiples of the denier (silver coin), which allows some kind of comparison. As they were all paid by the king of France, we can assume that they were all paid according to the same system of money of account. Furthermore, they were all from within a ten-year period, so this might limit the effect of the declining value due to debasement, which was a real problem in the medieval period. In money of account a sou was the term for 12 deniers and the livre was 20 sous. This means that we can calculate the theoretical pay in deniers per day as a way of comparing incomes. However, practitioners would obviously not have been paid this amount in coin.

A number of factors limit the interpretation of these figures. They do not include the extras such clothing, regular meals, assistants, forage for horses and other items that were paid for by the court. Nor do they account for any other income they may have earned through private fee-for-service work once royal duties were completed,[196] or through other occupations such as law. Despite this, the figures do highlight the lower pay of the barber compared with physicians and surgeons, with Jean getting just a quarter of the salary given to surgeons at the same date. Another surprise is why the surgeon Pierre de Soissons and physician Hersende received just half the salary in 1251 that their colleagues Guillaume de Salu and Pierre de la Broce were to receive a decade later. Pierre de la Broce did not become chamberlain until 1266 so his extra post could not have been the reason. It is possible that the debasement of the value of the denier over this ten-year period might be involved, but this could not be so considerable as to explain an apparent doubling in the number of deniers per day. Another

---

[196] Hammond 1960; Rawcliffe 1988.

possible alternative is that the circumstances under which Guillaume and Pierre were expected to work for the the royal court might have changed in those ten years. Perhaps there was a decrease in the amount of free perks of the job, perhaps an increase in the workload or a limit to their other sources of income.

While I have tried to find out as much as possible about those participating in the crusades themselves, there were, of course, a significant number of medical practitioners who appear to have settled in the Latin East. While some might have gone east with a crusading expedition and stayed on, others would have travelled east in times of peace. When the evidence for their existence in the east does not indicate how they got there, it can be very difficult to be sure which catagory they belong to. In consequence I have merely classed them all as settlers. Nearly fifty individuals have been identified, largely from legal documents and contracts that are usually unrelated to their medical practice. The largest number are from the Frankish state of Cyprus, as the notarial records of Lamberto de Sambuceto are exactly the kind of records that would mention the dealings of this section of society. If only more such records had been preserved for all the Latin states and for their entire 200-year existence, we might theoretically have details of certainly hundreds, and perhaps thousands, of medical practitioners who settled in the east.

Of those forty-nine settlers that have come to light, seventeen (35 per cent) were barbers, twelve (25 per cent) were apothecaries, eight (16 per cent) were *medici*, seven (14 per cent) were surgeons and five (10 per cent) were physicians. Since the Lamberto records are a fairly complete collection (as medieval records go), it could be argued that this might give us a reasonable indication of the proportions of the different medical subspecialities at work in Frankish Cyprus at the end of the thirteenth century. While I am by no means suggesting that they are statistically accurate, I think this kind of information may well be more balanced than the records of crusading medical practitioners left us in the documents of the European royal courts. After all, we would expect to see more barbers and apothecaries in medieval towns than the more highly trained physicians and surgeons, and that is certainly the pattern seen here. Interestingly, six of the seven surgeons and four of the five physicians were masters. This is a strikingly high proportion and might at first suggest a bias in the sources once again. However, we must remember that these are notarial registers of the Genoese community in Cyprus, and that most medical practitioners mentioned had origins in Italy. Italy was a leading light in medical education in late thirteenth-century Europe, with several large universities. It was also the principal area in Europe where surgeons could study their course at a university and obtain the title of master, rather than merely following the apprenticeship training route. In consequence, the high proportion of masters in these two medical subspecialisms may not be quite so surprising after all if we remember that they were Italians.

It has also been demonstrated that there were a significant number of non-European doctors from different cultural groups within the Frankish states. These included those born to Latin parents who intermarried and settled in the east, oriental Christians, Jews and Muslims; twenty known individuals have been discussed. The vast majority of the individuals identified here are Christian. At first glance this might be interpreted to suggest that the majority of practitioners in the Frankish states were Christian. However, it is quite likely that a bias in the sources may also be a significant factor. Most of the sources for the Latin East were written by Christians for Christians. In consequence, few Jews and Muslims would have been asked to witness Latin documents, and Latin authors may not have mixed significantly with the Jewish and Muslim communities. Their cultural differences with Europe led to jealousy on the part of some Europeans, but also respect by a number of nobles who chose them for their personal physicians. The states reacted to the situation with special adaptations to Christian laws and statutes so that these different groups could still be allowed to practise their art, even if there was some later legislation prohibiting the treatment of Christians by Muslims and Jews. These laws covered medical licensing, clinical practice and also malpractice.

The evidence for the involvement of medical practitioners from Europe in successive crusades during the twelfth and thirteenth centuries gives an interesting glimpse of the structure, status, role and evolution of the medical profession at that time. It is now clear that a significant proportion of European practitioners were involved with the crusades at some time in their lives, but this is rarely mentioned in any of the modern secondary sources discussing medieval medicine. We might expect this period of travel, with consequent exposure to new ideas and treatments, to have profound effects on the careers of many individuals. There are also accounts of a thriving medical tradition among the indigenous inhabitants of those lands which became the Frankish states, and the interaction between these individuals and the invading Europeans is quite intriguing.

CHAPTER 2

Hospitals on the battlefield and in the towns

Some institutions in the Latin East were clearly hospitals as we understand them today, in the sense that they treated the sick by providing medical treatment to the standards of the period. It is these institutions showing evidence of medical care for the sick and injured that are the focus of this chapter. Some might argue that differentiating *hospitalia* by whether or not they provided conventional medical care may be irrelevant.[1] However, since the principal focus of this book is the treatment of wounds and injuries, and not *hospitalia* in themselves, it seems reasonable to concentrate on those Frankish hospitals where such treatment took place.

In some cases the records of treatments employed in these hospitals have been preserved, as in the hospitals run by the Order of St John. Occasionally documents written by people who actually stayed in such hospitals give an idea of what it must have been like to have been a patient. However, for many institutions little or no detail on their function has been preserved in the records and other approaches have to be employed. One stumbling block is the terminology used to refer to a hospital in the medieval period. The medieval Latin word *hospitale* was sometimes used to refer to a hospital providing medical care, but also for other residential charitable institutions such as alms houses, lodgings or hospices.[2] To make things more confusing, property of the Order of St John (the Knights Hospitaller) was often referred to by the same word. However, this did not necessarily mean that there was a hospital providing medical care at every one of their properties. The *domus infirmorum* or *firmaria* was a much less ambiguous medieval term and refers to an infirmary. The infirmary was a place where the sick were cared for, but it varied whether doctors were employed or if treatment was given just by a monk or someone with a rudimentary knowledge of a few medical treatments.

[1] Horden 1988.   [2] Niermeyer and van de Kieft 2002; Latham 1994.

Further information that may help differentiate the function of a *hospitale* includes the choice of terms for those who stayed there. The *peregrinus* was a pilgrim or crusader and the term did not imply any ill health, so where no further details are given the use of this term might imply that a *hospitale* functioned as a guest house or hostel. A pauper was poor or impoverished, and while care for these people shows philanthropy it does not imply any medical treatment. However, the *infirmus* was weak, invalid or unwell while the *egerlegrotus* was sick.[3] Clearly the presence of people in these latter categories is more compatible with the functions of a hospital in the modern medical sense. While there is considerable evidence for the perceived role of religious pilgrimage sites in the healing of the sick in the Latin East,[4] saints' relics fall outside the remit of this work. In consequence these pilgrimage destinations and also the charitable institutions for which there is as yet no evidence for medical treatment (such as the *leprosaria* of the Order of St Lazarus and the various hostels and food distribution centres) have not been discussed.

In order to fully assess the network of hospitals in the Latin East, it is necessary to study the contemporary crusader writings of pilgrims and professional chroniclers together with medieval maps and town plans, and to reconcile evidence from these sources with information derived from modern archaeological excavation. In this way it is possible to complement past studies of particular medical orders with discussion of newly excavated hospitals and recently discovered texts. This approach provides a relative comparison of the range of medical establishments that existed. It also helps to shed further light on the services they provided for the population and their interaction with one another. It is possible to calculate the approximate patient capacity of these hospitals by assessing their excavation plans, using our knowledge of the physical stature of the population of medieval Europe and of contemporary ideas on bed layout. The medical treatments used in these hospitals can also be compared with those known in Europe and the Near East at that time, in an attempt to assess the degree to which the various medical traditions of the medieval world might have influenced practice in the Frankish states.

THE HOSPITAL IN MEDIEVAL EUROPE, THE BYZANTINE EMPIRE AND THE ISLAMIC WORLD

In order to study crusader and Frankish hospitals we should be aware of the state of comparable institutions in neighbouring cultures. This allows the

---

[3] Niermeyer and van de Kieft 2002; Latham 1994.　　[4] Pringle 1998, II, pp. 52, 118, 220; Kedar 2001.

Frankish hospital to be seen against the background of the standard practice of the day. While the fundamental need to look after the sick means that some factors will be noted across all regions, certain aspects of hospitals in western Europe, the Byzantine empire and the Islamic world demonstrate interesting variation. It seems likely that these were a consequence of the differing religious beliefs, cultures and functional requirements of philanthropic institutions in the medieval period. Any Frankish practices for which no equivalent can be found in the contemporary hospitals in other cultures are clearly of particular interest, as they might suggest innovation on the part of the Franks. Any Frankish practices which are not known in medieval Europe but are known in Islamic or Byzantine institutions might suggest the adoption of new ideas.

Byzantine hospitals remain a hotly debated topic, as there are still large gaps in our knowledge. The Byzantine period, from the fourth to the fourteenth century, is over a thousand years long and there are significant chronological gaps between the sources of evidence that we do have, so that a certain amount of educated guesswork has been employed by some previous authors. Byzantine hospitals began to develop in the fourth century AD when caring institutions were established by Christian clergy. While some of these fed and clothed the poor or elderly, a proportion hired doctors to look after the sick.[5] In the following centuries a fair number of the latter type (termed *nosokomeia* or *xenones*) were founded. Some were created in association with monasteries which were responsible for funding and in a number of cases nursing the sick, but in later periods it became rare for monks to actually work on the wards. Some hospitals, such as the Sampson and Markianos *xenones* eventually severed their monastic connections.[6] From the seventh century onwards, staff were normally salaried laymen. While most of the *xenones* in the records appear to have been built in Constantinople, cities such as Alexandria, Antioch and Caesarea in Cappadocia possessed them as early as the sixth century. Early *xenones* frequently had a non-medical cleric as administrator, but in later periods it became more usual for senior doctors themselves to take on this role. It is not known how representative the institutions of Constantinople were of the rest of the Byzantine empire,[7] but reasonable detail is known of hospitals such as the Mangana, Sampson and Pantokrator *xenones*. There is evidence for a form of separation of patients by their diagnosis in some *xenones* from as early as the seventh century. The later Pantokrator *typikon* (c.1136) mentions a ward each for patients with fractures and wounds, ophthalmological and

---

[5] Miller 1984; Miller 1990; Allan 1990.   [6] Miller 1997 p. 135.   [7] Nutton 1986.

intestinal diseases, two wards for other illnesses and a ward for women. The Pantokrator employed a hierarchy of doctors, based on their experience, and sometimes surgeons specialising in certain problems such as hernias.[8] Staff worked seven days per week with medical ward rounds daily in winter and twice daily in summer.[9] Doctors worked alternate months in the hospital, leaving a total of six months each year for private practice in the city. This made up for the very poor pay they received for their hospital work, similar to that of a labourer. It is presumed that the prestige of working in the *xenon*, with the resulting increase in private practice fees, explained this system. Other staff described by the twelfth century include pharmacists, medical attendants/nurses, surgical instrument sharpeners, priests, cooks, pallbearers and latrine cleaners. In general Byzantine hospitals do not appear to have been large; often they had between ten and one hundred beds, with separate sections for men and women. The Pantokrator *typikon* mentions a female doctor and female nurses working on the female ward, but most doctors were male.[10] At least by the eleventh century some patients with less serious illness were treated in the outpatient clinic. For the inpatients, religion played an important role and prayers for the soul of the founder, especially if an emperor, were regarded as important. Few *xenones* left a record of the diet fed to the patients, but the standard meals in the Pantokrator appear to have been vegetarian. However, patients were allowed to buy other foods if they desired. Treatments other than dietary modification included bloodletting, baths, medicines and surgery.

Another area of debate is the clientele to be found in *xenones* and *nosokomeia*. The Pantokrator records suggest that only the acutely sick were cared for there, and that the frail and terminally ill were elsewhere. In theory other institutions were available to help the poor and hungry (*xenodocheia*) or elderly (*gerokomeia*) who were not actually sick, although the terminology may not always have been precise. However, it is unclear how representative the twelfth-century Pantokrator evidence is for other institutions in Constantinople, other cities of the empire and for that matter other centuries.[11] Medical education may potentially have been another role of the hospital in later centuries. In the Pantokrator *xenon* a doctor was employed to teach medicine to the children of other doctors on the staff and the most junior doctors were unsalaried, perhaps having a role equivalent to that of the modern medical student.[12] A few medical manuscripts of collections of prescriptions claim origin in hospitals as well as illustrated

---

[8] Miller 1999.   [9] Codellas 1942; Miller 1997 pp. 12–21; Gautier 1974.
[10] Miller 1997 pp. 141–66.   [11] Conrad 2001.   [12] Miller 1997 p. 156.

texts that may theoretically have been used for teaching in these *xenones*, suggesting the possibility of some kind of academic environment at least in the larger hospitals of medieval Constantinople.[13]

The earliest hospitals in the Islamic Middle East are thought to have been founded in the eighth or ninth centuries AD. While it has often been stated that the Umayyad caliph al-Walid founded the first hospital in Damascus during his reign (705–15 AD), recent reassessment has shown no sound evidence for this.[14] It seems that it was only from the end of the eighth century that the foundation of true hospitals began, with the Abbasid caliph ar-Rashid establishing one in Baghdad around 790.[15] Initial expansion in the ninth century was slow, but by the twelfth century most major cities in the Middle East possessed at least one hospital and large cities such as Baghdad possessed several.[16] Some of these cities subsequently became part of the Frankish states and it is possible that they may have acted as an example for the invaders. For example, the Eastern Christian practitioner Ibn Butlan supervised the construction of a hospital in Antioch in 1063, and this would have been functioning when the city fell in the First Crusade thirty-five years later.[17]

A number of scholars have speculated as to why Islamic hospitals were founded. It is possible that with the Islamic conquests there were fewer wealthy Christians who could afford to endow monasteries on a lavish scale, so that fewer monasteries were able to provide their traditional role of philanthropy and health care. Establishing hospitals was also seen as prestigious for rulers, who thereby hoped to gain popularity with their subjects.[18] There are many dubious stories in later Islamic historical texts about the very early Islamic era, and in consequence it is not at all clear if the inspiration came from the hospital (*nosokomeion*) developed by Orthodox Christians in the Byzantine empire or similar institutions of the Nestorian Christians in the Syriac-speaking Sassanian empire of Persia. Islamic hospitals were typically private, secular institutions funded originally by donations from rulers and rich benefactors, with further income from land and properties held in trust (*waqf*) for the benefit of the hospital. They were usually run by a government official in conjunction with the senior medical staff. Doctors of all religions worked in the hospital setting but only male doctors are recorded as working there, never women. It was usual to provide separate buildings or wings for male and female patients, with nursing staff of the same sex as the sick. By the close of the crusades these areas were

---

[13] Bennett 1999.   [14] Conrad 1994.   [15] Dols 1987.
[16] Ibn Jubayr 1952.   [17] Schacht 1937 p. 65.   [18] Dols 1987.

sometimes further divided to look after patients with similar conditions, as at the Mansuri hospital. Such wards included those for patients with fevers, gastrointestinal illness, ophthalmological conditions, mental illness, the wounded and those requiring surgery. Those most unwell were treated as inpatients while others were treated as outpatients. Some contemporary passages stated how hospitals were for the use of the rich and poor, locals and visitors. However, most people still paid for a doctor to treat them at home and it was normal to give birth at home, rather than go to the hospital.[19]

One pre-crusade example was the 'Adudi hospital in Baghdad.[20] This was founded in 982 AD with twenty-four medical practitioners, including physicians, oculists, surgeons and bonesetters. Medicine was taught to students there using manuscripts held in its library and many staff wrote medical texts themselves. Doctors were Muslim, Christian and Jewish and worked in the hospital some days and in the city other days. By 1068 twenty-eight doctors were employed and in 1184 we know they visited the patients twice a week, every Monday and Thursday.[21] Jerusalem was a major pilgrimage destination for the Muslim world and consequently had particular need for a hospital.[22] The hospital in Jerusalem was described in 1047 by the Persian traveller Naser-e Khosraw.

Jerusalem has a fine, heavily endowed hospital. People are given potions and draughts, and the physicians who are there draw their salaries from the endowment. The hospital and Friday mosque are on the eastern side of the city.[23]

When Saladin regained control of Jerusalem from the Franks in 1187, he founded a new hospital in one of the churches in the complex of St John.[24] By the time of the crusades the major cities in Asia Minor, Syria, Persia, Egypt and North Africa all possessed large and prestigious hospitals. The Nuri hospital in Damascus was founded by Nur al-Din b. Zangi in 1174, and according to al-Makrisi was paid with the ransom of an unnamed king of the Franks. The staff kept lists of all the patients' names, along with the prescriptions for their drugs and other treatment they required. Senior doctors would visit the sick in the morning, visit their private patients in the afternoon and then return in the evening to lecture on medical subjects.[25] In Egypt Salah al-Din founded the Nasiri hospital in Cairo. By 1183 this comprised large separate buildings for men, women and a secure block for mental health patients. The patients were reviewed morning

---

[19] Conrad 2001.   [20] Dunlop 1960.   [21] Elgood 1951 pp. 161–71; Ibn Jubayr 1952 pp. 234–5.
[22] Elad 1995; Bahat 2002.   [23] Naser-e Khosraw 1986 p. 23.   [24] Richards 1994.
[25] Dunlop 1960; Ibn Jubayr 1952 p. 296; Tabbaa 1997 fig. 143.

and evening and given special foods and drugs to improve their health.[26] A hospital specifically for strangers and foreigners in Alexandria was described in 1183. Doctors were employed to care for them and the hospital even sent people out on visits to those sick who were 'too modest' to attend the hospital. These would describe the patient's condition to the doctors at the hospital and organise treatment on the basis of their advice.[27] The most prestigious establishment in medieval Egypt was the Mansuri hospital. It was founded in 1283 AD when a Fatmid palace was converted to care for the sick. The hospital could look after several thousand people and was funded by endowed property providing nearly one million dirhams per year. It comprised four main buildings covering 10,000 square yards, with separate halls for patients with fevers, eye diseases, diarrhoea, surgical conditions and mental illness. Facilities also included a medical library, lecture room and pharmacy.[28] Mobile hospitals were also created, complementing the fixed institutions found in the cities. These had the advantage of intermittently visiting areas that had insufficient population to justify a normal hospital, but they could also cater for the sick in situations where the patients were themselves mobile, such as an army.[29] In 942 AD a mobile hospital was functioning from Baghdad, to treat those in outlying regions when epidemic disease occurred and to visit the sick in prison. In 1122 a field hospital was set up by Mustawfi 'Aziz al-Din of Baghdad. This accompanied the Seljuk Sultan Mahmud, transported on the backs of 200 camels. It was staffed with doctors and nurses and carried all the medical instruments, drugs and tents required to service the army on the march.[30]

In medieval Europe the word for a hospital (*hospitale*) referred to a broader range of institutions than was the case in the Middle East at that time.[31] One group housed the chronic and incurable sick such as leprosy patients (in *leprosaria*), the blind, the disabled or those otherwise unable to care for themselves. As these were not acutely unwell typically no medical care was felt to be necessary. Some *hospitalia* provided a retirement home for the frail as they grew older (alms houses), others housed and fed pilgrims and travellers overnight and only a small proportion of hospitals actively treated the acutely sick.[32] In the East these establishments were sometimes referred to with distinct terms that allow a reasonable understanding of their differing functions[33] but in Europe it is only by studying the documentary evidence for each particular *hospitale* that its true function can be ascertained. Up to the eleventh century monastic infirmaries are thought to

[26] Ibn Jubayr 1952 pp. 43–4.   [27] Ibn Jubayr 1952 p. 33.
[28] Dunlop 1960; Ibn Jubayr 1952 pp. 43–4; Dols 1992 p. 122.   [29] Elgood 1951 pp. 174–6.
[30] Levy 1929 p. 212.   [31] Jones 1983.   [32] Carlin 1989; Prescott 1992 pp. 1–2.   [33] Jones 1983.

have been the primary source of medical care for the sick poor in England, France, Italy and Spain, while the wealthy employed a doctor to attend them in their own home.[34]

From the eleventh century a number of *hospitalia* were founded, initially often still associated with monasteries but later established by rich merchants, guilds and lay fraternities.[35] It has been argued that this change came about to enable a stricter way of life in the monasteries while benefiting the rich founders of these secular institutions, as clergy and inmates were required to pray regularly for the benefactors' souls.[36] In England there were about 250 *hospitalia* by 1200 AD and roughly 500 by 1300 AD. Of around 1,000 institutions founded in England during the entire medieval period, less than 10 per cent were solely to care for the acutely sick.[37] These *hospitalia* were typically staffed by secular clergy with a rule based on that of St Augustine. Mass was said regularly and patients would repeat sets of prayers throughout the day.[38] They were funded by donations from the founder and other patrons, income from land, fees for long-term entry and some even participated in banking and loans.[39] They tended to be self-governing institutions rather than members of an organised network. Although some of the crusader orders did establish large numbers of *hospitalia* along the pilgrimage routes in twelfth-century Europe[40] most of these were hospices providing accommodation for pilgrims. There is little evidence for the presence of medical staff or treatment for the sick this early, and it remains unknown how much local practice may have changed before the thirteenth century.[41] In England the Order of St John founded twelve *hospitalia* for the general population and one for members of the order; the Order of St Lazarus had around thirteen *leprosaria* and St Thomas of Canterbury had just the one *hospitale* in London. Little is known of any actual medical care practised in these institutions and they were certainly not direct copies of the infirmaries in the orders' principal houses in the east. In England and Spain there is hardly any evidence for the activity of medical practitioners in any *hospitalia* earlier than the fourteenth or fifteenth centuries.[42] Ibn Jubayr commented on the presence of Christian churches that cared for the sick when he visited Sicily in 1185, but the only Christian institutions that he described as following the model of Muslim hospitals were to be found in the Latin East, in Acre and Tyre.[43]

---

[34] Orme 1995 pp. 21–3; Skinner 1997; Brodman 1998.   [35] Gilchrist 1995 p. 12; Rubin 1989.
[36] Orme 1995 p. 49.   [37] Carlin 1989; Gilchrist 1995 p. 10.   [38] Orme 1995 pp. 47–56; Bird 2001.
[39] Rubin 1989; Lorentzon 1992.   [40] Riley-Smith 1967 p. 40; Selwood 1999 pp. 50–6.
[41] Miller 1978; Epstein 1984 p. 178; Luttrell 1994.   [42] Rawcliffe 1999; Brodman 1998 pp. 86–99.
[43] Ibn Jubayr 1952 p. 346.

However, a number of institutions in France, the Netherlands, Italy and Germany were employing doctors by the thirteenth century.[44] In contrast to the situation the century before, we hear from an early thirteenth-century medical student who watched cranial surgery performed at the hospital of the Holy Spirit in Montpellier.[45] Similarly, the statutes of the hospital of the Order of St John at Altopascio in Italy showed that it employed medical practitioners at least by 1239.[46] Clearly medical intervention in hospitals had progressed by that time. Despite this, in those *hospitalia* where inmates were disabled, frail or acutely sick it was widely believed that medicine for the soul was much more important than medicine for the body. In consequence, treatment of bodily disease was often regarded as of much less importance than prayer, and may explain why we hear so little about doctors in the early *hospitalia*.[47]

It has been suggested that to study the institutional medical care of the sick in medieval Europe it is the monastic infirmary, not the *hospitale*, that should be under investigation.[48] Those monasteries that just treated the sick of their own order might make a good comparison for the infirmaries of similar Frankish institutions such as the Order of the Temple, while monastic infirmaries that treated the public might provide good comparisons for the more open orders of St John, St Thomas of Canterbury and the Teutonic Order. Infirmary halls usually followed a design of four to sixteen bays in England, but tended to be larger in mainland Europe. In those halls available to the public it was normal to separate men from women, either by inserting a partition down the middle of the hall or by having two separate floors or buildings. The chapel was typically at the east end of the hall or, less commonly, half way down one side and this was also divided into two by a partition. In France there was less distinction between the hall and chapel than in England.[49] There is some archaeological evidence for the practice of medicine in these infirmaries.[50] Fragments of urine flasks have been recovered from the fourteenth-century infirmary of St Mary Spital in London,[51] while a pharmacy jar with remains of an ointment containing poppy, cannabis, myrrh and rose was excavated at the medieval hospital of Soutra in Scotland.[52]

One useful comparison with the Frankish orders is the infirmary of the Benedictine Abbey of Westminster in England, as good records survive

---

[44] Agrimi and Crisciani 1998; Henderson 1989; Miller 1978; Skinner 1997.
[45] Demaitre 1975.   [46] Mencacci 1996.
[47] Rawcliffe 1998; Rawcliffe 1999; Bird 2001.   [48] Gilchrist 1995 p. 37.
[49] Gilchrist 1995 pp. 17–21; Prescott 1992 pp. 7–12.   [50] Gilchrist 1995 pp. 32–6.
[51] Thomas, Sloane and Phillpotts 1997 p. 111.   [52] Moffat, Thomson and Futton 1989 fig. 19.

from 1100 onwards.[53] This infirmary functioned just to care for those monks from the abbey who became unwell, not for the sick in the general population. At this institution the infirmary was a hall which extended west from the chapel. Tapestries and hangings were on the walls and the floor was covered with rushes. Several fires kept the sick warm and the beds had mattresses stuffed with either straw or feathers. Beds were arranged in two aisles, with space between for the infirmarian and his servants to perform their tasks. The infirmarian did have some basic medical knowledge but was not sent to university, as did other monks who left to study topics such as theology. Some medicinal plants were grown in the abbey herb garden, while others were purchased from nearby apothecaries. Doctors (*medici*) were hired to treat the sick in the infirmary, sometimes on a yearly contract and sometimes on a fee-for-service basis. Male and female surgeons were also employed and while their actual fees were high per operation, there is some evidence that they were regarded as having a lower social status than the *medici*, as they were not given ceremonial cloaks by the abbey. Surgical treatments recorded include manipulating fractured bones, operations on hernias, washing leg ulcers with white wine and giving enemas. Bloodletting was performed by a barber hired on an annual stipend. The actual procedure was performed outside the infirmary hall on account of the mess made if the blood was spilt. In the thirteenth century healthy monks were bled seven to eight times per year, eating a strengthening diet for the following two days. By no means all the monks in the infirmary were acutely ill, and a number of elderly and frail monks lived there long term. In 1297–8 only 40 per cent of inpatients in the infirmary were actually taking any syrups or drugs, which might suggest that they were not regarded as severely ill. On average 40 per cent of the monks were admitted to the infirmary as inpatients at some time each year, although most were there for a week or less.[54]

The battlefield hospital in medieval Europe is an institution about which little is known. However, one useful source of information has been preserved in a work of Arnold of Villanova. This Spanish medical practitioner wrote two works for his patron King James II of Aragon. One of these was a conventional *Regimen Sanitatis* but the other was more original, the so called *Regimen Almarie*.[55] It was thought to have been written in 1310 as King James besieged the Muslim city of Almeria in Granada, Spain. This was the time when the Franks still held Cyprus but had just lost the mainland Frankish states. Master Arnold's text summarises a typical approach

[53] Harvey 1993 pp. 81–109.   [54] Harvey 1993.   [55] McVaugh 1992.

to military medicine for the beginning of the fourteenth century, tailored
to the needs of a Spanish crusade.

The *Regimen* starts with advice on where to locate an army camp and
which areas of the camp might be the healthiest for the most important
individuals to place their tents. 'An army should not pitch camp in marshy
regions for a long period of time. Wherever the camp may be located,
the king should reside away from the side from which the land wind is
blowing off the mountains.' The water supply for a large number of people
was always a problem; even if it was pure when the army arrived it would
not have remained so for long if human and animal waste was allowed
to contaminate it. When first encountering a source of fresh water such
as springs, dead plants or logs were to be removed before it was used as
drinking water.

Make the same examination in cisterns and wells as in springs and always be careful
to see whether there is a gummy or greasy mass at the bottom, and take it out. If
you cannot make such an examination, then thoroughly moisten a fine white linen
cloth in the water and fold it loosely; once folded and tied with a cord, suspend
it in the sun or the air and when it has dried, unfold it. If stains appear in it, of
whatever colour, the water is sure to be diseased, but if it is not stained it is healthy.

This is a very practical way of determining how clear the water was. If it
was stained green or brown then algae, mud, animal dung or carcases may
have made the water unhealthy to drink.

Once the hostilities had commenced then the wounded needed special
care, not only so they might recover to rejoin the fight but also as large
numbers of wounded slowed an army down when on the march. Arnold
gave his recommendations for how to treat the wounds and what diet to
take to encourage healing.

All the wounded should use powder of lesser poligony daily as follows, taking a
spoonful of it with wine, fasting – or, if they are poor, with the aforesaid water; and
when the wound has been cleansed let the powder be sprinkled on externally too.
If someone is poisoned, by an arrow or something else, he should take, fasting,
one spoonful of the following powder with aromatic wine or the above mentioned
tisane: Rx one part of citron seed, three parts of hart's tongue fern and make a
powder. Such patients can also be given cabbages with oil as food.

Those who managed to avoid injury were always in danger of contracting an
infectious disease due to the poor sanitary conditions and the overcrowding in an army camp. This could kill as many as died in battle. Arnold
recommended, 'so that the army may be preserved from epidemic, let pits

be dug everywhere outside its lines, like trenches, where animal wastes and bodies can be thrown; and when they are half full, cover them with earth'.

Care of the sick in the medieval Christian infirmary or battlefield tent followed the conventional pattern of spiritual care, nursing care and then medical care. Where medical care was available, the doctor would assess the patient in order to make a prognosis and if possible a diagnosis. For diseases thought to result from humoural imbalance this was followed by treatment which traditionally commenced with the modification of diet, later complemented by drugs, baths and bloodletting if necessary and finally the use of surgery if the former techniques failed. Clearly in the case of trauma, on or off the battlefield, surgery was moved to the top of this list with the other techniques playing a supportive role to strengthen the patient.

CRUSADER FIELD HOSPITALS

The role of medical staff in maintaining the health of an army had been well understood since classical times,[56] and they were just as essential during the medieval period. Crusader armies sustained many thousands of casualties during the twelfth and thirteenth centuries and rulers in command had to develop ways to cope with them on campaign. The wounded not only slowed down the army but also weakened its fighting strength, and restoring the injured to fitness would have increased the likelihood of victory.

In the early years of the crusades there is no record of organised field hospitals, although doctors did accompany the armies on the march.[57] It seems that the injured were usually taken to the nearest friendly town after a battle to be cared for there. At the battle of Tell Danith near Antioch on 14 August 1119, Walter the Chancellor mentioned how those wounded who were unable to walk or crawl off the battlefield were helped.[58] King Baldwin II came back to the battlefield the next day and, 'he ordered that both those wounded on the field and the dead to be brought from there and all around', presumably to be given first aid and then returned to Antioch with him to recover. During the Third Crusade, King Richard I of England had so many wounded and sick by January 1192 that they were slowing down the army and limiting its effectiveness. It is also possible that he was concerned for the health of his soldiers as the chronicles suggest.

[56] Nutton 1969; Jackson 1988 pp. 112–37.   [57] Edgington 1994.
[58] Walter the Chancellor 1896 pp. 104–5; Walter the Chancellor 1999 p. 155.

An enormous number of the sick would have died if it had not been for King Richard, because they could not take care of themselves and had no one to look after them. Prompted by his regard for divine mercy he took care of everyone, sending messengers all around to seek out those who were ill. In his goodness he gathered together those who were dying, and when he had assembled them all he arranged from them to be brought with him to Ramle.[59]

If there was a public hospital in Ramle the records of this have not come to the attention of modern scholars, but it is likely that every town in the region would have had at least a hostel for pilgrim accommodation. We can only presume that the sick and injured were cared for in the town hostel, unoccupied houses or tents. It is unknown whether they merely received food and shelter or whether formal medical care was arranged. On other occasions no preparation could be made for casualties, as was the case for surprise attacks or small raids into enemy territory. A Frankish caravan taking supplies from Jaffa to King Richard I's army at Beit Nuba was ambushed by Muslim forces on 17 June 1192. Those who survived had to make their way to the camp as best they could. A record of the event tells how, 'they gently laid our wounded and fallen on horses and took them back to the army'.[60] On another occasion William Longspee attacked a Muslim caravan near Alexandria during the crusade to Egypt in 1250. We hear that, 'he lost only one knight and eight retainers who were slain; some, however, were wounded, whom he brought back to be restored by medical aid'.[61]

Sometimes the slow pace at which the sick could move put both themselves and others at risk. In December 1191 the injured crusaders who were recovering in the city of Jaffa were keen to rejoin the army of King Richard I as it was rumoured to be about to attack Jerusalem. Understandably, many were unable to walk and they were carried in the customary way.

Those who had fallen sick at Jaffa were carried to the army on pallets and litters, hoping to advance to Jerusalem . . . However, while the sick were being carried along like this the Turks rushed down on them, killing the bearers with the sick because they did not believe any of their enemies should be spared.[62]

This slow-moving caravan must have been a easy target for passing enemy troops. Some commanders took care to provide transport for the inevitable casualties so that they did not slow the army down. We have good details

[59] Richard de Templo 1864 p. 310; Richard de Templo 1997 p. 285.
[60] Richard de Templo 1864 p. 376; Richard de Templo 1997 p. 333.
[61] Matthew Paris [Luard] 1880, v, p. 132; Matthew Paris [Giles] 1853, II, p. 354.
[62] Richard de Templo 1864 p. 304; Richard de Templo 1997 p. 279.

of the preparations Emperor Frederick of Germany made for his crusade in 1189. With regard to the transport of the sick and wounded the *Itinerarium Peregrinorum et Gesta Regis Ricardi* noted that, 'a great many wagons were constructed for sick travellers so that the infirm should not delay the healthy and the crowd of sick and destitute should not perish on the way'.[63]

There are some early examples when it is known that the wounded were treated while the army was on the march, rather then just sent to the nearest town. In January 1126, King Baldwin of Jerusalem was engaged in battle with Tughtegin near Mergisafar on the Plain of Medan. William of Tyre[64] recounted that 'they sent the wounded back to the baggage train to receive care'. In the confusion of battle it must have been difficult to know exactly where to take the injured for medical care. In the Third Crusade we are told that Richard I of England had his banner hoisted up on a tall wooden pole. To allow it to be moved about with the army the pole was placed on a wooden platform on wheels. This was surrounded by a force of soldiers whose job it was to prevent it falling into enemy hands. It is recorded that 'the infirm and wounded are brought there to be cared for',[65] protected by the knights while the battle raged on around them.

The first evidence for an actual field hospital in the Frankish armies dates from the 1180s. A text written by an anonymous cleric about his experiences as a patient in the hospital of St John in Jerusalem also recorded information regarding the medical facilities provided by the Order of St John on the battlefield.[66] He mentioned that those soldiers of the army who were wounded were attended to in mobile hospitals set up in tents of the order. Those who needed further treatment were transported to the Jerusalem hospital, or closer towns if necessary, using camels, horses and donkeys kept for this purpose. The four surgeons working for the hospital of St John in Jerusalem at that time[67] are known to have been attached to this field hospital. Usama described the type of large tent used in Frankish armies on the march.[68] The particular tent he claims he saw was actually for use as a church by the patriarch, but it is plausible that a field hospital might be similar, with the addition of beds or mattresses. The floor was covered with bulrushes and grass to prevent the ground becoming muddy in wet weather. Unfortunately many fleas and other insects lived in the floor covering, which caused a nuisance to those inside. In 1190 during the long siege of Acre by Christian forces in the Third Crusade merchants and

[63] Richard de Templo 1864 p. 43; Richard de Templo 1997 p. 55.
[64] William of Tyre 1986, I, pp. 608–10; William of Tyre, 1943, II, p. 29.
[65] Richard de Templo 1864 p. 250; Richard de Templo 1997 p. 237.   [66] Kedar 1998.
[67] *Cartulaire Général* 1894–1906, I, p. 458, cart. 690.   [68] Usama ibn Munqidh 1929 p. 116.

sailors from the Baltic Sea, Bremen and Hamburg established an improvised field hospital made out of wood from dismantled ships and roofed with sail canvas.[69] The knowledge that they had to break up ships to build this suggests that the troops had not brought a field hospital with them on the crusade, but that circumstances had triggered the foundation. A similar field hospital was established by the English troops at Acre at the same siege. This was organised by a priest named William and was dedicated to the martyr St Thomas Becket.[70] It has been suggested that military medicine at in the crusades was unstructured and of poor quality, with only the wealthy nobles receiving appropriate medical care.[71] However, the presence of such field hospitals from the late twelfth century onwards shows a coordinated and practical approach to the care of the sick and wounded on campaign.

TOWN HOSPITALS

It was principally the poor and pilgrims who tended to use those Latin hospitals that were open to the public. The wealthy of the kingdom could hire the services of a doctor who would come to their own home or castle and who was in a position to give his undivided attention to the well-being of his client. When Conrad of Montferrat, the ruler of Jerusalem, was stabbed by two of the Assassin sect in April 1192 at Tyre, he was carried to his own palace[72] rather than to one of the town's hospitals, as might happen today. Likewise, as a child in the early 1170s Prince Baldwin, the son of King Amalric of Jerusalem, did not go to a hospital for treatment of his leprosy but had physicians brought to him.[73] There are a few examples of nobility using the services of these hospitals and these were typically those from Europe without property or family in the kingdom on which to rely. Count Henry of Rodez made his will while in the hospital of St John for the sick in Acre during October 1222.[74] In 1190 Clarembaud, seigneur of Noyers, gave the Order of St John at Tyre a gift of 100 sous every year in gratitude for the care he received at the time he fell ill in the Holy Land.[75] The poor inhabitants of the Frankish states certainly did not have the money to obtain the services of a personal physician. Pilgrims from Europe may have been unwelcome in their lodgings if there was a perceived risk of their spreading disease to others in their dormitory. Members of these

---

[69] Prawer 1972a p. 119; Mayer 1988 p. 142; Sterns 1983.   [70] Ralph of Diceto 1876, II, p. 80–1.
[71] Gabriel and Metz 1992 pp. 207–8.   [72] Ambroise 1897 p. 235; Ambroise 1939 p. 119.
[73] Mitchell 2000a.   [74] *Cartulaire Général* 1894–1906, II, pp. 308–9, cart. 1760.
[75] *Cartulaire Général* 1894–1906, I, p. 571, cart. 900.

three groups might have stood a better chance of survival if cared for in one of the public hospitals.

Hospitals in the Frankish states developed from a variety of sources, with origins back in the early Islamic period or newly built during the Latin occupation. Some were run by carers with purely religious motives while others involved a more calculated functional approach, by healing wounded soldiers to keep the army up to strength. All the hospitals for which there is evidence of medical care were run by military orders, and funding came from pilgrim gifts and legacies as well as from the profits from the farming land owned by these orders. One possible reason for the range of different hospitals was the linguistic diversity found between different areas of the Frankish states. While the social and cultural dominance of the Franks made French the verbal language of the Latin East (although much written correspondence was in Latin), different groups which formed up the original armies naturally spoke differently. In the kingdom of Jerusalem people tended to speak the dialect of northern and central France, in the county of Tripoli the language was often Provençal or Occitan, and in the principality of Antioch it was Norman.[76] This was quite apart from the confusion added by those from England, Spain, Italy, Germany, Hungary and Scandinavia who used their native languages among themselves. The sick would naturally seek someone who spoke their own language or dialect at a time when complete clarity might be extremely beneficial to their health. This helps to explain the presence of hospitals run by the French, English and Germans in the same town.

THE ORDER OF SAINT JOHN (KNIGHTS HOSPITALLER)

In the second half of the eleventh century Amalfitan merchants refurbished the decaying monastery of St Mary in Jerusalem, then under the tolerant control of the Fatmid caliph al-Mustansir (reigned 1036–1094). Along with this they renovated the old hostel which had been dedicated to St John the Baptist by the Byzantines in the fifth century.[77] They staffed the complex (Figure 3) with Italian Benedictines who in return provided accommodation to Amalfitans on business or pilgrimage in the area. A convent of nuns was also founded to cater for women in the hostel of St Mary Magdalene. The name of the first abbess was Agnes and the nuns wore an eight-pointed white cross on a red habit.[78] A third hostel was then built for the benefit of

---

[76] Prawer 1972a p. 199.
[77] Jacques of Vitry 1611 p. 1082; Jacques of Vitry 1971 pp. 46–8; Saewulf 1994 p. 67; Luttrell 1997.
[78] Delaville 1904.

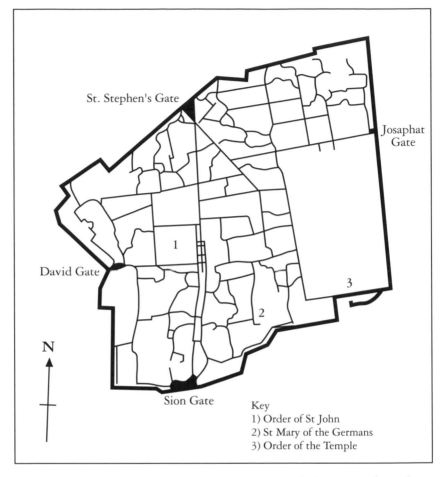

St. Stephen's Gate

Josaphat Gate

David Gate

1

2

3

N

Sion Gate

Key
1) Order of St John
2) St Mary of the Germans
3) Order of the Temple

Figure 3.   Map of twelfth-century Jerusalem, marked with the location of several
Frankish hospitals

non-Amalfitans and this was entrusted to lay brothers, whose counterparts were later to be the Knights Hospitaller, and for distinction they wore white crosses on their black mantles. After the First Crusade, with the Levant now in Frankish hands, many crusaders and pilgrims decided to join them in caring for the poor and needy and numbers swelled. It is likely that this was influenced by religious fervour associated with the pilgrimage to Jerusalem. The institution became a self-governing body by 1113 when it was recognised as such by Pope Pascal II in the bull *Pie Postulatio Voluntatis* dated 15 February.[79] The order developed complexes in several other major cities such as Acre, Antioch and Jaffa,[80] at an early stage although the presence of a *hospitale* is not necessarily mentioned.

In a few years the *hospitale* of St John in Jerusalem gained considerable fame through the caring activities of brother Gerard, sister Agnes and others,[81] so that gifts and legacies from pilgrims, crusaders and nobility enabled its expansion. After a battle with the Egyptians on the plain of Ascalon in September 1101 one-tenth of the captured plunder was given to, 'the Hospital and Christ's poor'.[82] Roger I, count of Sicily, sent an envoy to the patriarch of Jerusalem in 1101 with 1,000 gold bezants. These were to be divided equally between the Holy Sepulchre, the king's army and 'the Hospital for the feeble and other sick'. Unfortunately the patriarch kept the lot for his own personal use, as he had done with a number of other donations. With this evidence he was proved guilty of fraud and was deprived of his powers, while many of his staff were thrown into prison.[83] Raymond de Puy succeeded brother Gerard following his death in 1118[84] and became the first master of the Order of St John. Some time between 1125 and 1153 he added a chapter to the original rule of Gerard[85] concerning the care of the sick, which described a caring approach to the patients in a strongly religious setting.[86] This rule was an adaptation of the rule of St Augustine,[87] as was so common in European *hospitalia*, rather than the Benedictine rule of the original founders. In article 16 of his rule it is written,

in the obedience in which the master and the chapter of the hospital shall permit, when the sick man [*malade*] shall come here let him be received thus, let him partake of the Holy Sacrament first having confessed his sins to the priest, and afterwards let him be carried to bed, and there as if he were a Lord, each day before the brethren go to eat, let him be refreshed with food charitably according to the ability of the house.

This confession of sins on arrival is fully in agreement with religious views at that time. In the slightly later Fourth Lateran Council of 1215, it was stated that,

as sickness of the body may sometimes be the result of sin . . . we by this decree order and strictly command physicians of the body, when they are called to the

---

[79] *Cartulaire Général* 1894–1906, i, p. 29–30, cart. 30.
[80] *Cartulaire Général* 1894–1906, i, p. 9, cart. 5; p. 21, cart. 20.
[81] Jacques of Vitry 1611 p. 1082; Jacques of Vitry 1971 p. 48; Hume 1940; Barber 2000.
[82] Albert of Aachen bk 7, ch. 70.   [83] Albert of Aachen bk 7, ch. 62.
[84] *Cartulaire Général* 1894–1906, i, pp. 38–9, cart. 46.
[85] *Cartulaire Général* 1894–1906, i, pp. 62–8, cart. 70; King 1934 pp. 20–8.
[86] Sinclair 1978.   [87] Riley-Smith 1967 p. 48.

sick, to warn and persuade them first of all to call in physicians of the soul so that after their spiritual health has been seen to they may respond better to the medicine for their bodies; for when the cause ceases so does the effect.[88]

This concept is echoed in later documents of the Latin East too. In 1252–7 the Latin Church of Cyprus recorded just the same order of treatment, priest before doctor, for the Franks living there who became sick.[89]

One Frankish pilgrim guide from 1128–37 used the terms *xenodochium* and *nosokomeion* to differentiate the functions of the hospital in Jerusalem.

In Jerusalem is the xenodochium or the nosokomeion. The Greek word xen-odochium translated into Latin is a refuge for travellers and poor people. Nosokomeion is the hospice [*hospitale*] which cares for the sick people [*egrotantes*] taken into it from the squares and alleys.[90]

The use of the words *egroti* and *nosokomeion*, especially when distinguished from *xenodochium*, is an important early indication of the function of the hospital and the type of clientele who stayed there. Certainly the Frankish writer regarded the hospital of St John of Jerusalem as looking after acutely sick people. Furthermore, it was looking after them in the way a *nosokomeion* would, namely by providing them with medical treatment. This is the earliest indication of such a function that I have been able to identify. Before this time, the hospital is typically referred to as being for the poor. However, a document of Roger of Sicily from 1136[91] refers to those in the hospital at Jerusalem as the poor and sick (*infirmis*), and Pope Innocent II similarly mentioned the sick in the hospital between 1139 and 1143.[92] Strictly speaking, the word *infirmis* refers to the disabled and the weak, but the term sick is often used as these groups must have had a disease of some kind to incapacitate them, even if it was just arthritis or malnutrition. The earliest use of the word *egroti* in the order's own archives is from 1175, when referring to the hospital of the order at Acre.[93] However, other than the use of the term *nosokomeion* mentioned above there is no reference to provision of medical treatment by that time, just food and lodging in a strongly religious setting. Theodorich[94] was a pilgrim who saw the hospital in 1169, some time after Raymond de Puy's chapter. He wrote,

---

[88] Decrees of the Ecumenical Councils 1990, I, p. 245.   [89] *Synodicum Nicosiense* 2001 pp. 96–7, XII.
[90] Work on Geography 1860 p. 427; Work on Geography 1988 p. 200.
[91] *Cartulaire Général* 1894–1906, I, p. 100, cart. 119.
[92] *Cartulaire Général* 1894–1906, I, p. 107, cart. 130.
[93] *Cartulaire Général* 1894–1906, I, p. 323, cart. 471.
[94] Theodericus 1994 pp. 157–8, Theodorich 1988 p. 287.

I would not trust anyone to believe it if I had not seen with my own eyes how splendidly it is adorned with buildings with many rooms and bunks and other things poor people and the weak and the sick can use. What a rich place this is and how excellently it spends the money for the relief of the poor and how diligent in its care for beggars. Going through the Palaces we could in no way judge the number of people who lay there, but we saw a thousand beds.

The fact that Theodorich did not know how many patients were in the hospital, despite counting how many beds there were, is perplexing. It is possible that there were fewer patients than 1,000 if not all the beds were full at that time, or that there were more than 1,000 if the extra patients were lying on the floor.

John of Würzburg[95] was present in Jerusalem around the same time (c.1170), and wrote,

in various houses a great crowd of sick people is collected, some of them women and some men. They are cared for and every day fed at vast expense. The total number of persons at the time when I was present I learned from the servitors talking about it, and it was two thousand sick persons. Between night and day there were sometimes more than fifty corpses carried out, but again and again there were new people admitted. What more can I say! This house feeds so many human beings outside and within.

Clearly he regarded the hospital to have been for sick people, rather than just the poor and hungry, and this is supported by the claim that a significant number died each day (perhaps 1–5 per cent). Even more interesting is that he describes that they were made well again at great expense. He could have merely meant that the food and bed provided by the order allowed many of the sick to cure themselves, but he might also be implying that doctors and were employed and medicines given. The dietary supplementation of the poor inhabitants of Jerusalem, distinct from the patients, should have been an effective form of preventative medicine for the time. It is well known that the undernourished are more susceptible to many diseases.[96] Even apart from the specific nutritional deficiency syndromes, insufficient intake of energy, certain vitamins and minerals has been associated with an impaired immune function and the reduced ability to resist infection. Maintenance of an adequate diet for the poor would be expected to reduce the numbers subsequently requiring the services of the hospital. Of course, the order would have been unlikely to see it that way and probably just thought of it as another way to express their charity. The estimates of 1,000 beds

---

[95] John of Würzburg 1994 p. 131; John of Würzburg 1988 p. 266.
[96] Chandra 1986; Gross and Newberne 1980; Watson 1984.

by Theodorich and 2,000 patients by John of Würzburg were enormous numbers for a hospital at that time. The figures immediately provoke the response that this must have been medieval exaggeration,[97] but it is known that the building was very large. After the battle of Montgisard in 1177, 750 wounded were taken to the Jerusalem hospital despite there already being 900 patients in it at the time.[98] A study of patient capacity in this hospital is outlined in a later section, to see if medieval exaggeration can indeed be blamed.

The statutes of Master Roger des Moulins (1177–87) incorporated a number of decrees[99] at the Chapter-General of March 1182. He records 'that for the sick in the hospital there should be engaged four wise doctors [*mieges/medici*] who are qualified to examine urine and to diagnose different diseases and are able to administer appropriate medicines'. The beds of the sick were to be as long and wide as was most convenient to lie on, but exact measurements were not given. Each person was to have a sheepskin cloak, boots and a cap of wool for going to the toilets. Interestingly, the toilets at the complex of St John in Acre have now been excavated and it has been shown that many of those who used the latrines were infested with parasitic intestinal worms such as roundworm, whipworm and fish tapeworm.[100] Brethren of the order were to guard and watch the sick poor day and night, serving them 'with enthusiasm and devotion as if they were their Lords'. Other decrees included the use of cradles for babies born in that part of the hospital reserved for women, so that they should not be disturbed by their mother's restlessness. Nine sergeants of the order, not of noble birth like the knights, were assigned to each ward to wash feet, change sheets, give food to the weak and be at the service of the sick. Also recorded were details of the tribute Hospitaller priories outside the area had to send for the benefit of the sick at the hospital in Jerusalem. The Frankish bailiff of Tiberias and the prior of Tripoli each had to send two quintals of sugar for syrups and medicines for the sick, as these areas had considerable sugar cane plantations.[101] From Europe the priors of France and St Gilles each had to send 100 dyed sheets to replace those worn out with use, while the Frankish bailiff of Antioch sent 2,000 ells of cotton cloth for coverlets. The prior of Constantinople was required to send 200 felts for the sick, while the priories of Italy, Pisa and Venice, each had to contribute 2,000 ells of coarse twilled fabric of diverse colours.

---

[97] Miller 1978; Luttrell 1994.   [98] *Beiträge* 1874 p. 128.
[99] *Cartulaire Général* 1894–1906, I, pp. 425–9 cart. 627.
[100] Mitchell and Stern 2000.   [101] Ibn al-Furat 1971, II, p. 113.

Two years later, in 1184, Pope Lucius III mentions the presence of four *medici* and the same number of *cyrurgici* at work in the hospital for sick poor.[102] Not only did this show an increase in the number of doctors in the Palais des Malades to eight, but it also shows a perceived need for the treatment of injuries and other surgical conditions. It has been suggested that the surgeons were underworked compared with the general doctors, particularly in times of relative peace.[103] However, the injuries from falls and other accidents would still have occurred, elective surgery was still needed for chronic surgical conditions such as abscesses, hernias and bladder stones, and it should not be forgotten that medieval surgeons also treated a wide range of pathologies today seen by physicians, such as a number of skin and venereal diseases and ascites.[104] It is unlikely that the order would have spent money on employing unnecessary doctors as more could always have been contracted from the community in times of need, such as after battles. It seems more logical to interpret this text to show that there must have been a need for these four surgeons in the hospital working at a typical workload.

A manuscript containing a valuable set of regulations of the order that were not published in Delaville le Roulx's *cartulaire* has recently come to light.[105] They are dated to between 1177 and 1183 and were entitled, 'Concerning food for the sick, doctors and the organisation of the Palace of the Sick in Jerusalem'. The admission procedure began with the confession of sins to the chaplain followed by a meal. Clothes were then exchanged for the bed clothes used in the hospital and the pilgrim was given eating and drinking utensils. The daily routine comprised of mass every morning and a procession through the wards every evening saying prayers. Patients ate at tables and the linen was changed every two months. Details of food given included white bread, wine twice a day, meat such as poultry, young goat and lamb, and vegetables such as vegetable broth and barley-meal gruel. If the doctors advised it further foods were given. Boar (male pig) could also be served between Michaelmas and Lent but never the meat of the sow (female). The same advice on the time of year that pork could be eaten is found in Eastern texts on dietetics, such as the fourth-century work of Oribasius of Pergamon.[106] The sick were also given fruits such as pomegranates, apples, pears, plums, figs and grapes and other treats such as almond milk. Interestingly, cereal grains and pollen of wheat, barley and rye along with fig seeds have been recovered from excavation of the latrines

[102] *Cartulaire Général* 1894–1906, I, p. 458 cart. 690. [103] Edgington 1999.
[104] Theodorich Borgognoni 1498; Theodorich Borgognoni 1955–60.
[105] Edgington 1998b; Edgington 1999. [106] Oribasius 1997 p. 37.

of the Order of St John in Acre. However, it is not known whether these particular latrines were used by the patients, or just the soldiers and staff of the order.[107] Foods forbidden in the hospital included lentils, beans, eels and cheese. A discussion of the dietary regime in hospitals of the Orders of St John, of the Temple and the Teutonic Order is given later in this chapter and comparisons made with dietary advice in medical texts from Europe and the Middle East. This comparison allows an assessment of the dominant influences upon Frankish hospitals, to see if they followed European or Eastern ideologies. Fascinatingly, the findings suggest that previous ideas as to the principal influences of medical care in Frankish hospitals may have been entirely wrong.

There were twelve sergeants per ward in the day and two at night, to make beds, wash the patients, bring them fresh water and take them to the toilets. The weakest patients were under the care of a *fisicien* while other patients were looked after by the *mieges*. A new doctor was required to take an oath when he started work in the hospital and 'would swear by the saints or would vow to do all in his power to look after the sick'. It has been suggested that these two alternative versions of the oath enabled doctors of all religions to work in the hospital.[108] Christians would be expected to swear by the saints while non-Christian doctors would choose the latter oath. A parallel can be found in records of the order's hospital on Rhodes in 1445, when a Jewish doctor named Jacuda Gratiano was employed after swearing his oath on Jewish holy scriptures.[109] The sum of 1,500 bezants was allocated each year to hire doctors and buy almonds for the sick. While it is not clear what proportion of this figure was for doctors rather than almonds, it does suggest that the pay was probably generous. The Italian master Robertus *medicus* was paid 100 bezants a year in 1220 to treat the Bolognese troops on the Fifth Crusade to Egypt.[110] If it is assumed that all eight doctors in the hospital of St John in the 1180s received this salary then that would still only account for 800 bezants, leaving enough money to buy an awful lot of almonds. When the effects of medieval inflation and coin debasement are borne in mind it can be seen that 100 bezants would have bought much more in the 1180s than the 1220s. Clearly this approach has its limitations, as not all doctors would have received the same wage, it depending on their experience and qualifications. The *fisicien* may well have received more than the *mieges*, for example. However, it does suggest that wages for doctors in the hospital would have been generous.

[107] Mitchell, Huntley and Stern, in press.   [108] Edgington 1998b; Edgington 1999.
[109] Luttrell 1994.   [110] *Annali Bolognesi* 1789, II, part 2, p. 442.

Another highly informative manuscript discovered recently dates from the 1180s, in which an anonymous cleric wrote of his experiences as a patient in the hospital of St John in Jerusalem.[111] This eye witness says that it was not only Christians who stayed in the hospital but also Jews and 'pagans' (Muslims). This is particularly interesting bearing in mind the high profile of religious ceremonies in the daily life of the hospital, which might be expected to have put off people from non-Christian religions from attending. The section of the hospital for men was divided up into eleven wards and if all the beds became full then the brethren gave up their own beds to create new wards for the hospital. The section for women was also divided up into wards but no information was given as to the number, presumably as the male writer would not have been allowed into these areas. There were apparently 143 male nurses for the eleven male wards which equate to thirteen per ward, not that different from the evidence in the statutes.

The doctors (both *medici* and *cyrurgici*) were salaried and employed exclusively in the hospital. Accompanied by two servants, they visited the sick twice each day and checked their urine and pulse.[112] One of the servants would hold up the urine flasks for the doctor to examine them and then discard the contents once they were no longer needed. The other carried 'syrups, oxymel, electuaries and other medicines'. Medical texts of the period were full of praise for oxymel, a liquid made from vinegar and sugar syrup. The contemporary Arabic book of pharmacy by al-Samarqandi (died 1210) wrote, 'oxymel is a syrup which is beneficial in acute fevers as it calms the heat, prevents putrefaction, stops the confusion of humours and opens obstruction'.[113] The doctor's dietary instructions were recorded for each patient and arrangements made for bloodletting as required. Like the doctors, the bloodletters (*minutores*) were also paid a regular salary by the hospital. The section *De cyrugicis hospitale* described how surgeons from the hospital accompanied the Christian army into battle and treated the wounded in tents. There was also reference to 'the strength in stones and the power in herbs' and to the fact that all the medicines requested by the doctors were provided by the order's treasury. It is not clear if the stones mentioned were ground and then used topically as poultices or taken orally, or whether the stones were used whole as amulets.[114] While there is no direct evidence for the names of doctors who worked in the hospital, a number did sign documents of the order at locations where a hospital was known

---

[111] Kedar 1998. [112] See Wallis 2000. [113] Al-Samarqandi 1967 p. 62.
[114] Spier 1993; Meaney 1981 pp. 66–105.

and some of these were wills, suggesting that the individual concerned may have been a patient. Master Bertrandus and master Petrus Maurinus signed the will of Count Henry I of Rodez in 1221 as he lay in the hospital of St John at Acre[115] and master Johannes *medicus* witnessed a document written in the Acre complex in 1244.[116] It is possible that these practitioners may have been employed by the order to work in the hospital at those times.

At last firm evidence for the medical treatment of the sick in the hospital of St John is found, eighty years after the foundation of the Frankish states. While there are references to the presence of sick in the hospital since the 1130s, it is only in the 1180s that doctors are mentioned. Not only were doctors employed then, but there are references to medicines and the sugar cane to make them with. This implies that the hospital prepared many of its own drugs rather than buying them all ready made from apothecaries in the town. This information does not prove that the hospital did not provide medical care before the 1180s, but it is safe to say that evidence for this is scanty at present. However, it does suggest that back in the times of the Amalfitans or brother Gerard the institution should not be thought of in the same way as the hospital that had evolved by the 1180s.

An idea of the location and structure of the hospital for the sick in Jerusalem can be gathered from the account known as the *Travels of John Mandeville*. Since Schick's original excavation report of the Hospitaller complex,[117] Mandeville has often been quoted as it appears to give the exact location of the hospital for sick poor within the complex. However, this text was written in the mid-fourteenth century, and most of it was copied from earlier texts, with much of the rest comprised of imaginary tales; it is quite likely that the author never went to the east to see the hospital himself.[118] In consequence, we must ask ourselves just how reliable Mandeville really is. However, he does contain some details that closely match the archaeological findings, such as the number of columns in the hospital for the sick. This is not found in those other pilgrim accounts that survive today, such as the Estat de la Cité de Iherusalem,[119] and suggests that some kind of eye witness source was consulted while he was preparing this section of his work.

In it are one hundred and twenty four pillars of stone, and in the walls of the house, besides the number aforesaid, there are fifty four pillars which support the house. From that hospital going towards the east is a very fair church, which is called Our Lady the Great, and after it another very near, called Our Lady the Latin.[120]

---

[115] *Documents Historiques* 1900 p. 19.   [116] *Regesta Regni* 1893, 1, p. 299 doc. 1122.
[117] Schick 1902.   [118] Denny 1973 pp. 9–14; Kohanski 2001 p. xx–xxviii.
[119] L'Estat de la Cité de Iherusalem, 1882, pp. 34–5; *The City of Jerusalem* 1897, p. 7.
[120] John Mandeville 1848 p. 168; John Mandeville 1983 p. 80.

If we are still sceptical about Mandeville, the recently identified manuscript by the anonymous cleric who stayed in the hospital in the 1180s also confirms the location.[121] This text mentions that the part of the hospital for men was divided up into eleven wards. If we consult the excavation plans of Schick, it is seen that in the east–west alignment there are eleven halls in the building suggested to be the hospital. Each of these sources of information seems to corroborate the others.

Archaeological excavation of the complex of St John in Jerusalem took place at the very end of the nineteenth century (Figure 4). The report[122] gives important structural information.

Being all erected about the same time, the buildings were all according to one plan and style, massive with square piers, supporting vaults and arches . . . The whole area of the place formed one building, although consisting of various parts and often divided by narrow lanes, containing some open, but small, courts for light and air.

The location of the hospital for sick poor in the complex is identifiable on comparing the information from Mandeville and the anonymous cleric with the excavation plan. It was situated in the north-west corner of the complex, to the west of the Church of St Mary Major and north of the church of St John. The building is supported by fifty-four pillars, exactly the number mentioned in Mandeville. The internal dimensions of this hall were 230 feet (70 m) by 120 feet (36.5 m) with its long axis approximately north–south. The arches were about 18 feet high (5.5 m). The roof of the main part of the hall was supported by three rows of seven piers, creating thirty-two bays. Three more piers supported a six-bay extension to the south, resulting in a total of thirty-eight bays in the hospital. Some pillars in the complex were noted to be particularly thick, which suggests that originally there would have been upper floors to a number of buildings. Unfortunately it is not known if the section of the hospital for women was in the same block as the men but on a different floor, or perhaps in a separate part of the complex. A considerable number of cisterns underneath the complex collected rain during the winter, ensuring an adequate water supply, and effluent was removed via a network of drains. The west entrance of the church of St Mary Major opened directly to the fifth east–west vault of the hospital, so providing the medicine for the soul typical of Latin hospitals. It has been suggested that the part of the hospital for women was located in the east of the complex.[123] However, the building proposed is not adjacent to any of the churches in the complex, nor does it contain its

---

[121] Kedar 1998.   [122] Schick 1902.   [123] Boas 2001 p. 87.

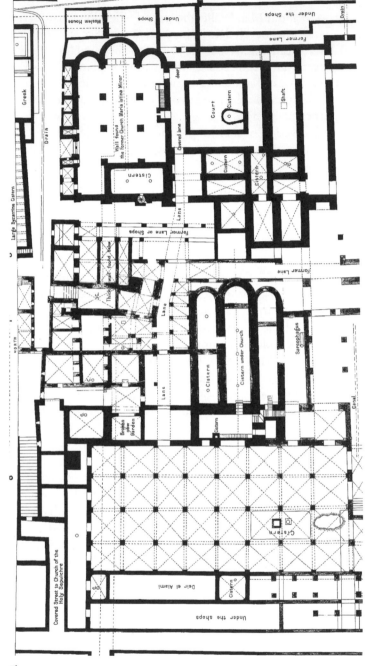

Figure 4. Plans of the hospital of St. John in Jerusalem (after Schick 1902). (a) Plan of Muristan complex; (b) East–west section through hospital and adjoining church of Maria Latina Major

Reproduced with the permission of the Palestine Exploration Fund.

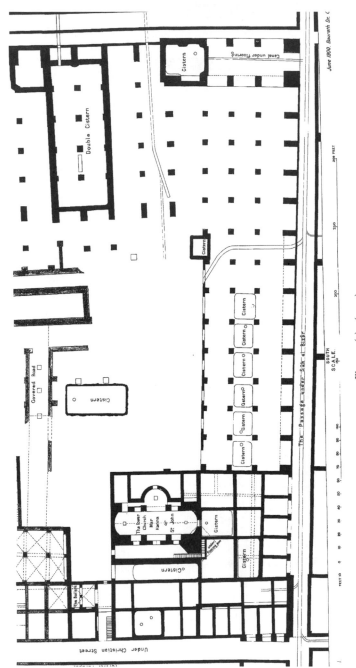

Figure 4(a). (*cont.*)

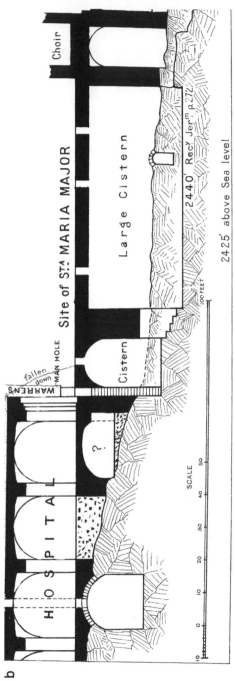

Figure 4(b).

own chapel. In consequence this building is highly unlikely to have been a hospital, as the intimate association with a church is not present.

The dead mentioned by John of Würzburg and others would have been buried in the communal cemetery for deceased pilgrims at the Hospitaller church of St Mary in Aceldama, to the south of the city walls.[124] The church and surrounding land was given to the Order of St John in 1143 by William I, Patriarch of Jerusalem.[125] Theodorich[126] wrote that,

In the field of Aceldama, which is separated from Mount Zion only by a valley, is the burial place of strangers. In it is the Church of the Saint and Virgin and Mother of God Mary. It is also where, on the Holy Day of Palms, we buried a brother who had died. His name was Adolf and he was born in Cologne.

Burials did not only take place on the hillside but also deep underground in an unusual building. The nineteenth-century excavation report[127] described the structure at Aceldama as a

building 78 feet long and 57 feet wide, erected over rock-cut caves and a deep trench . . . situated on a steep slope of a rocky hill. At the southern part the roof consists of rock and is level with the hillside and the northern part, being 20 feet lower, is walled up as a rectangular building, roofed with a vault just over the deep rock-hewn trench, which is 63 feet long and 21 feet wide . . . From the top of the roof to the accumulation is 44 feet . . . The depth of the accumulation is not known.

There was a central pier of rock and masonry to support the roof. The masonry work of the walls in the west, north and east, standing on perpendicular rock scarps, seems to be crusading. In the centre of the arch are in one line, at equal distances, nine openings or holes of a square form, nearly two feet wide, which could be covered by flat stones. There were four more square holes 3 foot 4 inches across.

The reason for all these holes was certainly to give light and allow access for air; but they may also have served, as many writers say, for letting down the dead bodies.

Another Jerusalem hospital which came under the control of the Order of St John was that of St Mary. The *hospitale* of St Mary of the Germans was established as an independent institution in the early years of the Frankish states. At that time it did not develop into a religious order, as had been the case for the Hospitallers and the Templars. This may have been because the founders were married. In his *History of Jerusalem*, Jacques of Vitry[128] said of its origins that,

[124] Pringle 1990–1; Boas 2001 p. 185.   [125] *Cartulaire Général* 1894–1906, I, pp. 121–2, cart. 150.
[126] Theodericus 1994 pp. 146–7; Theodorich 1988 p. 277.   [127] Schick 1892.
[128] Jacques of Vitry 1611 p. 1085; Jacques of Vitry 1971 p. 55.

many Teutons and Almayns who went to Jerusalem on pilgrimage could not speak the tongue of the city, so the divine clemency inspired an honourable and religious Teuton, who dwelt in the city with his wife, to build a hospice at his own cost, wherein he might entertain poor and sick Teutons . . . For a long time, in great poverty, he ministered to the sick and needy.

In 1143 a German *hospitale* in Jerusalem, presumably the one described by Jacques de Vitry, was shown to be subordinated to the Order of St John by Pope Celestine II in a letter of 9 December to Master Raymond of the Hospitallers.[129] The point that this institution was under the control of the Knights Hospitaller may suggest that the complex of St Mary in Jerusalem provided medical care for the sick, rather than just performing the role of a pilgrim hostel. This is confirmed by a document of 26 March 1173 from King Amalric which referred to *infirmis* in the German hospital,[130] and a later charter of Amalric from 1177 confirmed a number of properties and farmland owned by the hospital, including sugar cane from Nablus which was for the sick. This suggests the use of syrups and electuaries for the treatment of the sick just as in the main hospital of Order of St John around that time.[131] However, no references to the employment of doctors have come to light for this early period. John of Würzburg noted the complex of St Mary in Jerusalem as it was around 1170,[132] positioned in the south of the city. He wrote,

On the way down the same street, which goes to the gate by which one reaches the Temple, and on the right, is a cross street with a long portico. In this street is a hospital with a church, which has been newly built in honour of Saint Mary, and is called the House of the Germans.

Based on this description the compound has been identified (Figure 3) and subsequently excavated.[133] It has been proposed that from north to south the structures represented a hostel for pilgrims, the church of St Mary and the hospital for the sick, each adjoining and aligned on an axis approximately east–west. However, evidence for the exact location of an infirmary for the sick within this area is debatable since there are no chronicles detailing the internal layout, as was the case for the main hospital of the Order of St John in Jerusalem, nor were any medical debris excavated, such as broken pharmacy jars or urine bottles. In consequence it is arguable where the infirmary might have been located, or even whether the sick would have been separated from pilgrims boarding there in the

---

[129] *Regesta Regni* 1893, I, pp. 54–5, no. 214.   [130] *Tabulae Ordinis* 1869 pp. 7–8, doc. 6.
[131] *Cartulaire Général* 1894–1906, I, pp. 425–9, cart. 627.
[132] John of Würzburg 1994 p. 133; John of Würzburg 1988 p. 267.   [133] Ovadiah 1993.

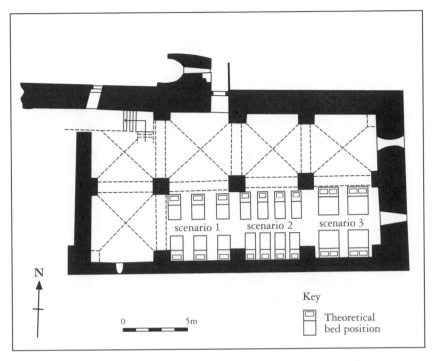

Figure 5. Plan of the hospital of St Mary of the Germans in Jerusalem (after Ovadiah 1993), with possible bed layout options added. Scenario 1: six single beds per bay; scenario 2: eight single beds per bay; scenario 3: four double beds per bay
Plan reproduced with the permission of Professor Ovadiah.

early years. The excavation confirmed that the complex was on a street corner, with a 3-metre wide paved road covered with arches, as noted by John of Würzburg, lying adjacent to the hospital. An ornate painted ceremonial hall was built above the area suggested to be the hospital. The entrance to the north-western corner of this lower hall was down a set of stairs from the south side of the church.

The hall was rectangular in plan, being 25 m long and 12 m wide, with an eight-bay ribbed vaulted roof construction and three supporting central piers (Figure 5). At the eastern end were two narrow windows and originally all four bays in the southern wall had a window (Figure 6). The floor was of flagstones while there was a plaster ceiling and there remain small areas of plaster on the walls today. Despite the compound's proximity to an aqueduct, five cisterns had been dug to collect rainwater. Discarded thirteenth-century glazed pottery fragments were recovered from these cisterns and

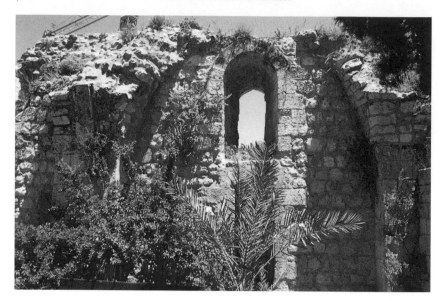

Figure 6. Southern bay of the hospital of St Mary of the Germans in
Jerusalem, looking east

may have been dishes used by the pilgrims. All were of local manufacture
or imported from the east, with no imports from Europe. While it is not
known for certain whether these sherds originated during the Latin occupation between 1229 and 1244,[134] it may be that they were dumped after
the sack of the city. It is presumed that the complex was evacuated in 1187
when Jerusalem fell to Saladin, but it is not clear what happened after that.
Jacques de Vitry wrote in the thirteenth century that this German hospital later evolved into the Teutonic Order after the Third Crusade.[135] It is
perhaps understandable that he might make this connection, as both institutions named their hospitals after St Mary. However, modern assessment
has concluded that that the institutions were actually unrelated, and that
the Teutonic Order developed spontaneously in response to the need to
care for the sick during the long siege of Acre.[136] It is possible that the
hospital of St Mary disbanded after the loss of Jerusalem in 1187, and
that its staff were incorporated into the main hospital of St John from
then on.

[134] Ben Dov 1993.   [135] Jacques of Vitry 1611 p. 1085; Jacques of Vitry 1971 p. 55.
[136] Favreau 1975 pp. 95–161.

The order ran further hospitals throughout the Latin East and played a major role in the treatment of the sick in the Levant. The medical nature of the order means that wherever they had a large complex, it is highly likely there would have been facilities for caring for the sick, even if only an infirmary for the brethren themselves. Changing fortunes and Islamic victories occasionally led to evacuation of these hospitals, as happened in Jerusalem following Saladin's victory at the battle of Hattin on 4 July 1187. Saladin did, unusually for the period, allow ten Hospitallers to stay to care for those sick too unwell to travel. The rest moved to Tyre along with many of the Latin population[137] and then to Margat, which was a town near to the northern boundary of the county of Tripoli.

The hospital of St John the Baptist was run by the Order of St John in Nablus in the twelfth century. The order had possessed property there at least since 1110, shown by the donation of houses and a mill by King Baldwin I on 28 September of that year.[138] At some time in the next fifty years the order had set up a *hospitale* for the poor. King Baldwin III mentions the institution's name as St John the Baptist in a record of 7 June 1156.[139] In 1166 King Amalric confirmed the Order of St John's possession of the *hospitale* in Nablus and of the alms given by previous monarchs, 'on the condition that this hospital always serves the sick'.[140] This reference to the sick shows that this was not merely a pilgrim hostel but a hospital. The complex of St John in Nablus is thought to have been located on what is now the street of the Prophets. Only the western one-third remains, but plans and photographs of the town before the demolition[141] suggest that there was a barrel vaulted structure 50–55 m long and 15–16 m wide. This barrel vaulting ties in well with an early construction date for the complex and contrasts with the romanesque vaults of the later complex of the order in Acre. The surviving part of the vault is 7.8 m wide internally, is constructed from rubble and supported with an ashlar-built transverse arch. Originally the entire surface would have been covered with layers of plaster. The north wall of the vault is 4 m thick and possessed a tower, suggestive of an outer wall, while the much thinner southern wall had three doorways. However, it is not known whether this particular part of the complex housed the sick, lodged pilgrims overnight or was for use by members of the order for other functions. The hospital complex was lost to the Frankish states along with the rest of Nablus after the battle of Hattin in 1187.

---

[137] Ibn al-Athir 1969 p. 180; *Cartulaire Général* 1894–1906, I, pp. 531–2, cart. 858.
[138] *Cartulaire Général* 1894–1906, I, p. 21, cart. 20.
[139] *Cartulaire Général* 1894–1906, I, pp. 183–4, cart. 244.
[140] *Cartulaire Général* 1894–1906, I, p. 245, cart. 355.   [141] Pringle 1993–, II, pp. 104–7.

The order's hospital at Acre was functional at least by 1175,[142] and was located in the northern part of the city (Figure 7). The Hospitallers had property in Acre as early as 1110[143] and since their principal role in the early years was to care for the poor and infirm, it is likely that there was at least a hostel for these people in this large port even then. Statutes of the order[144] show that the hospital for sick pilgrims was in the actual Hospitaller complex, not separate, as some had suggested,[145] in the northern suburb of Montmusard. The hospital of St John for sick poor was known as the *Palais des Malades* while the *hospitale* written on contemporary maps refers to the fortress of St John with the residence of the Grand Master. Much of the site of the Hospitaller complex in Acre has been excavated and remains have been found that are thought to represent several towers, a refectory, dormitory, cloister, reception hall, latrines, barracks and bath house.[146] However, the various buildings previously identified as the hospital of sick pilgrims have since been reassessed and now are believed to have performed other functions. The search for the hospital for sick pilgrims and the infirmary is at present continuing. These are thought to have been located in the south of the complex, as the plan of Frankish Acre by Paolino Veneto (Paulinus de Puteoli) locates the *domus infirmorum* to the south of the other buildings.[147]

In 1200 the bishop of Acre gave the order a cemetery by the walls of the city,[148] which may have been the church of St Michael where the masters of the order were buried by the middle of that century, as recorded in a statute of 1263.[149] Before that time it seems that the dead from the hospital were buried in the public cemetery of the city. In the summer of 1250 Lord John of Joinville stayed at the church of St Michael while sick himself. He mentioned that, 'there was no day on which twenty or more dead were not carried into the church and from my bed, as each was carried in, I heard the chant of "*Libera me Domine*" '.[150] He may well have been watching those who had just died in the nearby hospital of St John for the sick poor. By 1263 a priest and an acolyte were continuously looking after the spiritual welfare of the sick in the hospital at Acre. At the church of St Michael another priest, again assisted by an acolyte, said repeated masses for the

---

[142] *Cartulaire Général* 1894–1906, I, p. 323, cart. 471.
[143] *Cartulaire Général* 1894–1906, I, p. 21, cart. 20.
[144] *Cartulaire Général* 1894–1906, II, pp. 731–2, cart. 2612.   [145] King 1934 p. 104, n. 4.
[146] Goldmann 1966; Goldmann 1994.   [147] Prawer 1953; Jacoby 1979.
[148] *Cartulaire Général* 1894–1906, I, pp. 689–90, cart. 1113.
[149] *Cartulaire Général* 1894–1906, III, pp. 75–7, cart. 3075, stat. 6.
[150] John of Joinville 1874 p. 226; John of Joinville 1955 p. 129.

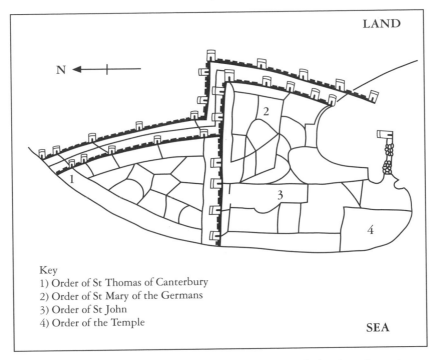

Figure 7. Map of thirteenth-century Acre, marked with the location of several
Frankish hospitals
The ground plan used is based on the early fourteenth-century map of Pietro Vesconte
(see Prawer 1953 and Jacoby 1979).

dead.[151] The competition between the order and the secular church led to
conflict over donations recorded in the wills of the sick. Legislation was
introduced in 1175 to prevent disputes, so that if any sick person with a
will in favour of the church at Acre entered the order's hospital and died
within seven days, the Hospitallers were not entitled to his money unless
he changed his will during his stay there.[152]

While the Order of St John founded some *hospitalia* and renovated
derelict ones, it also took over a number of functioning institutions throughout the Latin East which were run by smaller organisations. These were not
always specifically referred to as caring for the sick but the medical function
of the order suggests that these *hospitalia* may have performed a medical
role as well as just feeding the poor. However, it could also be argued that

---

[151] *Cartulaire Général* 1894–1906, III, pp. 75–7, cart. 3075, stat. 5.
[152] *Cartulaire Général* 1894–1906, I, pp. 323–4, cart. 471.

since the order did provide pilgrim hostels, the *hospitalia* discussed here may have merely provided food and accommodation. For example, a *hospitale pauperum quod est* in Monte Peregrino (Tripoli), to the north of the kingdom of Jerusalem, was founded by Count Raymond of Saint Gilles and extended by his successor Bertrand of Tripoli. On 28 December 1126 Count Pons put an end to the independence of the *hospitale* by transferring it to the Order of St John.[153] The church and cemetery of Mont Pelerin have been excavated and lay a short distance to the south-east of the city.[154] Unfortunately it is unclear exactly where the hospital lay. Likewise, in the county of Edessa there was a *hospitale* attached to the church of St Romain at Turbessel. This was endowed by Joscelin I of Courtnenay and King Baldwin II, but given to the Order of St John in 1134 by Joscelin II with the agreement of the archbishop responsible for the diocese.[155] It has also been tentatively suggested that the order's property at Aqua Bella near Jerusalem may have been an infirmary for sick, aged or wounded members of the order[156] but the evidence for this suggestion is rather weak.

Over time a structural hierarchy developed for those responsible for the caring activities of the order. The Hospitaller was head of these activities, with his office appearing by 1155.[157] His seal was made in black wax, in contrast to the comparable seals of the Grand Commander and Marshal, which were in green. The contemporary thirteenth-century manuscript *Ci Dit des Bulles que le Maistre et les Autres Baillis del Hospital Bullent*[158] described the seal of the Hospitaller 'with a bed, having on it a sick man, with a brother who gives him (food) to eat'. Under him were the seneschal of the *Palais des Malades*, the almoner and the infirmarian. Supervised by the seneschal of the *Palais des Malades* were those taking care of the sick in the hospital. By the end of the 1180s the principal hospital employed four physicians and four surgeons (laymen not members of the order), nine sergeants per hospital ward (brethren of the order) and by the 1260s a priest and acolyte. During the twelfth century the almoner was responsible for distribution of clothes and food to the poor. The post of infirmarian, who ran the infirmary for sick members of the order, is not recorded before 1235. However, the early references to infirmarian do not imply that the post was a new one and it would be expected that someone would have been responsible for similar duties before this time. As well as the brethren of the order, there appear to have been volunteers who helped care for the sick but were not full members. Sancia, the daughter of King James I of Aragon, is

[153] *Cartulaire Général* 1894–1906, I, pp. 74–5, cart. 79.   [154] Salame-Sarkis 1980 pp. 95–119.
[155] *Cartulaire Général* 1894–1906, I, pp. 89–90, cart. 104.   [156] Pringle 1992.
[157] *Cartulaire Général* 1894–1906, I, p. 178, cart. 234.   [158] King 1932 pp. 42 and 127.

believed to have helped care for those in the Acre hospital anonymously up until her death in 1275.[159]

The infirmarian was a brother sergeant, subordinate to the Hospitaller. In November 1235 the post was held by brother Johann, in December 1238 by brother Andrew and in August 1248 by Bernard Corbel.[160] The infirmary was distinct from the hospital for sick pilgrims, at least in thirteenth-century Acre, and cared for members of the Order of St John who were ill. Master Hugh Ravel in the General Chapter of September 1262 tells us[161] that in the infirmary, the doctor's rounds were twice daily, as it is recorded that 'at all times at which the doctor [*miegel medicus*] shall visit the brethren the brother of the infirmary should go with him, that is to say in the morning and in the evening'. The use of the term in the singular might imply that just one doctor was responsible for the infirmary in contrast to the eight who worked in the hospital for sick poor. By 1300 the statutes of Master Guillaume de Villaret record that doctors working in the infirmary in Cyprus had to take an oath of allegiance to the order before the infirmarian and seven other brother representatives of the order.[162] Records of 23 November 1304 clearly describe the spatial separation of the Hospital for the Sick Poor and the infirmary at Limassol.[163] This confirms the approach of the order that sick brothers should be cared for separately from pilgrims, which is implied by earlier references to doctors' rounds specifically in the infirmary at Acre.

Passing references to the use of bloodletting by members of the order confirm its frequency in the infirmary. In the *Esgarts* (judgments) of 1239 it is recorded[164] that 'if any brother have himself bled without leave, unless it be in case of illness . . . let him undergo seven days penance'. The *Usances* (customs of the Hospital) of the same year also include information[165] on the prophylactic use of phlebotomy as 'in the house of the Hospital it is customary that the brethren should be bled on Saturdays'. If we recall the evidence discussed earlier for the use of bloodletting in the hospital for sick poor, these references demonstrate how widely phlebotomy was employed. The procedure was used by the order both to treat disease and also prophylactically to maintain health, as would be expected in Galenic medical theory.[166]

[159] Jaspert 1997; Luttrell 1998.
[160] *Cartulaire Général* 1894–1906, II, p. 493, cart. 2126; p. 536, cart. 2212; pp. 673–4, cart. 2482.
[161] *Cartulaire Général* 1894–1906, III, pp. 43–54, cart. 3039, art. 33.
[162] *Cartulaire Général* 1894–1906, III, pp. 810–16, cart. 4515, stat. 5.
[163] *Cartulaire Général* 1894–1906, IV, pp. 93–4, cart. 4672, stat. 1 and 2.
[164] *Cartulaire Général* 1894–1906, II, p. 546, cart. 2213, stat. 78.
[165] *Cartulaire Général* 1894–1906, II, pp. 548–61, cart. 2213, stat. 105.
[166] Brain 1986 pp. 67–99.

The Order of St John first took on its military role in the 1130s and 1140s, around the same time as the Order of the Temple began taking on the defence of castles. The Hospitallers received the important castle of Bethgibelin in the south of the kingdom of Jerusalem from King Fulk in 1136[167] and by 1180 held twenty-five castles.[168] The papal bull *Quam Amabilis* of Innocent II in 1139–43 mentions the protection of pilgrim routes by the knights of St John.[169] It seems they saw armed protection of pilgrims an extension of their care for the poor in their hospitals.[170]

To summarise, in the early years the hospitals of the Order of St John functioned to care for poor, weak and old pilgrims by providing food and a bed in a religious environment. This was very similar to a typical *hospitale* back in Europe. After a number of decades the function evolved so that by the 1180s there is firm evidence for the medical treatment of sick pilgrims in the order's *hospitalia* at Acre, Jerusalem and Nablus. However, the exact time when medical activities were added to the earlier supportive care of the poor is not clear. By 1235 there was an infirmary for sick members of the order at Acre and later at Limassol, which were distinct from the *Palais des Malades*. Other establishments referred to as *hospitalia* where medical practice is suspected, but not proven, include Tripoli and Turbessel. Medical practitioners working in the main hospital included a *physicus*, several *medici*, *cyrurgici* and a number of *minutores*. Conditions managed there ranged from weapon injuries to the delivery of babies. Treatments known to have been employed include dietary modification, drugs such as oxymel and electuaries, bloodletting and surgery. They also provided a mobile field hospital which accompanied the army into battle, where surgeons from the hospital in Jerusalem worked in tents on the battlefield.

It has been suggested that the hospital of St John was backward, even Third World, compared with equivalent institutions in the medieval Middle East, since it had only eight doctors for perhaps a thousand people, while Islamic and Byzantine hospitals typically had a much better doctor to patient ratio.[171] However, it must be remembered that the majority of patients in this hospital were poor and hungry pilgrims rather than people who were acutely unwell with a specific illness. Most just needed rest, shelter and plenty of food to allow them to regain their strength after an arduous journey east; without family there was no one else to care for them. These people would not have needed the attention of a doctor. Consequently, using the doctor to patient ratio in different institutions to compare the

---

[167] *Cartulaire Général* 1894–1906, I, pp. 97–8, cart. 116.   [168] Prawer 1972b p. 265.
[169] *Cartulaire Général* 1894–1906, I, pp. 107–8, cart. 130.   [170] Forey 1984.   [171] Kedar 1998.

standard of care in Frankish and non-Frankish hospitals is not very reliable as it does not compare like with like. The patients in the hospital of St John were a different group from typical hospitals elsewhere in the eastern Mediterranean, and the hospital performed a rather different role. In view of this it is not really possible to say whether the hospitals of the order of St John in the Latin East were any better or worse than their equivalents in neighbouring countries. However, it would be safe to say that at least by the 1180s they appear to be far in advance of most European *hospitalia*, having evolved to both care and attempt to cure on a large scale.

THE ORDER OF THE TEMPLE

The Templars were founded in 1120 by a group of knights led by Hugh of Payns.[172] Their aim was to protect pilgrims from brigands, Muslim raids and wild animals. These were a real problem in the early years of the Frankish states, and some chroniclers mention how human bodies were left to decompose by the side of certain roads after attacks as people were too scared to stop and bury them.[173] The order received its name from the position of its headquarters, as the knights were given space by King Baldwin II at the south of the former Jewish Temple in Jerusalem, in and around the Aqsa mosque (Figure 3).[174] Originally attached to the regular canons of the Holy Sepulchre, they were formally recognised by the pope as a military order in 1129. The knights wore white mantles with a red cross while sergeants and squires wore black or brown mantles and their rule was based on that of the Cistercians.[175] While no Templar infirmary has ever been excavated, the complex of the order in Jerusalem was surveyed during the repairs to the Aqsa mosque of 1938–42.[176] Unfortunately, those areas around the Aqsa mosque that were not of Muslim origin have been removed since that time. New buildings constructed by the Templars stretched to both east and west of the mosque building, and the infirmary is likely to have been located in one of these halls. While the presence of a church is often a good guide to the location of a monastic infirmary, churches and chapels are thought to have been located to both east and west of the Aqsa[177] and consequently the exact position of the infirmary remains unclear.

This infirmary was not established to serve the sick or poor in general, but was founded purely for members of the order who were unwell. While the

---

[172] Partner 1987 pp. 1–23; Barber 1994; Luttrell 1996. [173] Saewulf 1988 p. 100; Saewulf 1994 p. 64.
[174] Ibn al-Athir 1969 p. 144. [175] *Rule of the Templars* 1992 p. 3. [176] Hamilton 1949.
[177] Boas 2001 p. 91.

Templars did provide food for the hungry[178] and a few hostels to house the poor, such as at Valania in the county of Tripoli,[179] their medical activities were for the sick of their own order. This was an example of a specialist hospital at the opposite extreme from that of the Order of St John. It is unknown just how many infirmaries the Order of the Temple ran in the Frankish states.[180] In the whole of England there were just two infirmaries, and only one in the kingdom of Aragon in Spain.[181] It could be assumed that the headquarters of the order would have contained an infirmary and this would have been Jerusalem in the twelfth century and Acre for most of the thirteenth century (Figure 7). Several early fourteenth-century maps mark the complex of the Templars in Acre in the south-west part of the old city, against the sea.[182] In the thirteenth century the order is thought to have comprised 600 knights and 2,500 sergeants in the Frankish states.[183] The military function of the order resulted in many injuries and the evidence for weapon injuries from Templar sites such as Le Petit Gérin[184] and Jacob's Ford illustrate this. It would have been sensible for the order to provide an appropriate medical service for them so that they could be fit for active service as quickly as possible. The order's soldiers would also have been at risk of contracting any of the infectious diseases present in the Near East at that time, just as the general population were, and supportive treatment may have helped them to recover. Segregation of the sick in an infirmary may also have lessened the risks of transfer of some conditions to healthy members of the order. The geography of the Frankish states meant that many sick brothers in the north of the region would have had an arduous journey travelling south to the headquarters of the order, one that many may not have survived. In consequence it is possible that they may have run infirmaries at other large cities further north, such as Tripoli and Antioch. There is reference to the presence of the sick together in a room in the Templar Castle of La Fève in 1187[185] and this might suggest that any Templar stronghold was able to look after its sick or wounded, at least in the short term, by calling in local doctors as required.

The hierarchical statutes are thought to date from around 1165. The section 'The Retrais of the Infirmarer Brother'[186] gives valuable information about the diseases, treatments and general approach found in the infirmary.

[178] *Rule of the Templars* 1886 pp. 208–9; *Rule of the Templars* 1992 p. 102; Barber 2000.
[179] *Regesta Regni* 1904 p. 40, no. 614(b).   [180] Mitchell, in press (a).
[181] Parker 1963 p. 41; Forey 1973 pp. 292–3.   [182] Prawer 1953; Jacoby 1979.
[183] Barber 1994 p. 2.   [184] Mitchell 1997.
[185] Kedar and Pringle 1985; Continuation of William of Tyre 1982 p. 40; Continuation of William of Tyre 1996 p. 33.
[186] *Rule of the Templars* 1886 pp. 138–41; *Rule of the Templars* 1992 pp. 65–6.

All members of the order who were ill for longer than one day were required to go to the infirmary except the Master, who had special dispensation to stay in his own room. Just as with the Order of St John, those entering the infirmary were to confess their sins and receive communion before they did so. If they were severely ill, the chaplain could perform extreme unction as well. While most conditions were treated within the infirmary hall itself, those with diseases which would have caused distress or annoyance to other patients were given a separate room as close as possible to the infirmary. One group included under this section were those with vomiting and diarrhoea. In the hot weather of the eastern Mediterranean it is likely that most diseases causing these symptoms would have been bacterial or viral infections such as gastroenteritis and dysentery. A patient with this kind of illness would have been both noisy and smelly and this would have explained the segregation. An alternative theory is that it may also have been noticed that these conditions could be transmitted from one person to the next, although the role of pathogenic microorganisms in this process would not have been understood. Segregation should have made this spread less likely and even in modern hospitals it is normal to manage patients with infective gastrointestinal illness in side rooms.

The other conditions treated separately were those with serious wounds and those who were delirious. Even if a Templar knight or sergeant survived the immediate effects of wounding in battle, it was by no means certain that he would recover. The potential for wound infections and gangrene was significant and many would have died in the days following wounding. Flies are numerous in the Middle East and these are attracted to wounds and decaying unviable flesh. Any wound left uncovered for even a few minutes would have run the risk of flies landing on it and laying their eggs. While maggots in the wound may have helped some aspects of healing by removing the unviable tissue,[187] flies have a cocktail of bacteria on their feet from their habit of landing on waste and these bacteria would have been transferred on to any open wounds, so making infections more likely. If the groans of pain from these patients did not keep everyone else awake at night then the foul smell from gangrenous wounds would have done so.

Delirium is an acute confusional state resulting from reversible functional impairment of the brain and may be triggered by infection or trauma.[188] The fevers accompanying a range of infectious diseases from malaria to wound infections may cause delirium. Both malaria and wound infections are referred to in the statutes. The confusion associated with delirium could

---

[187] Baer 1931; Goldstein 1931.   [188] Meagher 2001.

have led to the patient wandering about the infirmary, calling out at night or otherwise creating disturbance and this may well be the reason why such patients were nursed separately. This separation was as close a scenario to the Eastern practice of separating patients into wards by their diagnosis as I have yet found in Frankish hospitals. Patients with diarrhoea, fevers causing delirium and those requiring surgery were each nursed in their own separate wards in some of the wealthier Eastern hospitals, such as the Mansuri hospital in Egypt[189] and the Pantokrator *xenon* in Constantinople.[190] However, in contrast to Byzantine and Islamic hospitals, such patients do not seem to have been actively placed together in discrete groups by their diagnosis, but this was rather a blanket exclusion from the principal ward. When patients with these conditions were improving they could join the others in the infirmary once 'the other brothers could tolerate their presence'.

The bulk of the statutes cover diet in the infirmary. This is not surprising as dietary modification was seen as the basic starting point for the treatment of any disease. A number of foods were regarded as good or bad and therefore encouraged or excluded, just as in the hospital of St John. Interestingly, statutes showed that the infirmarian was required to ask the patient himself what he could and could not tolerate, rather than recommending that a doctor should determine the dietary regime for the patient in each case. Foods thought to be bad for the patients included certain plants (lentils, broad beans and cabbage), particular meats (beef, goat, mutton and veal) and some fish (trout and eels). Cheese was never to be given in the infirmary.

Medicines were referred to and the commander was required to give the infirmarer 'the means with which to buy the medicines they need'. The infirmarer was put in charge of the garden, but it is not clear if this was just so that food plants suitable for patients could be grown or whether medicinal herbs were grown there too. Syrup from sugar cane was also mentioned in the statutes and it was to be given to those patients who asked for it.

The functions of the barber were also included in the rule, although there was no mention of an actual barber. The infirmarer was able to give permission for patients to have their heads shaved or undergo bloodletting but the master of the house had to give permission for surgery to take place for a serious weapon injury. It is possible that this was to prevent the barber from undertaking surgical procedures that were too complicated, and so enable a surgeon to be brought in. There were a number of references to the practice of bloodletting, on both the healthy and the sick. Healthy

[189] Dunlop 1960.	[190] Codellas 1942; Miller 1997 pp. 12–21; Gautier 1974.

brothers were allowed to eat three meals in the infirmary after undergoing bloodletting, presumably as the special diet was thought to help them recover their strength. It is not recorded if bloodletters or barbers were hired on a regular basis to perform these tasks, if they came in just when called for or if the infirmarian or members of the order themselves were able to perform bloodletting. The infirmarian was a brother of the order and not a trained medical practitioner. However, since he organised the appropriate food for the patients, bought medicines from town and perhaps grew them in the garden and also decided when bloodletting could take place, this does suggest that he needed reasonable medical experience. It is possible that he would have gained this by working in the infirmary for a number of years and receiving on-the-job training from the previous infirmarer.

It is presumed that the sick were washed and nursed while in the infirmary but there is no evidence to say who did this. It may well have been members of the order, but since the Templars were not a medical order themselves outside help is theoretically possible. There was also reference to the work of actual doctors in the infirmary. Just as was the case with other orders, these were laymen and not Templars. The master of the house was responsible for finding 'a doctor for the sick brothers so that he may visit them and advise them on their illnesses'. The only named medical practitioner that I have been able to identify as working with the sick of the order is a Master Theodorus. He is referred to in 1300 Famagusta in Cyprus as the *medicus* of the Templars.[191] From this I assume that he was employed by the order to treat the sick in their infirmary. It is significant that the Templars chose a master *medicus*, rather than a cheaper, less qualified practitioner, as the rule did not actually specify the level of skill the *medicus* was required to possess. There is also some evidence that the order owned medical books that might have been of great use to doctors treating the injured. On the dissolution of the Order of the Temple in 1308 a list of those books held by the order in Aragon was sent to King James II. A copy of the *Chirurgia* of Theodorich Borgognoni was included, written in the vernacular rather than Latin.[192] While there is no way of knowing if this text was specifically for reference use in a Templar infirmary, the choice of such a practical book on the treatment of weapon injuries[193] held by a military order, written in the local language, means that this possibility should be considered. It is a shame that no similar lists for other Templar commanderies have come to light that might show whether this practice was more widespread.

---

[191] Lamberto de Sambuceto [Polonio] 1982, doc. 148, pp. 170–1: *magister* Theodorus, *medicus* Templi.
[192] *Viage Literario* 1806, v, pp. 200–2.
[193] Theodorich Borgognoni 1498; Theodorich Borgognoni 1955–60.

This evidence shows how the Templar infirmary performed two very different roles. First, it was similar to a closed monastic infirmary in Europe,[194] in the sense that it was just for members of the order and provided a place for the sick to go until they died or recovered. They were treated with the standard approach of prayer, dietary modification, medicines, bloodletting and surgery. The healthy members who underwent their regular prophylactic bloodletting in the infirmary also ate a special strengthening diet for a short period. In contrast to the monastic setting, the military function of the Templars resulted in members of the order sustaining significant weapon injuries in battle. Operations on these wounds were alluded to and the master was responsible for ensuring that they were managed by the most appropriate practitioner. Such records show that these unusual infirmaries were able to provide a medical service with all the components available in the medieval period.

THE TEUTONIC ORDER

This German medicomilitary order developed from the siege of Acre during the Third Crusade. In 1190 merchants and sailors from the Baltic Sea, Bremen and Hamburg established an improvised field hospital made out of wood from dismantled ships and roofed with sail canvas. After the siege was over they moved inside the city (Figure 7) near the gate of St Nicholas where they built a *hospitale*, church and other buildings.[195] It has been suggested that a field hospital was originally established because the Hospitallers at the siege favoured the French and English nationals, and left the Germans to fend for themselves when sick.[196] However, I have been unable to find any evidence to substantiate this claim. The Ospital des Alemans was later mentioned in Matthew Paris's description of Acre,[197] and the complex was marked in the eastern part of the old city on the early fourteenth-century map of Pietro Vesconte, which accompanied the treatise of Marino Sanudo Torsello.[198] By February 1192 the brothers of St Mary were under the leadership of Gerard. At that time a charter of the German hospital was witnessed by members of the Order of St John, and the wording implies that the German institution had some degree of independence from them.[199]

---

[194] Harvey 1993.   [195] *Tabulae Ordinis* 1869 p. 22, doc. 25; p. 23, docs. 26–7.
[196] Urban 2003 pp. 11–13.   [197] Matthew Paris [Michelant] 1882 p. 136.
[198] Prawer 1953; Jacoby 1979.   [199] *Tabulae Ordinis* 1869 p. 23, doc. 26.

The narrative known as the Old French Continuation of William of Tyre mentions the tension between the two orders in Acre from 1190 onwards.[200]

At that time the German order could not cater for the sick because they did not yet have a hospital. For the Hospitallers of Saint John said that they had a privilege from Rome that said no one should have a hospital in the city of Acre unless they were subject to them. It used to happen that when a great man died in Acre, particularly if he died in the house of the Germans, they would go and seize him and bury him in their cemetery. At that time the German hospital did not have great power as it does now. The device that they wore on their mantles was a wheel with a half cross in black. The brother knights had mantles of Stamford cloth. They did not dare wear white mantles because of the Templars. But since the Damietta campaign [1217–21] they have had their white mantles with the cross without the wheel.

We can perhaps understand the viewpoint of the Order of St John on this issue. In twelfth-century Jerusalem the German hospital of St Mary was subordinate to them, so from their perspective it might seem reasonable for the newly founded German hospital in Acre to be subordinate to them too. However, unlike the earlier German hospital in Jerusalem, this new foundation strove to remain independent and attain the status of a medicomilitary order in its own right.

On 19 February 1199 Pope Innocent III confirmed the organisation as a religious order, the Teutonic Order. Their rule incorporated statutes from the Order of St John regarding the care of the poor and sick (*infirmis*) and statutes of the Order of the Temple concerning the activities of clerics and soldiers.[201] At first glance this decision is rather perplexing. Since the Order of St John was a major military force as well as a medical order, it might have been more sensible for the Teutonic Order to adopt the entire Hospitaller rule than cobble together an ill-fitting combination of the two rules. One reason for their choice may have been that they were striving to become distinct from the Hospitallers, and adopting their rule in its entirety would hardly have helped their case for independence. Another possibility is that they adopted statutes from the two most powerful military orders in the Latin East to avoid making enemies of either.

The statutes of the order stated that 'in the principal house, which is the head of the order, doctors [*medici/mires*] are to be employed as the finances of the house allow and as the numbers of the sick require'.[202] While the number of doctors hired was not stated, as was the case for the Order of St John, the use of the plural does suggest that several may have been

[200] Continuation of William of Tyre 1982 p. 99; Continuation of William of Tyre 1996 p. 90.
[201] *Tabulae Ordinis* 1869 p. 266, doc. 297.   [202] *Die Statuten* 1890 p. 32, art. 6.

working there at any one time. The infirmarian in charge of the care of
the sick was known as the *spetelier/hospitalarius*.²⁰³ The first Spittler known
by name was Henry, a knight brother, in 1208.²⁰⁴ He was responsible for
ensuring that the diet in the infirmary was beneficial to the sick. Just as
with the other medical orders, certain foods were prohibited for the sick
and the list is very similar to that followed by the Order of St John and
the Templars. Beef, salt meat, salt fish, salt cheese, lentils and unpeeled
beans were all avoided.²⁰⁵ Women were also engaged in caring for patients
as 'some work with the sick in hospitals . . . is more suited to the female
sex'.²⁰⁶ It is likely they spent their time in the areas of the hospital which
would have been reserved for women who were sick or in labour. Drugs
and medicines were clearly used in the infirmary as the statutes referred
to the electuaries and syrups.²⁰⁷ A document of King Aimery dating from
February 1198 mentions sugar for the hospital of St Mary.²⁰⁸ Although actual
surgical procedures were not mentioned in the statutes, wounds from the
dagger, sword and lance were²⁰⁹ and the kind of doctors employed to work
in the hospital (*medici* rather than *physici*) should have been able to treat
these injuries. Bloodletting was referred to indirectly as the rule specifies
certain days of the year when the procedure was forbidden,²¹⁰ since it was
widely thought that illness or even death could result if performed with the
moon in the wrong phase.²¹¹

As the order was often referred to as l'Ospital des Alemans in the thirteenth century, it is hard to determine whether a particular site included a
hospital that treated the sick or merely provided accommodation for pilgrims. While the rules of the order stated that every house had an infirmary
for members of the order, only the principal house was obliged to have a
hospital for the treatment of the sick in the general population. The order
was able to accept hospitals donated to them, but the consent of the master
of the order was required before a new hospital could be built; this may
well have been due to the heavy cost of running a hospital.²¹² The Teutonic
Order had bases in the major cities of the Latin East, such as in Tyre where
the complex lay within the city near the postern of the Boucherie.²¹³ It
is quite possible that property of the order in larger cities may also have
included a hospital for the general public as well. In Europe the order had

---

²⁰³ *Die Statuten* 1890 p. 36, art. 6.   ²⁰⁴ Militzer 1998.   ²⁰⁵ *Die Statuten* 1890 pp. 66–8.
²⁰⁶ *Die Statuten* 1890 p. 52, art. 31.   ²⁰⁷ *Die Statuten* 1890 p. 66, art. 7.
²⁰⁸ *Tabulae Ordinis* 1869 pp. 27–8, doc. 34.   ²⁰⁹ *Die Statuten* 1890 p. 83, art. 38.
²¹⁰ *Die Statuten* 1890 p. 165.
²¹¹ Voigts and McVaugh 1984; *Regimen Sanitatis Salerni* 1953 p. 85.
²¹² Demel 1998; Forey 1992 p. 110.
²¹³ Philippe de Navarre 1887 p. 131; *Tabulae Ordinis* 1869 p. 26, doc. 31.

been given at least twenty-six hospitals by 1230 and had the potential to become a major source of charitable care there.[214] However, it is thought that the order gradually lost its caring credibility, and perhaps competence, over the rest of the thirteenth century. The numbers of hospitals donated fell off significantly and the medical statutes inherited from the Order of St John were not adapted or augmented, as was the case in other medical organisations, which suggests little interest in their medical role.[215] There is limited evidence to evaluate the medical capability of the order in the Frankish states themselves. However, the knowledge that it employed lay doctors would suggest that the level of competence for this aspect of patient care would have remained the same regardless of how well trained the order's own staff in the hospital might have been.

It seems the Teutonic Order initially attempted to perform a similar function to the Order of St John, but presumably for German-speaking pilgrims. It undertook a medical role alongside its military activities and treated both the general public and its own knights and brothers. Lay doctors were contracted to work in the hospital, drugs and electuaries were referred to and there were separate sections in the hospital for male and female patients, each nursed by members of their own sex. The Teutonic Order was given a number of hospitals, especially in Europe, but for various reasons its medical activities appear to have declined in importance while its military function continued to develop.

THE ORDER OF ST THOMAS OF CANTERBURY

The *Opera Historica* of Ralph of Diss,[216] the archdeacon of Middlesex, records that this English order resulted from a vow taken by his own chaplain during the Third Crusade. The priest, named William, dedicated himself to nursing the sick and burying those who died from wounds or illness during the siege of Acre in 1189–91. This was a very similar process to their German counterparts, the Teutonic Order, who were also founded at this time. William named the resulting organisation after the recently martyred St Thomas Becket. The saint evidently appeared in a vision to English crusaders during a storm in the Atlantic on their sea voyage to the east,[217] which may contribute to explaining his choice as patron by Father William. Following the surrender of Acre to the crusaders, a charter shows that the *hospitale* of St Thomas was located in the east of the old city close to the

---

[214] Militzer 1998.   [215] Van Eikels 1998.   [216] Ralph de Diceto 1876, II, pp. 80–1.
[217] Ralph de Diceto 1876, II, p. 116; Roger of Howden 1853, II, p. 146; Roger of Howden 1870, III, p. 42.

Teutonic Order.[218] The small community followed the monastic rule of St Augustine and was under the protection of King Richard the Lionheart. After the London house of the order was founded in the Parish of St Mary Colechurch, a *hospitale* of St Thomas was opened there too. A number of *hospitalia* were then donated to the order in England and Ireland.[219] On 13 October 1207, under Richard's successor King John, the *hospitale* in Acre had to send some members to England to beg for money for the redemption of prisoners[220] as their European houses were not making sufficient profit to fund this. In the early part of the century the order acquired the churches of St Mary and St Nicholas de Campo Anglorum in Acre, but they were still far from well off.

In 1227–8 their financial position improved when Peter des Roches, the bishop of Winchester (1204–1238), accompanied a contingent of English crusaders who crusaded with Frederick II during 1227–31.[221] The writings of Matthew Paris record that, at his own expense, the bishop transferred the order to a better position near the sea at the extreme north of Montmusard on the Vicus Anglorum (Figure 7) where most of the English lived. Peter des Roches built them a new church and left a legacy of 500 marks to assure the subsistence of his protégés.[222] The regulations of the order were also changed so that members followed the rule of the Teutonic Order, which means that they would have followed the medical statutes of the Order of St John and the military statutes of the Templars.

While records specifying medical practice have not survived, the order's origins as a field hospital and the decision to adopt the rule of a medical order rather than one of the purely military organisations demonstrates that they must have been treating the sick. Officials of the order mentioned in documents include the master, preceptor and commander, and distinction was made between the soldiers and priests. In 1236 Pope Gregory IX gave members permission to wear a half-red, half-white cross on their habits to distinguish them from the Templars.[223] The order is marked in the north of Montmusard on the mid-thirteenth-century map of Acre by Matthew Paris, identified with the words 'la maisum de seit thomas le m'.[224] This is confirmed by a deed of 1240 concerning the Order of St Lazarus. This

[218] *Regesta Regni* 1893, I, p. 187, doc. 701; *Tabulae Ordinis* 1869 p. 24, doc. 27.
[219] Page 1925, III, p. 486; Brooks 1956–7.   [220] Dichter 1979 p. 110.
[221] Roger of Wendover 1887, II, p. 2; Vincent 1996 pp. 229–58.
[222] Matthew Paris [Luard] 1876, III, p. 490; Matthew Paris [Giles] 1852, I, p. 133; Matthew Paris [Michelant and Raynaud] 1882 p. 136.
[223] Forey 1977.   [224] Cambridge, Corpus Christi MS.

states that the property of St Thomas of Canterbury lay to the north of the house of St Lazarus, with both lying between the public road and the sea in northern Montmusard.[225] When Prince Edward, son of King Henry I of England, arrived in Acre with a large company of crusaders in 1271 he paid for renovation of one of the towers in the outer wall of the old town (Edward's Tower) and confided its defence to the Order of St Thomas. The order's establishment is again referred to in pilgrim descriptions of Acre from the 1280s[226] and it left for Cyprus at the fall of the city in 1291.

POSSIBLE FURTHER SITES OF MEDICAL CARE

A number of institutions are referred to in the texts as running a *hospitale*, but no further information is given to help us interpret the meaning. The term might have been used in the medical sense but could just as easily have been referring merely to a hostel where pilgrims stayed. Some institutions were run by organisations with a reputation for looking after people with specific diseases, such as the Order of St Anthony, which was established to care for those with ergotism, and the Order of St Lazarus for those thought to have leprosy. While these orders are known to have run *hospitalia* in the Latin East, the paucity of records means that it is not clear if these patients were merely fed and washed or if they received any medical treatment. Examples of *hospitalia* founded by the military orders include those of the Order of St Stephen at Jerusalem and the Order of St Catherine of Campobelli at Acre. References among the religious orders include the Order of Crociferi at Acre and Nicosia, Our Lady of Jehosaphat at Tiberias and Acre, St Mary Latina at Jerusalem, St Martin of Tours for Poor Bretons at Acre and the Order of the Trinity at Acre, Beirut and Caesarea. Latin churches which ran *hospitalia* include the church at Bethlehem, Hebron, Nazareth and the Holy Sepulchre. Eastern churches also possessed *hospitalia*, such as the Armenian monastery of St James at Jerusalem, the Greek Orthodox monasteries of St Catherine at Acre, Jerusalem and Laodicea and also the Orthodox monasteries of St Theodosius at Ascalon, Gibelet, Jaffa, Jerusalem and Nicosia.[227] As there is as yet no firm evidence that any of these institutions did provide medical care in the Frankish states, they are not discussed in detail here.

[225] Comte de Marsy 1884; *Regesta Regni* 1893, 1, p. 285, no. 1096.
[226] Pelrinages et Pardouns 1882 p. 236.   [227] Amouroux 1999; Coureas 2001; Richard 1982.

CAPACITY OF FRANKISH HOSPITALS

Since two Frankish hospitals have been excavated, an interesting approach is to attempt an assessment of their patient capacity. Medieval estimates of inpatients in Frankish hospitals vary quite considerably and none of the chroniclers actually counted the numbers accurately. Estimates of numbers in the hospital of St John for sick poor in Jerusalem include 1,000 by Theodorich in 1169[228] and 2,000 by John of Würzburg around the same time.[229] There may also have been a tendency for chroniclers to overestimate numbers in their grandiose descriptions, to make their accounts more exciting for those hearing the details back in Europe. There are two areas in which some meaningful investigations can be made. The first is the maximum number of patients which a building could physically cope with in extreme circumstances, such as during epidemics or after nearby battles. The second is the approximate number of patients a hospital might have been able to comfortably accommodate in normal circumstances. Two excavated hospitals are to be studied. The first is the small, relatively simple hospital of St Mary of the Germans in Jerusalem. The other, also in Jerusalem, is the much larger and more elaborate hospital located in the complex of the Order of St John. These two hospitals provide an interesting comparison because of their differing size and role. This also allows an assessment of the accuracy of inpatient numbers recorded in contemporary chronicles.

One method of estimating the hypothetical maximum number is by determining how many times an average medieval person could fit into the available floor space. This presupposes a number of factors, not least that beds were not used in these circumstances, as they would tend to be a less efficient use of floor space. It also presumes that any equipment or belongings were either stored elsewhere, on the walls, or were slept upon so that they did not take up any extra floor space. This is limited to estimates of the numbers which could be housed in the hospital building itself. It may well be that any overflow might have been accommodated in adjacent buildings such as the associated church, hospital staff accommodation or function rooms. Furthermore, it is unknown how much of the hospital floor space would have been taken up by fixtures which have decayed with time and left no evidence of their existence. There may have been areas for the storage of medical equipment or documents, fireplaces, perhaps

---

[228] Theodericus 1994 p. 158; Theodorich 1988 p. 287.
[229] John of Würzburg 1994 p. 131; John of Würzburg 1988 p. 266.

tables from which food was taken to patients and even an equivalent of the modern nursing station from which the sick could be observed. The size of these areas cannot be accurately calculated, but they must be taken into account when interpreting any figures.

It might be expected that in situations of extreme overcrowding people would lie on the floor wherever they could find space. In order to find out how much space each person would occupy, it is necessary to determine how large the average medieval adult was. Those who have hit their head on the top of a thirteenth-century doorway might presume that the population in the medieval period were significantly smaller than today. However, study of medieval human skeletal remains from various parts of Europe has shown that average height was only a little less than in modern times. The length of the long bones in the limbs has been shown to correlate with reasonable accuracy with the overall body height. A number of formulae have been derived which allow inference of total body height from this long bone length.[230] Using this approach, values for average estimated height in medieval Franks in Europe are in the region of 1.66 m (5 ft 5½ inches) for males and 1.56 m (5 ft 1½ in) for females.[231] Anglo-Saxons are thought to have been of comparable size, with averages estimated at approximately 1.68 m (5 ft 6 in) for males and 1.57 m (5 ft 2 in) for females.[232] In comparison, the average height of modern adults in the United Kingdom is 1.74 m (5 ft 8½ in) for males and 1.61 m (5 ft 3 in) for females.[233]

For the hospital of St Mary of the Germans, my calculations based on efficient use of the floor area (Figure 5) suggest that the maximum capacity in extreme circumstances might have been up to 195 adult patients. Bearing in mind the range of factors which would tend to reduce this, an estimate of the true figure which this hospital could physically accommodate in extreme circumstances might be nearer 100 to 150 adult patients. However, the hospital would obviously for most of its life have functioned under less strain than in the case discussed above. Patients would have been in beds with sufficient space between them to allow access by those taking care of their medical, nutritional, hygienic and spiritual requirements. If there were six single beds in each bay with only three by the stairs, then up to forty-five patients might have been present. If there were eight smaller single beds, or four double beds, in each bay, then up to sixty patients might have been cared for. The confounding factors already mentioned would make these

---

[230] Trotter 1958.   [231] Martin 1959, II, p. 787.   [232] Munter 1936; Kunitz 1987.
[233] Knight and Eldridge 1984 p. 7.

figures smaller, so that patient numbers in the region of thirty-five to fifty might be more realistic.

Using the same approach as was applied to the hospital of St Mary of the Germans can give an idea as to the capacity of the ground floor of the hospital for sick poor of the Order of St John in Jerusalem. This building was very much larger than St Mary, so the margins of error associated with any estimation will be correspondingly larger too. Even after the calculations for this thirty-eight-bay area (Figure 4), the true capacity of the entire hospital remains a mystery. The site itself has long since been covered with buildings and our only records are from plans of 100 years ago with inexact measurements. The report describes a number of large, robust piers capable of supporting at least one upper floor, but there is no evidence for its function, if it did indeed exist. Further confounding the calculations is the evidence in contemporary texts,[234] which record that the women were cared for in a separate building to the men. However, a crude assessment of the part of the complex of St John that we believe was used as a hospital can give an indication of its patient capacity.

In extreme circumstances the available floor area could in theory accommodate anything up to 2,500 recumbent adults. In practice this figure would obviously be reduced with inefficient use of space, so that perhaps 1,500–2,000 might be a reasonable estimate. Further complicating the issue, it is known that members of the order gave up their beds for the sick in times of overcrowding, increasing capacity further. The figure of 1,500–2,000 adults in extreme circumstances is by no means claimed to be accurate, but is merely an approximate figure, which gives a rough idea as to the capacity of the structure. Using the same bed sizes and also the same preconditions applied to the German hospital of St Mary, the crude estimate of patients in this building under normal conditions raises some interesting points. This suggests a capacity in the region of 400–650 beds for this building. Bearing in mind the location of women elsewhere and the possibility of other floors, estimates by contemporary chroniclers of 1–2,000 beds in the hospital altogether are by no means out of the question and should not be dismissed as wild medieval exaggeration.[235] Indeed, this figure was comparable with a number of Islamic hospitals of the time. Independent assessment of this same problem has been undertaken by Benjamin Kedar,[236] who published his own figures after these calculations were performed. He employed a slightly different technique by using the floor area reserved per pilgrim travelling by ship to the Latin East in the thirteenth century, rather

---

[234] Kedar 1998; Edgington 1998b.   [235] Miller 1978; Luttrell 1994.   [236] Kedar 1998.

than using measurements derived from the people themselves. His findings are broadly similar and suggest about 900 single beds, the figure being slightly higher as the calculation only allowed for 18 inches between each bed (which would have been extremely cramped) as opposed to the metre I have allowed.

DIETARY MODIFICATION

Dietary modification was a ubiquitous treatment in the medical management of the sick. In medieval medical texts it was regarded as a fundamental technique when attempting to correct the humoural imbalance believed to be responsible for most disease. To understand how Frankish hospitals modified the diet of their patients it is necessary to be aware of the normal foodstuffs in the everyday Frankish diet. Archaeological excavation of sites such as the Red Tower,[237] Caymont,[238] Belmont castle[239] and the complex of St John in Acre[240] has found remains of the seeds and pollen of wheat, barley, rye, peas, beans, chick peas, lentils, cherries and figs. Animal bones with charring and butchery marks included chicken, goose, pigeon, fish, sheep, goat, cattle, pig, donkey and deer. Historical evidence demonstrates the export of many foods from Europe to the kingdom of Jerusalem by sea. Foods of vegetable origin included wheat, barley, legumes, chick peas, walnuts, wine and oil, while animal products included salt meat, fish, cheese and livestock such as hens and pigs.[241]

The dietary advice found in the statutes of the Hospitallers, Templars and Teutonic Order is very similar (see tables 2.1 and 2.2). All forbid the sick to be given cheese, lentils, unshelled beans and eels or salt fish. Some of the orders also forbid further foods, mainly meats, but no list contradicts that of another order. None of the foods encouraged for the sick in the Hospitallers' statutes is forbidden by other orders. Past research on diet in Latin hospitals[242] has noted a similarity in the dietary rules of the military orders and the *Regimen Sanitatis Salerni*.[243] This was a text derived from selectively editing and adapting information in those larger medical texts written in the Islamic world that had been translated in Italy during the eleventh, twelfth and thirteenth centuries.[244] For example, the Salerno *Regimen* is in agreement with the Frankish medical orders in forbidding the sick to eat cheese, lentils, unshelled beans and eels/salt fish. In consequence, it has been argued that European/Salernitan medical philosophy was dominant

---

[237] Hubbard 1986.   [238] Horwitz 1996.   [239] Croft 2000.
[240] Mitchell, Huntley and Stern, in press.
[241] Pryor 1988.   [242] Sterns 1983.   [243] *Regimen Sanitatis Salerni* 1953.   [244] Sotres 1998.

Table 2.1 *Foods forbidden to the sick in medicomilitary orders and medical texts*

	Hospitallers	Teutons	Templars	Salerno	Oribasius	Maimonides
Fish	eels	salt fish	eels	eels	–	salt fish
	–	–	*trout*	–	–	–
Meats	pork (summer)	–	–	–	pork (summer)	–
	–	beef	beef	beef	–	–
	–	–	*veal*	–	–	–
	–	–	mutton	–	–	mutton
	–	–	goat	goat	–	old goat
	–	salt meat	–	salt meat	–	–
Dairy	cheese	salt cheese	cheese	cheese	–	–
	–	–	–	*milk*	–	–
Vegetables	lentils	lentils	lentils	lentils	lentils	–
	beans	unshelled beans	broad beans	unshelled beans	beans	–
	–	–	cabbage	–	–	–
Fruit	–	–	–	*apples*	–	–
	–	–	–	*pears*	–	–

Note: Italicised text indicates a contradiction between Frankish statutes and any medical text.

in Frankish medical practice, with little influence from Byzantine or Islamic traditions.[245]

However, a considerable number of these regimens of health had been written by the medieval period[246] and the study did not assess comparable dietary advice in Eastern medical texts from Byzantine and Islamic regions adjacent to the Frankish states. If the Frankish hospital diet is compared not only with the Salernitan text but also other that of Western authors such as Theodorich Borgognoni and Eastern authors such as Moses Maimonides and Oribasius of Pergamon, a more balanced assessment is possible. The dietary advice in the *Chirurgia* of Theodorich Borgognoni discusses foods that encourage wound healing.[247] While this was written in Italy in the 1260s, the author states that it is record of the views of his mentor, master Hugo of Lucca, who lived from about 1160–1257. This period spans the time when the Frankish records on diet originate. Maimonides wrote his *Regimen of Health* in Cairo between 1193 and 1198[248] and gives plenty of

---

[245] Sterns 1983.   [246] Mauron 1986; Sotres 1998.
[247] Theodorich Borgognoni 1498 pp. 113r–v; Theodorich Borgognoni 1955, I, pp. 92–3.
[248] Bar-Sela, Hoff and Faris 1964.

Table 2.2 *Foods encouraged for the sick in medicomilitary orders and medical texts*

	Hospitallers	Theodorich	Salerno	Oribasius	Maimonides
Fish	–	–	*trout*	–	–
Meat	poultry	poultry	poultry	–	poultry
	lamb	–	–	sheep	lamb
	boar (winter)	–	*all* pork	pork (winter)	–
	kid	kid	–	kid	kid
	–	*veal*	*veal*	–	–
Dairy	*milk*	–	–	–	–
Vegetables	barley broth/gruel	–	broth	–	barley broth
	white bread	–	–	white bread	bread
Fruit	*apples*	–	–	apples	–
	pears	–	–	pears	–
	plums	–	–	plums	–
	figs	–	figs	figs	–
	grapes	–	raisins	grapes	currants
	pomegranate	–	–	pomegranate	pomegranate
	almonds	–	–	–	almonds
Drink	wine	wine	wine	–	white wine
	syrups	–	–	–	syrups
	oxymel	–	–	–	oxymel

Note: Italicised text indicates a contradiction between Frankish statutes and any medical text.

advice on the use of diet to treat disease. This text is also from an identical time period to the manuscripts of dietary regulation in the Order of St John. The Byzantine example used for comparison is the earlier (fourth century AD) text of Oribasius of Pergamon,[249] which was a standard text in the Byzantine world for many centuries. It was also hoped to use the *Tacuini Sanitatis* of Ibn Butlan, the Eastern Christian practitioner who settled in Antioch in the late eleventh century.[250] Unfortunately, his dietary recommendations do not systematically specify whether a particular food should be given to or avoided by the sick, which makes the text of little use for this investigation.

While not all manuscripts mention all foods and Theodorich only mentions beneficial foods, a careful study of the four medical texts for items

[249] Oribasius 1997.   [250] Ibn Butlan 1990; *Tacuinum Sanitatis* 1976; Elkhadem 1990.

specified in the Frankish order statutes gives an idea of their compatibility with each source. Bearing in mind the shared origins of the various regimens it seems sensible to pay more attention to the ways in which advice differs between regions, rather than their similarities. With regard to foods for the sick, it is found that both Oribasius and Maimonides gave broadly similar recommendations to the Frankish orders. Of particular interest is the fact that there is no contradiction between these Eastern authors and the hospital statutes, but a number of Salernitan recommendations are completely contradictory to the Frankish statutes. For example, the Salerno *Regimen* forbids the sick to consume milk, fresh pears and apples but these are encouraged in the statutes of St John. Similarly, the Salerno *Regimen* encourages trout, veal and pork for the sick. However, trout and veal were forbidden by the Templars, and most kinds of pork (sow at any time and boar in the summer) were forbidden by the Order of St John. Interestingly, the details on pork in the St John statutes specify that boar may be eaten in the winter and the same seasonal recommendation is found in the text of Oribasius, but there is no mention of this in the Salerno *Regimen*. It is understandable that Maimonides, being Jewish, did not mention pork.

In summary, Maimonides agrees with the Frankish statutes on fourteen items and contradicts them on none. Oribasius agrees with the Frankish statutes on eleven items and contradict them on none. The Salerno regimen agrees with that of the Franks on thirteen items but contradicts it on five items, nor does it mention a time of year to eat pork. Theodorich is very similar to the Salerno advice but goes into rather less detail. It seems clear that dietary statutes in Frankish hospitals did not directly follow the advice in the Salerno *Regimen*. While the Frankish statutes followed Eastern ideas much more closely, it can be seen that they were not copied directly from Oribasius either and Maimonides could not have been the source as it was only written 10–20 years after the relevant statutes of St John were written. It is accepted that only a limited number of works on diet have been examined and by no means every text from the period has been consulted, but the findings from those discussed are very interesting. The variation between statutes suggests that each institution may have evolved its own regulations and did not merely copy them from other previously established orders. This is surprising as the Teutonic Order is supposed to have adopted the medical statutes of the Order of St John. It is possible that the doctors working in the hospitals at the time the statutes were drawn up were asked to record their recommendations. It is known that both European and Eastern doctors worked in these institutions. The greater similarities between these statutes and recommendations found in the Eastern authors compared with those from the West might suggest that it was local Eastern medical ideas, rather than those popular in Europe at that time, that were more dominant in determining diet in the hospitals. If that was the case, then it is just as possible that these Eastern influences were dominant in determining other forms of medical and surgical treatment in these hospitals too.

INFLUENCES ON FRANKISH HOSPITALS

A number of authors have speculated on the predominant traditions which provided the basis for the routine in those Frankish hospitals that provided medical care. Some have proposed the Islamic *bimaristan*,[251] others Byzantine *xenones*[252] and others still favour European influence from Salerno.[253] An impartial comparison between Frankish hospitals and each of these traditions may help to clarify this question.

Byzantine *xenones* shared a number of similarities with Frankish hospitals. Both were religious Christian institutions attached to monastic orders. Patients confessed their sins on admission while prayer and ceremonies took place regularly. They both provided food, nursing and medical care. Male and female patients were kept separate in different areas of the hospital. In those cases where sufficient records are known to us (the Pantokrator and the Hospital of St John), the doctors visited the patients every day. While these similarities might at first sight suggest a conclusive link, there are many contrasts between the Byzantine *xenon* and the Eastern Frankish hospital. In the early years of their foundations, the function of most Frankish *hospitalia* seems to have been to provide food and accommodation to the poor and medical treatment appears to have evolved only after a number of decades. This would suggest that they were not founded to emulate the *xenon*, but were more similar to the *xenodocheion*. Once medical treatment did become standard in the Frankish hospitals, there were considerable differences between Frankish and Byzantine practice. The patients in the Pantokrator appear to have been just those who were acutely unwell and in need of active treatment, but only the minority of patients in Frankish hospitals were in this state. Most were poor, hungry, feeble and weak but not necessarily acutely sick. In consequence, the doctor patient ratio in the Pantokrator was much higher that in the Order of St John, which employed just eight doctors for perhaps a thousand people in the 1180s. Doctors in the Hospital of St John did not work alternate months in the hospital for poor

---

[251] Hamarneh 1993; Toll 1998.   [252] Miller 1978; Amouroux 1999.
[253] Sterns 1983; Riley-Smith 1999b p. 30.

pay and make up for it with a month of private work, as was the case in some *xenones*, but worked exclusively for the hospital for a generous wage. By the twelfth century *xenon* directors were often doctors, but the administrators of Frankish hospitals were not. Monks from monasteries that possessed a *xenon* did not themselves work with patients as hired employees did this, but brothers of the military orders were required to nurse the sick. There is evidence that some *xenones* did not function to care long term for untreatable patients, but the Order of St John prided itself on giving equal care to hopeless cases as to those who were recovering. Some *xenones* (such as the Pantokrator) appear to have allocated patients to wards depending on the condition from which they suffered. While the Order of St John did have distinct wards and the Templars did temporarily segregate patients whose illness made them noisy, smelly or disruptive, there is no evidence that an organised approach to patient distribution took place on admission. It seems that despite sharing some similarities, Frankish hospitals were certainly not a direct copy of the Byzantine *xenon*.

Islamic hospitals also share a number of factors with their Frankish counterparts. They both provided food, nursing and medical care to the sick. Male patients were kept separate from female. Funding was often from a combination of income from lands granted to the hospital and gifts from wealthy patrons. Ibn Jubayr must have also noted these similarities as when he saw the Frankish hospitals at Acre and Tyre in 1184 he thought that they were 'after the model of the Muslim hospitals'.[254] However, he did not comment on how similar the Frankish institutions were to those existing in the Byzantine world or Latin Europe at that time, so it is not possible to conclude from this that the Islamic hospital was the original inspiration. In any case, there are a number of marked contrasts between Muslim and Frankish hospitals. While Islamic hospitals were fundamentally secular institutions, Frankish hospitals were typically run by a monastic religious order. Sometimes a *bimaristan* (such as the Mansuri) allocated patients to a certain area by their type of illness, while Frankish hospitals typically did not. Where evidence exists, such as for the 'Adudi and Nuri hospitals, Islamic doctors were not employed exclusively in the hospital but saw their patients intermittently during the week between visits to their other patients in their homes. However, doctors in the Order of St John performed daily ward rounds and worked exclusively in their hospital. With such differences between Frankish and Islamic hospitals, it is hard to

[254] Ibn Jubayr 1952 p. 346.

propose that the Frankish institutions were a direct copy of their Islamic counterparts either.

Hospitalia and infirmaries in Europe again share many characteristics with Frankish hospitals. In the early years of the Latin East the Order of St John provided spiritual and nursing care to weak, frail and hungry pilgrims and poor locals in just the same way as *hospitalia* did in Europe. At this stage the hospital cannot be said to be a unique institution as seen from European eyes. By the second half of the twelfth century it had became very large and could house perhaps as many as 1–2,000 people and would therefore have been considerably bigger than the typical European hospital. Perhaps by 1128–37, but certainly by the 1180s, doctors were employed to treat the bodily illnesses of the patients, complementing the spiritual and nursing care given previously. This would have been surprising if it was a secular institution, but since the hospital was part of a monastic organisation hiring doctors for intermittent visits was common back in Europe and so not too unexpected. In contrast to the situation in Europe, however, these doctors worked full time rather than just visiting the sick when requested by the infirmarian. The dietary advice for the sick recorded in the statutes of Frankish orders demonstrates the common heritage between European, Byzantine and Islamic philosophies on the ideal diet but details are more compatible with Eastern influences than that of Salerno.

It appears that the Frankish *hospitalia* and *infirmaria* were similar to their European equivalents in the early years after conquest, but as the decades passed they evolved to meet the needs of their unique situation.[255] The belief in medieval Europe that Jerusalem was the place where heaven and earth intersected meant that many went there to die as they thought that their salvation would be thereby assured.[256] Indeed, this idea was also stated in some medieval Muslim texts. In his spiritual guide to pilgrims visiting Palestine, Ibn al-Firkah (1262–1329) wrote, 'who is buried in Jerusalem shall not be punished . . . who is buried in Jerusalem has escaped from the calamity and misfortunes of the grave'.[257] The range of establishments may in part be explained by the mixed racial composition of the Latin East, where many languages were spoken and the sick needed to be able to communicate clearly in their own tongue. Some became very large to cope with the sheer volume of people, such as the Order of St John. A number hired doctors either part time or full time, such as the Order of St John, the Templars, the Teutonic Knights and the Order of St Thomas of Canterbury. The significant number of weapon injuries sustained by the Franks may

[255] Edgington 1999.   [256] Ward 1982 pp. 124–5; Friedman 2000.   [257] Ibn al-Firkah 1949 p. 25.

well have been the reason for the employment of specialist surgeons in the hospital of St John by the 1180s. The doctors employed were not just from Europe but also included those indigenous to the eastern Mediterranean, and these were not necessarily all Christian. Details of dietary advice varied slightly between Frankish orders, showing that they did not all copy the statutes of the oldest institution, while the overall pattern appears to be more similar to Eastern dietary principles than those of the West. One possibility that might explain this is if the doctors employed by each institution at the time the statutes were drawn up were responsible for giving the advice recorded.

Frankish hospital infirmaries certainly did evolve from merely giving food and spiritual care to the sick to providing a more substantial medical service, and it seems most plausible that it was influence from local indigenous doctors that was responsible for this. While this cultural exchange of knowledge is certainly an exciting concept, this is by no means the only example we have for such exchange in Frankish health care. *Leprosaria* in the Latin East also evolved away from the role typical for Europe to one more applicable for life in the Frankish states.[258] In the early twelfth century Frankish *leprosaria* were built on the roadside outside towns as in Europe, but by the thirteenth century there are examples of their presence inside towns such as Acre and Caesarea. While knights with leprosy were not able to perform military service in Europe, the medicomilitary order of St Lazarus was founded in the Frankish states to allow those with leprosy to still fight with the main army. There are many other examples of how the attitudes of the Franks to disease and health care changed with their life in the east. This exchange of ideas between local and European medical practitioners was certainly complex, and is discussed in more detail in a later chapter. The general evolution noted in Frankish hospitals probably resulted from the social and religious need to care for the large numbers of sick pilgrims, coupled with easy access to local medical practitioners who would have been able to suggest the military orders adopt the relevant practices employed in Eastern hospitals at the time. Those aspects of Byzantine and Islamic hospitals not adopted were either culturally or religiously irrelevant to the Franks. Those practices that were incorporated into hospital life were regarded by contemporaries as being for the practical benefit of the pilgrims and Frankish settlers.

[258] Mitchell 2000b.

CONCLUSION

The medical care of the sick and wounded in the Latin East within institutions is one of the most interesting aspects of Frankish life. These hospitals and infirmaries were recognised by contemporaries both in Europe and the Middle East for the good work they performed. In the early years they mirrored the services back in Europe, concentrating on providing food and a bed with nursing care in a religious environment often referred to as medicine for the soul. As the decades went by the function evolved to include medical treatment of the sick by trained practitioners. The ideological significance of these Frankish hospitals must have been profound for the population who lived in the Latin East. They were a clear sign to those visiting the Holy Land that the settlers there took philanthropy very seriously, in the very place where Jesus had walked and encouraged the selfless caring for those in need. The political significance of the hospitals was not only to impress those visiting from abroad, but also to satisfy the general population by providing services they had not known back in Europe. The Frankish medical *hospitalia* discussed here might perhaps be thought of as hybrid institutions that evolved from those aspects of hospitals from the three cultures that were most useful to their society. This novel combination gradually fused out of necessity rather than following a preconceived design, as was the case in so many aspects of Frankish life in the Latin East.

CHAPTER 3

Archaeological evidence for trauma and surgery in the medieval period

The study of disease in excavated human skeletal remains, termed palaeopathology, has provided useful information as to the nature of injuries sustained both during warfare and also in daily life in the past. It allows researchers to look at the Middle Ages from a modern viewpoint rather than through medieval eyes, as is the case when reading written texts. This helps to counter the bias found in many chronicles, from both Christian and Muslim sources, that arises from the tendency to exaggerate enemy losses in battle while playing down the injuries sustained by troops on the side of the author. It also removes the bias in some chronicles towards documenting only the lives of important individuals, as archaeology allows the study of the poor villager crushed under his cart as well as the noble lord who falls from his horse while hunting for boar. We can look for the types of injury sustained, their location on the body, whether they have healed or become infected, whether they received medical treatment, the proportion of the population who suffered injuries and which sex or age groups were most affected. The findings from communities who lived in well fortified cities can be compared with those from poorly defended villages and similar comparisons can be made between groups with different ethnic backgrounds.

Palaeopathology is clearly associated with some of its own biases, of course. One obvious drawback to this technique is that there is no evidence of injuries to soft tissues such as the abdomen, as these decompose within a few months of death. Similarly, it is unusual to know the actual identity of excavated individuals unless they are buried in a marked tomb, and so integrating the archaeological information with historical records normally has to take place at the population level. Furthermore, poor preservation of the remains may limit the amount of information available from the excavation, and erosion of bone in the soil may leave changes that might be mistaken for pathology to a inexperienced eye. In consequence, even now many historians still have concerns as to how accurate palaeopathology really is. However, great advances have taken place since the 1970s, making it a much more reliable approach. One particular strength is that we are able to utilise evidence from modern medicine and forensic science to ensure that we are correctly interpreting the effects of weapons and disease upon bone. If we know that a particular modern individual suffered a certain injury before death, and the resulting bony lesion is identical with the changes seen on an excavated medieval skeleton, we can conclude that a similar event may have affected that medieval individual too.[1] This is how we can differentiate the effects of a wide range of weapons in excavated human skeletal remains. Furthermore, we no longer have to rely just on the visual inspection of bone to make a diagnosis. Other techniques from clinical medicine and forensics which are often found helpful in palaeopathology include imaging with X-rays and computerised tomography scans, light and scanning electron microscopy, mineral isotope analysis and DNA studies.

A discussion of the evidence for trauma in medieval Europe and the Frankish states helps to give an extra dimension to the study of injuries in the past and fills in many of the gaps that remain if only written sources of evidence are used. If it is considered how many battles have been fought in Europe and the Middle East through the ages, surprisingly few battlefield cemeteries have been excavated and none of these includes Muslim armies.[2] The injuries sustained would be expected to vary depending on the weapons used, the armour worn and whether the soldier was on horseback or fought on foot. Certain patterns of injury have been noted on the bones of individuals recovered with other evidence of their military role which further helps to explain the variation in wounds seen. Information suggesting the military role of a soldier can be present on the bones themselves[3] or from the grave in which they were placed. In optimal circumstances a knight may be excavated from a tomb carved with his name, allowing excellent identification, or the remains of an anonymous adult male may be found with his spurs. Sometimes horsemen were actually buried with their mounts.[4] A lifetime of riding may also sometimes be inferred by changes to the bones, an activity-related marker.[5] The adductor muscles of the inner aspect of the thighs become strong when a man fights from horseback as they are required to prevent him falling off – a real risk, bearing in mind the heavy weapons and armour horsemen would be wearing. As these muscles become stronger the site where they attach to the bones also becomes prominent and this can be seen on excavation as ridges on the bone. Archers using the

---

[1] Berryman and Haun 1996.   [2] Freeman and Pollard 2001; Pollard 2002.
[3] Knüsel 2000.   [4] Billard 1991.   [5] Molleson and Blondiaux 1994.

long bow are another group whose patterns of activity can sometimes result in altered growth and development in their bones. The force required to draw a medieval English long bow is huge and archers needed to be trained from a young age to enable them to draw the full-sized bow. This training as an adolescent would place different forces on the developing skeleton from other professions and result in asymmetry in the bones. It has been noted that archers may have had a great disparity in size between left and right elbow joint surfaces, that the left shoulder dimensions may have been enlarged and that they were prone to stress fractures at sites of growing bone in the shoulder (termed *os acromiale*) and lower spine (spondylolysis).[6] In modern times javelin throwers may develop changes to the olecranon at the elbow[7] and it is also possible that this may help to identify their military counterparts in the past. However, these changes show only patterns of activity and are not sufficiently specific to differentiate an individual soldier from the general public in a communal cemetery where occupations also placing heavy use on these bones might result in a similar pattern. Should these patterns be seen in the special examples of the battlefield cemetery or sunken warship then extrapolation of such findings to the type of soldiers present might be made with more confidence. Less specific activity-related markers may, however, still be of use in the interpretation of military activity. The spines of sailors drowned in the sixteenth-century English warship the *Mary Rose* were noted to have suffered degenerative changes at a much younger age than the bones of those in comparable cemeteries where the general population were buried.[8] This not only suggests that life on board ship caused considerable wear and tear to the spine, but also that the crew probably comprised professional, full-time sailors who were taken on at a young age. This was in contrast to much of the army at that time, who were called up in times of need, but then pursued other occupations in times of peace.

A small number of excavated medieval battlefield cemeteries have provided good archaeological evidence for weapon injuries, but all date from after the crusader period. The most complete study has been of the battle of Visby in Sweden.[9] This took place in 1361 between the Danes and the Gotlanders. Excavation of skeletal remains of over one thousand slain Gotlanders has given good insight into the techniques of battle in Scandinavia at the time. The majority of blade injuries were located on the head and lower leg, with smaller numbers on the thighs and arms. Injuries to

[6] Stirland 1984; Stirland 1993; Stirland 2000.   [7] Miller 1960.
[8] Stirland and Waldron 1997.   [9] Ingelmark 1939, 1; Courville 1965.

the head and shoulder were located more commonly on the left side of the body, which would be the natural side for the blows to land from a right-handed attacker. Wounds on the legs were mainly located on the right shin, which for a right-handed soldier would be closest to the opponent, both on foot and horseback. Interestingly, most of the limb wounds were on the lower leg and only a small proportion on the arms. At first glance this might seem surprising as there are no vital organs in the lower leg and it would be unusual to kill an opponent by wounding him there. A plausible interpretation is that a blow to the legs was a common method used to bring the opponent to the ground before finishing him off. There were also penetrating wounds compatible with the crossbow bolt, lance or spiked mace and depressed skull fractures compatible with the club or round mace. More recent work has taken place on the human remains from the battle of Aljubarrota in Portugal.[10] This took place on 15 August 1385, between Castilian and Portuguese armies. Bones in the ossuary were commingled so it was not possible to differentiate individuals, but it is known that over four hundred sets of remains were there. Common lesions were blade injuries to the limbs, either partial thickness or complete amputations, and to the front of the skull. Surprisingly, the majority of wounds were actually old, healed lesions rather than fresh cuts made at the time of death. This suggests that they were sustained in previous battles and that the soldiers survived their injuries. This is a finding noted in other series as well.[11] The battle of Towton in England occurred on 29 March 1461 during the War of the Roses.[12] The battle was followed by the rout of the Lancastrian army and apparently more died in flight than during the battle itself. Analysis of one mass grave from this rout found that the majority of wounds were to the front and back of the skull. Injuries elsewhere were less common but the majority were to the forearms, suggestive of defence injuries.[13] This highlights the fact that the distribution of wounds in fleeing soldiers is very different from that in those facing their enemy.

Since so few battlefield cemeteries have been excavated, much of the evidence for medieval injuries comes from town or monastery cemeteries. Before the medieval period, across much of Europe many soldiers fought without effective body armour. The distribution of perimortem blade injuries was noted on a series of skeletons from an Anglo-Saxon cemetery at Eccles in England.[14] While the expected skull and forearm injuries were found, there were also a significant number of cuts on bones of the

---

[10] Cunha and Silva 1997.   [11] Boylston 2000.
[12] Boylston, Novak, Sutherland, Holst and Coughlan 1997; Fiorato 2000.   [13] Novak 2000.
[14] Wenham 1989.

trunk such as the ribs, vertebrae and pelvis. This highlights the vulnerability of the chest and abdomen to weapon injuries if they were not protected by the armour of later times. A comparable sixth- to eighth-century series of over three hundred skulls from village cemeteries in southern Germany is illuminating for its evidence of trauma.[15] At a time when helmets were rarely used 10 per cent had cranial fractures, and interestingly 76 per cent of these had healed, indicating survival. Sword blows were more likely to be fatal if they crossed the saggital sinus, a major collection system for venous blood from the brain that lies in the mid-line. Only 12 per cent of wounds showed evidence of infection and 10 per cent of the fractures were treated with trepanation. In some excavations iron arrow heads used in battle remain *in situ*[16] but usually they have rusted away.

Contemporary with the crusades are a group of well-made tombs from Evora in Portugal and these have been identified as the burials of knights from one of the Spanish military orders.[17] They are dated to between the eleventh and thirteenth centuries and two knights were even buried with their spurs. One adult male sustained a major perimortem blade wound to the sternum, on the front of his chest, and in total four of the nine adults excavated demonstrate traumatic lesions. In 1312 AD the Catalans attacked and sacked Frankish Corinth in Greece. A number of bodies from the massacre of townspeople have been recovered from a well,[18] a common place for victors to throw bodies if they were leaving and wished to contaminate the local water supply. Injuries noted on nine apparently unarmed inhabitants were mainly located on the backs of the lower legs (presumably as they ran away), the forearms (defence injuries) and skull. An elegant interpretation of the injuries of a single adult male from medieval Cox Lane in Ipswich, England exemplifies this approach[19] and describes how a horseman might have been overcome by footmen. The individual was suggested to be a horseman, as excess bone was noted at the site of insertion of the adductor muscles of the thigh on to the femur bone. Blade injuries were sustained to the fibula of the right lower leg, the femur of the left thigh and the front of the pelvis. These would be expected injuries for a horseman attacked by men on foot as these would be the areas within reach of a sword. With his legs greatly weakened it would have been easy for the attackers to pull him from his horse, if he had not fallen off without their assistance. Once on the ground he would have been an easy target with both legs injured. The blade injury at the right shoulder and amputation of

[15] Weber and Czarnetzki 2001.   [16] Manchester and Elmhirst 1980.
[17] Santos, Umbelino, Goncalves and Pereira 1998.
[18] Williams, Barnes and Snyder 1997; Barnes 2003.   [19] Wells 1964.

the right forearm would have prevented his last attempts to defend himself with his sword and the sword blow to the skull should have knocked him unconscious. Cuts on two adjacent ribs are compatible with a final stab to the chest to finish him off.

Safed is one of the few medieval sites in the Middle East where skeletal remains have been studied. This was a large town with a castle which was built by the Franks and lay about 12 kilometres north-west of the sea of Galilee in Israel.[20] A series of skulls were excavated back in 1912 from a cave cemetery to the west of the town and radiocarbon dating has shown people were buried here from the thirteenth to the seventeenth centuries, the Mamluk and Ottoman periods.[21] Sixty-eight skulls provide plenty of information regarding disease and injuries sustained. The clearest example of an arrow injury was a healed, diamond-shaped lesion on the top of the skull of an adult male and this position shows that the arrow was not fired directly at the man, but high into the air to fall on him almost vertically. Sending up such a shower of arrows was common practice in medieval battles. Arrow heads have been excavated from a number of nearby medieval castles and cities, including Acre, Belvoir and Jacob's Ford.[22] Another adult male had a depressed fracture most compatible with a rounded mace or stone projectile from a sling. The injury was on the left side of the frontal bone (forehead) and was oval in shape. It was sustained at the time of death as there are radiating fracture lines but no evidence of healing. The inner table of the skull is significantly displaced indicating that the injury would have compressed the left frontal lobe of the brain. The arterial grooves on the bone were interrupted by the fracture, showing that the frontal branches of the middle meningeal artery would have been torn. This would have resulted in an extradural haemorrhage. If the contusion to the brain from the original blow did not immediately kill this man, the developing blood clot would have further compressed the brain and led to his death. The head of a spiked mace has been excavated from the nearby twelfth-century Frankish castle of Jacob's Ford in Galilee[23] and gives a good idea of how the rounded version (without the spikes) would have looked.

Archaeological evidence for accidental trauma, unrelated to combat, has also provided an interesting glimpse into life in the medieval period. It has been found that fracture patterns in males are markedly different from those in females, which would fit with the differing roles of men and women at that time. Women were more likely to fracture their forearms, an injury

[20] Pringle 1985.   [21] Mitchell 2003; Mitchell 2004b.
[22] Raphael 1999.   [23] Raphael 1999.

which today happens most commonly from falling forwards, while men suffered a variety of injuries to their legs and collar bones. Interestingly people in towns, the merchants and craftsmen, experienced fewer fractures than those farming in the country.[24] Ironically, it was the towns where most of the doctors lived and so many people with injuries from farming would have had to rely on friends or family for treatment. People with certain diseases also appear to have been more prone to accidental fractures. Those with leprosy have been noted to experience more fractures in the medieval period than those who were free from the disease.[25] It is possible that symptoms of the disease such as impaired vision, loss of skin sensation, muscle weakness and loss of joint position sense might all increase the likelihood of falls and other traumatic accidents. Severe injury to the lower limbs often leads to impaired function with a leg which could give way or cause pain when used. Interestingly, skeletal evidence for the use of crutches to allow mobilisation has been identified in individuals with severe deformity in the legs.[26] The role of the courts in executing criminals may also be apparent from skeletal material. Hanging is one punishment which may be inferred from the type of fracture in the cervical vertebrae in the neck.[27] Amputation of part of a limb is suggestive of a punishment when evidence for this is found in legal records for the period of the burial, especially if the cut is at right angles to the bone and more than one limb is amputated in a symmetrical manner.[28] A small number of prosthetic limbs have also been identified from the medieval period, either through excavation or in artwork. Some of these appear to be for people who underwent amputation for various reasons, but others were designed for those with an intact, but malformed, limb.[29]

Evidence for the surgical treatment of fractures can be in the form of cut marks on bone, the preservation of metal implants used to keep fractures still while they healed, and by comparing the angulation of healed long bone fractures in individuals who had access to differing standards of medical care in their lifetime. The cemetery of St Margaret Fyebridgegate in Norwich, England, was in use between 1245 and 1468.[30] The church was situated in a particularly poor area of the town. As well as being the burial place for the local population it was where the entire town's criminals were interred since it was next to the gallows. This produced a cemetery with a very high proportion of murderers and villains. Excavation has shown a correspondingly high prevalence of trauma in the remains. Most injuries

---

[24] Judd and Roberts 1999.   [25] Judd and Roberts 1998.   [26] Knüsel, Kemp and Budd 1993.
[27] James and Nasmyth-Jones 1992.   [28] Brothwell and Møller-Christensen 1963; Mays 1996.
[29] Bliquez 1996; Romm 1989.   [30] Stirland 1996.

were healed and not the cause of death. The majority of the healed forearm fractures were noted to be healed at an angle, and had not been returned to the natural position by manipulation. This would be consistent with limited access to medical care as this was a poor area of town. The cemetery of St Helen-on-the-Walls at York, England was in use from 1100 to 1550.[31] In contrast with the previous example at Norwich, the forearm fractures were usually healed straight rather than angulated, suggesting that they had been manipulated and a splint applied, as recommended in surgical texts of the period.[32] The manipulation of long bone fractures to improve the final healed position has been noted in archaeological cases from the earlier Anglo-Saxon period as well.[33] A small number of medieval examples of treatment for fractures indicate that padded metal plates had been applied in an attempt to stabilise the break and lead to healing in a good position. One case from York (England) dates from between the early thirteenth and mid-fourteenth centuries.[34] Copper alloy plates, padded with leather and held in place with twine or thongs, had been used to support an injury at the knee. Other medieval examples include the use of copper plates applied directly to the bone at an operation.[35]

If fractures of the skull were to be treated at all, medical texts advised the cleaning of the wound and removal of potentially harmful bone fragments. A good example has been recovered during the excavation of the twelfth- to thirteenth-century cemetery at Jewbury in York.[36] The skull of an adult had suffered a large blade injury, but it can be deduced that the individual did not die immediately, as there were signs of bone regrowth around the wound. More interestingly, the distribution of bony changes on the skull around the wound suggested that the scalp had been stripped back to allow a better view of the fracture itself. Scratch marks around the wound had the appearance of a surgical tool being used to explore the wound and widen it, which would have been useful to remove any deeper splinters of bone. Trepanation was a surgical procedure which involved actual removal of a section of the skull by scraping, cutting or drilling and could be used to remove damaged areas of bone. Depending on the technique employed, this would have resulted in the removal of either a rounded, oval or square piece of bone. The operation has been performed since prehistoric times, both for skull fracture and other conditions[37] and

---

[31] Grauer and Roberts 1996.
[32] Theodorich Borgognoni 1498 pp. 118v–119r; Theodorich Borgognoni 1955, I, p. 161.
[33] Wells 1974.   [34] Knüsel *et al.* 1995.   [35] Hallback 1976–7; Janssens 1987.
[36] Lilley, Stroud, Brothwell and Williamson 1994 p. 480–6.
[37] Brothwell 1994; Capasso and Di Tota 1996; Parker, Roberts and Manchester 1985–6; Lunardini, Caramella, Mallegni and Fornaciari 2000.

a number of examples have been found in the eastern Mediterranean.[38]
This was a more significant procedure for the patient than merely cleaning
up the wound edges by removing splinters of bone, as it necessitated the
removal of adjacent healthy bone to leave a defect in the skull. However,
the presence of many excavated skulls which show a well-healed edge to
the trepanation does demonstrate that it was not unusual to survive the
procedure. In most parts of Europe at this time trepanation in skulls is
usually found in less than 1 per cent of the total population. In a sixth-
to eighth-century series from south-west Germany 10 per cent of cases
of cranial fractures were treated with trepanation, 1 per cent of the total
excavated sample.[39] A series of trepanations from the medieval period have
been identified from Tiermes (Old Castilla) in Spain,[40] where 5 per cent of
individuals underwent the procedure, a slightly higher proportion than is
usually seen. In some medieval European cases large sections of bone were
removed[41] and the presence of healing at the bone edges show that this
could still be compatible with long-term survival. It seems that from the
archaeological perspective, cranial surgery in its various forms was a widely
used technique in medieval Europe.

Surgery also took place for reasons other than trauma, but understandably it was only those operations affecting bone that survived the centuries
for us to identify in modern excavations. A series of twenty-four skulls
from medieval Oslo in Norway have smooth, oval-shaped indentations in
the outer table of the skull, with an inflammatory reaction around them.
Most are in the same position on the skull, in the mid-line at the top of the
forehead (the bregma). The majority of skulls possessed just the one indentation but some possessed two, with the second lesion at either the front
or back of the skull. As it is highly unlikely that all would have sustained
depressed fractures in an identical position, these have been interpreted as
changes to the bone from cautery to the skull.[42] Certainly the application
of a heated cautery iron to the head was advocated in medieval medical
texts in the treatment of a whole range of conditions.[43] Furthermore, the
sites of these indentations were typical locations for applying the cautery.
If applied firmly for long enough, the iron might well have damaged the
underlying bone and caused such an indentation.

In summary, the evidence from these medieval excavations suggest that
weapon injuries in battle were most common in the skull, the forearms
and the outer aspect of the lower leg. It is not possible to determine from

---

[38] Barnes and Ortner 1997; Mogle and Zias 1995; Zias and Pomeranz 1992.
[39] Weber and Czarnetzki 2001.   [40] Reverte 1980.   [41] Thurzo, Lietava and Vondrakova 1991.
[42] Holck 2002.   [43] Albucasis 1973 pp. 16–18.

excavations how commonly injuries to the abdomen were sustained. It has been proposed that the legs were a target to incapacitate a footman and allow an easy kill as he lay on the ground. Forearm injuries are known as 'defence injuries' and occur when the arm itself is used to fend off a blow to the head or body. This may suggest loss of the shield or sword normally used to fend off such a blow. The head was clearly a target in battle and it is easy to understand why. Even if the blow did not penetrate the mail or helmet the opponent was wearing, there was a good chance that he might be disorientated or knocked unconscious by a heavy blow, allowing a subsequent easy kill. Horsemen may theoretically have been more prone to leg wounds as that part of the body was easiest for foot soldiers to reach and, likewise, footmen may have been more prone to head and forearm wounds as these areas were most accessible to horsemen. Soldiers in an organised battle line were more likely to sustain injuries on the left side of their bodies, from right-handed opponents, while loss of this pattern may suggest commingling of the two sides as the ranks broke formation. Those in flight were more prone to injuries to the back of their bodies, especially the head and lower legs. Importantly, a significant proportion of soldiers appear to have survived serious injuries to fight another day. The most common fracture sustained in peacetime appears to have been in the long bones of the arms. There is evidence to suggest that doctors of the time manipulated fractured long bones back into their correct position and held them there with external splints.

THE CRUSADES

A considerable number of crusader period tombs and cemeteries have been identified at various times in the past,[44] but no serious study of their con-tents has been performed until recently. For example, in the nineteenth century a grave was discovered under the south wall of the church of St Mary Latina in the complex of St John in Jerusalem. Skeletal remains were present in the grave, and apparently other unspecified material believed to date from the crusader period. One of the skulls in the grave was described as having a deep sword cut across it.[45] However, there were no illustrations of the wound, no further details of the description of the bones and no one knows where the remains are today. In consequence it is impossible to know whether the interpretation of the skull as having sustained a weapon injury is correct. It may well have been a sword cut, but similarly it may

[44] Boas 2001 pp. 180–8.   [45] Warren and Conder 1884 p. 255.

have been a split in the bones of the skull resulting from the pressure of overlying soil acting unevenly on softened, waterlogged bone after a period of rain. Sadly, it is only in the last ten years that thorough analysis of human skeletal remains from the Frankish states has taken place. However, study of remains from the Templar fortification of Le Petit Gérin has been completed and sites currently under investigation include the royal castle of Castellum Vallis Moysis,[46] the coastal city of Caesarea and the Templar castle of Jacob's Ford. These have demonstrated a range of weapon injuries and are starting to clarify the effect of wounds on the health of the Franks.

The first settlement studied was that of Le Petit Gérin (now Tel Jezreel, Israel) which lay 15–20 kilometres south of Nazareth. In the twelfth century this was a village of local Syrian Christians who lived under the protection of the fortified tower which was manned by the Order of the Temple.[47] Written sources show that the settlement was sacked by Muslim forces on at least two occasions.[48] While only part of the crusader period cemetery has been excavated, thirty-four immature and six mature individuals were recovered. There was no evidence of weapons, spurs or other finds to suggest a particular occupation or high status for these individuals and it is presumed that they were farmers and craftsmen. One of these six adults was a male aged about 20–30 years old exhibiting a sword wound to the left shoulder.[49] The acromion of the left scapula (shoulder blade) was cut through by a blow which also destroyed much of the shoulder joint beneath. The angle of the cut suggests that the blow came from the left side and would be compatible with a right-handed attacker. Interestingly there is evidence of early new bone formation at the injury, which shows that the victim did not die during the attack but lived at least one or two weeks after. It is not known whether he eventually died from the shoulder injury, perhaps if it became infected, or whether he sustained soft tissue injuries elsewhere. One possibility is that he was actually attacked at Le Petit Gérin as he farmed the fields or while defending the village. However, the period of time between the injury and his death means that he could alternatively have been injured elsewhere while serving in the army of the king of Jerusalem or with another military expedition and survived long enough to return home.

An interesting case was also discovered from the late twelfth-century Frankish castle at Paphos in Cyprus.[50] The castle was destroyed in an earthquake in 1222 and while systematic palaeopathological study of the bones has not taken place, the excavation did discover the remains of one poor

---

[46] Rose, Taani, al-Houroni and Vannini 1998.   [47] Mitchell 1994; Roger of Wendover 1886, I, p. 33.
[48] Ralph de Diceto 1876, 68(ii), p. 28; Roger of Wendover 1886, I, p. 133.
[49] Mitchell 1997; Mitchell 1999a.   [50] Rosser 1986.

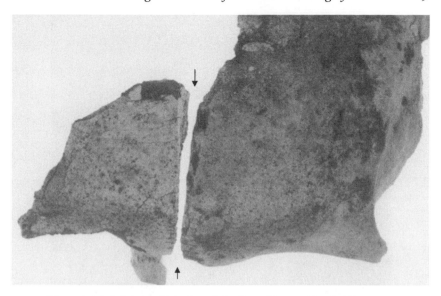

Figure 8. Blade injury which cleaved the frontal bone of the skull into two Member of the Frankish garrison who died at Jacob's Ford castle in 1179. Arrows on the illustration highlight the injury.

individual. He appears to have climbed down the hole of a latrine into the castle's main drain during the earthquake in an attempt to escape with a beautiful glass bottle. The falling masonry resulting from the earthquake then blocked the exits to the drain and he was trapped and died with the bottle beside him.

The castle of Jacob's Ford (Vadum Iacob) is a Frankish excavation with great future potential. This was a Templar fortification in Galilee stormed by the forces of Saladin in 1179.[51] Textual sources describe how several hundred Frankish soldiers were killed either in the battle for the castle or executed after its fall. The remains are under study by Yossi Nagar and the author. The first few soldiers to be found demonstrate non-fatal perimortem blade injuries to the left shoulder, face and mandible, along with fatal injuries such as penetrating blow to the skull (Figure 8) and amputation of the left arm (Figure 9). Arrow heads found where the soft tissues would have been suggest that the soldiers had been wounded by these prior to the blade injuries that caused their death. This is the earliest large-scale medieval battlefield excavation, predating Visby, Aljubarotha and Towton[52] by several centuries. It is also the first to investigate the

[51] Ellenblum, Marco, Agnon, Rockwell and Boas 1998; Ellenblum 2003.
[52] Ingelmark 1939, 1; Cunha and Silva 1997; Fiorato, Boylston and Knüsel 2000.

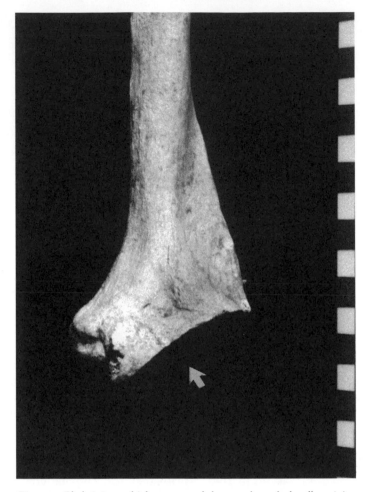

Figure 9. Blade injury which amputated the arm through the elbow joint
Member of the Frankish garrison who died at Jacob's Ford castle in 1179. Arrow on the
illustration highlights the injury.

wounds resulting from medieval Islamic weapons and military tactics, and
so promises to be highly informative.

Crusader period municipal cemeteries from the coastal city of Caesarea[53]
in the kingdom of Jerusalem have also demonstrated cases of trauma. A
recent study[54] found fractures of the tibia with a prevalence of between
10 and 20 per cent in adults. None of these cases was complicated by

[53] Bull 1987 ch. 5, pp. 7–8; Rowsome and Yole 1999.   [54] Smith 1999.

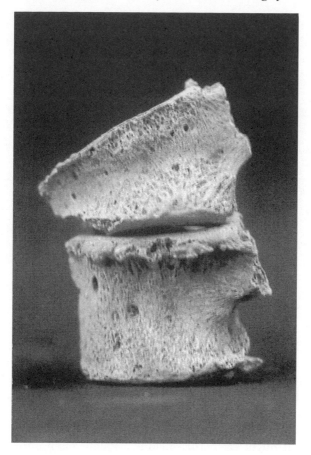

Figure 10. Compression fracture of a lumbar vertebra in the spine
Wedge-shaped, crushed vertebral body, positioned above normal shaped vertebral body
for comparison. From an adult male in a Frankish cemetery at Caesarea
(twelfth–thirteenth century).

osteomyelitis. They were not perimortem injuries and had typically healed straight well before death. Since fractures of weight-bearing long bones in adults often heal at an angle if not treated medically, this could be interpreted to suggest that medical treatment was practised in the town. It is plausible that surgeons performed manipulation of such fractures to an anatomical position followed by holding the bones with a splint until healed. This would certainly be compatible with the medical legislation of the kingdom of Jerusalem (see ch. 8). More recent study of later excavations of crusader cemeteries from Caesarea by the author has demonstrated

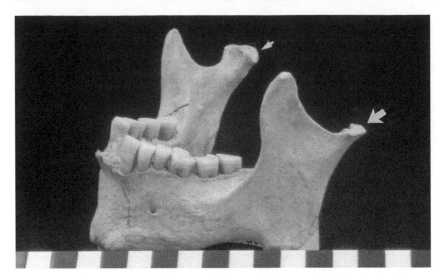

Figure 11. Fracture to left side of the mandible, probably due to a blow on the chin
From an adult male in a Frankish cemetery at Caesarea (twelfth–thirteenth century).
Broad arrow shows site of injury, while thin arrow shows normal side.

further evidence of trauma. A healed, oval depressed fracture was noted on the top of the skull of one adult male. This could have originated from a weapon injury from a mace or stone projectile, or from a fall. Another individual had two healed wedge fractures of lumbar vertebral bodies in the spine (Figure 10). Such an injury often follows a fall from a height and typically results in angulation of the spine, known as a kyphosis. Medieval scenarios that might cause this include a knight falling from a horse, a farmer falling from his cart or even a disturbed burglar jumping from an upper window of a house to escape arrest. An interesting case is a man with an old, but poorly healed, fracture of the left condyle of his mandible (Figure 11). Such a fracture to the jaw tends to result from a blow to the chin and is often sustained during a fist fight. Perhaps this man was one of the less upright members of society in Frankish Caesarea. The absence of fresh, perimortem weapon injuries from such a town cemetery is not too unexpected, as such injuries would be more likely to be found in remains from the battlefield or castles on the borders of the kingdom.

It is hoped that as more sites from the Latin East are studied then a clearer picture of weapon injuries at this time will become available.[55] The total

---

[55] Mitchell 1998.

number of individuals from all crusader sites studied so far is not large, which makes statistical analysis difficult and limits comparison between groups, but this should improve in the future. One significant question still in need of an answer is how the differing weapons, armour and style of combat between Muslim and Christian forces may have affected the distribution and type of injury sustained by each side. At first glance this might seem difficult, as no Muslim army casualties have been excavated from the battlefield. However, by comparing the lesions on crusader bones (which were caused by combat with Muslim forces) with the patterns in Europe (caused by other Europeans) this difference may become apparent. Other areas of interest include the percentage of soldiers who sustained injury or were killed in each campaign, what proportion of soldiers survived their wounds in the long term and whether city inhabitants sustained fewer weapon injuries in their lifetime than rural populations, where fortifications were often smaller and may have offered less protection. A much more complete understanding of injuries in the Frankish states will doubtless result from the ongoing analysis of further sites.

CHAPTER 4

Torture and mutilation

Torture and mutilation appear to have been common during the crusades and were used by almost all military and racial groups. Sometimes torture was employed to extract information, a confession or money, but often it was just to punish captives or demoralise their relatives or friends who remained free. Mutilation was also an option with which to punish those found guilty of a crime or to incapacitate rivals for power so they could no longer pose a threat. In many parts of Europe torture occurred regularly by the time of the crusades, and in 1252 Pope Innocent IV went as far as to issue a decree confirming the use of torture in canon-law procedure.[1] While such practices were commonplace in many countries at that time, they were by no means universal. For example, in twelfth- and thirteenth-century England the amputation of a limb was used only rarely and tended to be reserved for those who displayed open contempt for the king's court by interfering with its proper function. Torture as a punishment or method of gaining a confession is also thought to have been unusual in England at the time of the crusades. Poor treatment in prison certainly did occur but the use of instruments of torture appears to have started in the fourteenth century.[2] The use of torture by mankind has a long history,[3] and the examples noted here dating from the crusades might be thought of as mere cases within this wider setting. However, if they are seen in the context of the crusades and the settled Latin East then it helps us to understand the mistrust between many cultural groups, the fear of capture of crusaders and pilgrims, and the hardships faced by the general population of the Frankish states.[4]

In order to appreciate what medieval torture was all about, it is helpful to understand what kinds of torture were in use in Europe at that time. Typical tortures employed by the Inquisition from the thirteenth century onwards included the pulley, the rack and the fire.[5] Torture by pulley consisted of

[1] Langbein 1977 p. 7.   [2] Bellamy 1973 pp. 139, 182–3.
[3] DuBois 1991, pp. 47–62; Scarry 1985, pp. 27–59; Friedman 2002, pp. 118–29.
[4] Mitchell in press (d).   [5] Scott 1940 p. 67; Peters 1985 pp. 40–73.

attaching weights to the feet and then suspending the prisoner from a rope tied to the wrists behind his back. The pulley was used to raise and suddenly drop the person until the shoulders dislocated. The rack was a frame on to which the prisoner was strapped by the wrists and ankles. The length of the frame was gradually increased so that the joints of the limbs and back became distracted and dislocated. A number of techniques employed fire to torture a victim. One of the more common involved fixing prisoners in stocks and roasting their hands and feet until they confessed to whatever crimes they were alleged to have committed. With the loss of the mainland Frankish states between 1291 and 1302 some soldiers in the military orders returned to Europe and found they had leapt from the frying pan into the fire. Members of the Order of the Temple in Europe were tortured in 1308 to obtain confessions that would support attempts by the king of France to dissolve the order.[6]

THE FIRST CRUSADE

Right from the start of the crusades the Frankish commanders were prepared to use torture and it does not appear to have been an activity learnt from their enemies. There are many examples in the records where it is clear that torture was employed but where no further details are given. For example, on the First Crusade a man was sent by Kilij-Arslan, the sultan of Rum, to spy on the crusading army as it crossed Asia Minor. When he was captured by the Franks he was led before the leaders of the expedition.

> Bohemond, Godfrey and the rest used threats of torture to force the man who had been caught to explain without any lies the reason why he had come. He, moreover, terrified by the threats of so many excellent princes and realising his life hung in the balance, was insistently beseeching them for his life and safety with a tearful voice, a humble expression and a continuous flood of tears, trembling in every limb.[7]

While no details of the type of torture threatened were given it was clearly enough to make this man terrified.

Baldwin went on to take the fortress of Ravendel (modern Ravanda) in the autumn of 1097 and entrusted its care to an Armenian Christian named Pakrad. This man's brother was called Koch Vasil (Basil the Robber) but apparently this did not alert Baldwin to the character of the family. Perhaps unsurprisingly, Pakrad refused to let any of Baldwin's men into the castle

---

[6] Barber 1994 p. 301; Partner 1987 pp. 60–1.   [7] Albert of Aachen bk 2, ch. 26.

and set up his son as commander. Baldwin then resorted to torturing Pakrad in order to get his castle back.[8] Baldwin ordered that he should

be bound with chains and tortured until he was forced to give up the fortress. But he was still not driven to give it up by undergoing any method of torture or fear for his life. Baldwin, overcome by loathing of the man's tortures, finally ordered that he should be torn limb from limb while yet alive unless he gave him satisfaction concerning the fortress's return.

Not surprisingly, Pakrad then had a change of heart and gave the castle back to Baldwin. However, in the autumn of 1098 Pakrad's men were still causing trouble by robbing both crusaders and local Armenians in the region of Ravendel.[9] The crusaders stormed the castle he was using as a base and blinded twenty of the soldiers inside, 'in retribution and revenge'. Blinding was a punishment used both in Europe and the Byzantine empire; it prevented victims from causing trouble in the future but was favoured by the church as it allowed later repentance for their crimes.[10] Just when Baldwin hoped things would calm down there was an attempted coup by Armenians in his principal city, Edessa. Having rounded up the perpetrators he accepted bribes in return for their lives as he was short of money. However, he ordered some to be blinded and others were banished after having their noses, hands, feet or other parts cut off as a punishment.[11]

In December 1097, during the long siege of Antioch by the armies of the First Crusade, Count Raymond of Toulouse captured a young Turkish nobleman during a skirmish outside the city walls. He tried to persuade his family to surrender a tower in the city walls, which they were guarding, in return for their son. News of the negotiations between the family and the crusaders reached the city rulers and the family was moved to a different part of the city.[12] In consequence the crusaders

put the youth to death by beheading, dragging him before the city walls in full view of all the Turks; by this time he was wretched and scarcely breathing on account of torture, since for not much less than a month constant baiting and different torments had been inflicted on him.

Death must have been a relief after such an ordeal.

---

[8] Albert of Aachen bk 3, ch. 18.   [9] Albert of Aachen bk 5, ch. 14.
[10] Bruce 1941; Lascaratos 1992.
[11] Albert of Aachen bk 5, ch. 17; Guibert of Nogent 1996 p. 165; Guibert of Nogent 1997 p. 71.
[12] Albert of Aachen bk 3, ch. 56.

When the crusader army took the town of Ma'arrat-an-Nu'man near Antioch in the winter of 1098 they were desperate for plunder and food. Raymond d'Aguilers[13] recorded the treatment dealt out to the local inhabitants by the crusader soldiers when they entered the town.

In the meantime the pagans hid in subterranean caves and practically none appeared on the streets. The Christians filched all the goods above ground and, driven by hopes of Saracen wealth underground, smoked the enemy out of their caves with fire and sulphur fumes. When the plunder in the caves proved disappointing, they tortured to death the hapless Muslims in their reach.

In August of the following year the same army was at the coastal town of Ascalon and in need of intelligence about the enemy army as they were facing an imminent battle. They came across some local farmers looking after their sheep and cattle as they grazed. They rounded up as many as they could and then 'compelled the captives to reveal their plans, state of preparations and their numbers'.[14] We can only guess as to the methods they used to gain the information, but they were likely to have been unpleasant.

The earliest possible example of the use of the rack was recorded by William of Tyre. During the siege of Jerusalem by the crusaders in July 1099 the Frankish cleric Gerard, who ran the hospice that later evolved into the hospital of St John, may have been subjected to torture with this machine. William, writing some years later, claimed that 'they beat him and cast him into prison. There he was subjected to torture so terrible that the joints of both his hands and feet were wrenched apart and his limbs became practically useless.'[15] If William really did know what had happened to Gerard several decades before, it must have been from talking with survivors of the First Crusade. If that was the case then a version of the rack was being employed in the prisons of Jerusalem in 1099. If it is argued that William might have made up the details of Gerard's suffering to show how holy and meritorious this cleric was, then the reason why William chose this method of torture for his example is still of interest. If the rack was never used in Frankish prisons we might have expected him to suggest another form of torture better known to his readers. However, the use of this example would suggest that the rack was a form of torture used in the Frankish states of the late twelfth century, at the time William was writing.

---

[13] Raymond d'Aguilers 1969 p. 98; Raymond d'Aguilers 1968 pp. 78–9.
[14] Raymond d'Aguilers 1969 pp. 156–7; Raymond d'Aguilers 1968 p. 134.
[15] William of Tyre 1943, I, p. 335; William of Tyre 1986, I, p. 375.

THE EARLY YEARS AFTER THE CONQUEST

Punishment by mutilation, especially of the face, was a standard penalty once the Frankish states were established. After Jerusalem was taken in 1099 Duke Godfrey was elected ruler. He took the army to Ascalon on the coast in an attempt to take the city. However, the locals tried to tempt the soldiers into taking plunder rather than attacking the city and left herds of animals on the nearby plains. Godfrey pronounced an edict that 'whoever of the pilgrims touched booty before battle would be punished by having his ears and nose cut off'.[16] Later examples of nasal mutilation can be found in the canons of the council of Nablus. These were the earliest surviving laws of the kingdom of Jerusalem and were laid down in 1120. They are believed to have been based on Byzantine law as there are many close similarities in both layout and the punishments for each offence.[17] The penalty for a male Frankish settler who committed adultery or raped a Saracen women was castration, while a women who committed adultery was to suffer rhinotomy. Mutilation of the face was certainly not introduced to the region by the Franks. For example, at the town of Tursolt (modern Icel in Turkey) local Christians were treated poorly in the 1090s by the Turks who ruled the town at that time.[18] Once the town came under the control of Baldwin in 1097 the Christian inhabitants came to Baldwin to show their 'ears and noses which the Turks had cut off them because they did not find them willing to be defiled'.

In the following decades a number of independent cities were conquered. These had originally been bypassed by the crusading armies as their numbers dwindled from disease, injuries and the need to garrison those fortifications captured along the way. In July 1109 King Baldwin I accepted the surrender of the town of Tripoli which had until that time remained in Muslim hands in exchange for annual tribute. Some of the inhabitants who chose to remain in the city after the surrender were tortured by the crusaders for both information and money.[19]

The torture was by no means all dealt out by the crusaders to their Muslim captives and when the tables were turned they themselves often suffered just as badly. The battle of the Field of Blood took place between Antioch and Aleppo on 28 June 1119. The Muslim forces of Il-Ghazi of Aleppo soundly beat the Frankish troops under Roger of Salerno, the prince of Antioch. Large numbers were captured and those not executed underwent torture at

---

[16] Albert of Aachen bk 6, ch. 42. [17] Kedar 1999.
[18] Albert of Aachen bk 3, ch. 13. [19] Albert of Aachen bk 11, ch. 14.

the hands of Il-Ghazi. Knowledge of the situation is extremely detailed as one of those captured was the Walter the Chancellor of Antioch, who wrote of his experiences in his chronicle *The Antiochene Wars*.[20] The injured and poor footsoldiers were beheaded after a period in chains without water in the heat of summer. The nobles were transferred to Aleppo and underwent extremely unpleasant treatment. Many were whipped and beaten at the pillory in Aleppo before meeting their deaths. Often knights were forced to see their comrades die before them, so that by the time their turn came these battle-hardened soldiers were reduced to a state where 'their teeth chattered and their bowels trembled'. Some were flayed alive, some hung upside down by the feet and used as target practice for archers, some were buried up to their groin, navel or chin and speared with lances while others had every limb cut off before being thrown into the town square to die as a spectacle for the local population. A small number were ransomed and lived to tell of their experiences. In his chronicle Walter had to stop himself short while describing the disgusting tortures. 'I think it is better for me to keep quiet about the kind and quantity of their tortures than to express them, lest Christians hearing this bring the same to bear on Christians and turn them into accustomed usage.' Another example can be found in the case of Count Joscelyn of Edessa and King Baldwin II of Jerusalem. They had the misfortune to be held in prison in the fortress of Quartapiert, to the east of the Euphrates river. A group of Armenians bluffed their way in, took over the citadel and rescued them. Unfortunately Balak, who owned the castle, then retook it. He spared the life of King Baldwin but not the Armenians. William of Tyre[21] wrote how, 'Some were flayed alive, others sawn in two and others still buried alive. The remainder Balak handed over to his men to serve as targets in archery practice.'

THE LATER YEARS

As the decades passed there is little evidence that torture became any less prevalent. This may in part have been due to the continued influx of crusaders from Europe, who felt it reasonable to torture their Muslim enemies since they were not Christian. However, this theoretical distinction gave little protection when the two opposing sides were actually both Christian, as was the case for Pakrad in 1098. Sometimes the powerful lost their temper even with the most senior of the clergy and tortured them. In the 1150s

---

[20] Walter the Chancellor 1896 pp. 91–4; Walter the Chancellor 1999 pp. 132–6.
[21] William of Tyre 1986, I, p. 570; William of Tyre 1943, I, p. 544.

Reynaud of Chatillon fell out with the patriarch of Antioch. In a fit of rage Reynaud ordered the patriarch to be taken to the citadel of Antioch and forced

to sit in the blazing sun throughout a summer's day, his bare head smeared with honey. No one, for piety's sake, offered him any relief from the relentless rays of the sun or tried to drive away the flies.[22]

Baldwin of Ramla was a captive of Saladin in Damascus around 1180. When Baldwin explained that he could not pay his ransom it seems that Saladin lost his temper. He replied that

either he would pay up or he would pull every tooth he had in his mouth. Baldwin told him to go ahead as he could not pay. So Saladin ordered his teeth to be pulled out. They pulled two of them, at which point, so great was the pain, he cried for mercy and said that he would pay the ransom which amounted to at least 200,000 bezants.[23]

An early case of burning for witchcraft used torture to extract the required confession. In 1187 some sergeants from the Frankish army found an old woman from Nazareth travelling on a donkey and they suspected that she was running away from her Frankish lord. They tortured her to find out what she was doing. 'She revealed that she was a sorceress and had cast a spell on the men of the host . . . Then they collected brushwood and dry grass and made a big fire and pushed her on it.'[24] Of course the truth of what this woman was actually doing is likely to have been very different, and it is probable that admitting to being a sorceress was the only way she could see to stop the torture.

During the Third Crusade, King Richard the Lionheart of England annexed the Byzantine island of Cyprus from its ruler Emperor Isaac Ducas Comnenus. In May 1191 the inhabitants of Nicosia formally acknowledged Richard as their lord while Isaac was still trying to resist the Franks from the other end of the island. The *Itinerarum Peregrinorum et Gesta Regis Ricardi* recorded that

when the emperor heard this he was beside himself with fury. He had as many of our people as he could seized and had one of their eyes put out, or their nose cut off, or an arm or foot mutilated, exacting whatever revenge he could to soothe his rancour.[25]

---

[22] William of Tyre 1986, ii, p. 809; William of Tyre 1943, ii, p. 235.
[23] Ernoul 1871 p. 57; Ernoul 1996 p. 151.
[24] Continuation of William of Tyre 1871 p. 47; Continuation of William of Tyre 1996 p. 40.
[25] Richard de Templo 1864 p. 201; Richard de Templo 1997 p. 193.

In the same year the armies of the Third Crusade were besieging the city of Acre. That June the crusaders captured a Muslim ship trying to break the blockade and reach the city with supplies. Saladin's biographer, Ibn Shaddad,[26] wrote how the crusaders, 'picked up one of the crew, took him on board their galleys and saved him from drowning, but they mutilated him and sent him to the city to report the disaster'. This appears to have been done to demoralise the weakening defenders inside the city.

Shortly after this episode, the marquis Conrad was murdered at Tyre in 1192. He was stabbed to death by two Assassins. Most of the written records merely mention that they were caught and then killed, but do not give much detail as to how this was done. However, the English chronicler Roger of Howden is more specific. It is possible that he heard the details in person from an English participant in the Third Crusade, but it is hard to be completely certain that his version of the story is true. He recounted that 'one of them was immediately put to death while the other was flayed alive'.[27] Flaying alive was one of the most unpleasant methods used to torture someone to death in the medieval period.

After the battle of Gaza in 1244, Count Walter of Briene was tortured by the sultan of Damascus in front of the walls of Jaffa to encourage it to surrender.

They hung him by the arms from a gibbet and said that they would not take him down until the castle of Jaffa was in their hands. While he was so hanging, the count called out to those in the castle not to surrender the town, no matter what torture they might inflict on him.[28]

After the disastrous defeat of the Seventh Crusade in 1250, King Louis IX of France underwent interrogation and was threatened by his Egyptian captors.

The sultan's council tested the king in the same way as they had tested us, to see whether he would promise to surrender any of the castles of the Temple or the Hospital or of the Syrian barons. By God's will, the king gave them the same answer as we had done. They threatened him and said that as he would not agree they would put him in the bernicles. The bernicles are the most cruel torture that you can suffer. They consist of two pliable lengths of wood, armed at the end with teeth. They fit together and are lashed at the end with strong ox hide thongs. When they wish to put people in them they lay the victims on their sides and insert the legs between their teeth. Then they have a man sit on the planks. The result is that

---

[26] Ibn Shaddad 2001 p. 151.

[27] Roger of Howden 1853, II, p. 267; Roger of Howden 1870, III, p. 181.

[28] John of Joinville 1874 pp. 292–4; John of Joinville 1955 p. 160.

there is not six inches of unbroken bone in the legs. To make the torture as severe as possible, at the end of three days when the legs are swollen, they place them in the bernicles again and break them afresh.[29]

Luckily for the king, they did not use them on him in the end.

However, to encourage King Louis to swear the required oath that he would pay his own ransom, the Egyptians

took the Patriarch away from the king and tied him with his hands behind his back to a tent-pole, so tightly that his hands swelled to the size of his head and blood spurted out from his nails. The Patriarch cried out to the king, 'Sir, for the love of God, I beg you to take the oath.'[30]

If compression is applied to a limb the first blood vessels to be occluded are the veins as they have a thin vessel wall and the blood inside is at low pressure. The pressure in the arteries is much higher and it is not difficult to reach a point where blood enters the limb in the arteries as normal but cannot leave as the veins are occluded. This results in swelling of the tissues with the extra blood, as seen here. After a while the pressure in the tissues also increases so that the blood vessels rupture and this might explain the blood around the nails. After some hours of interrupted blood flow the tissues start to die, a state known as compartment syndrome.[31] This is an exquisitely painful condition and might be expected to break the resolve of the most determined prisoner. If bonds causing the compartment syndrome remained in place for sufficient time the tissues would have been so damaged that at best the prisoner would have been left with scarred, paralysed hands while at worst the soft tissues may have sloughed off and resulted in his death.

Following the possible use of the rack on brother Gerard in 1099, the rack is again referred to in thirteenth-century Cyprus. The Latin Church there was concerned by the rise in the use of flute players and hired female mourners who would wail at funerals. They claimed that this not only disturbed divine service but was also a pagan ritual. Archbishop Hugh of Fagiano ruled in 1252–7 that, 'if from this point on these [singing women] should go against our prohibition, we shall have them captured, beaten, put on the rack and then thrown into prison until they learn from the instruction of punishment how much they have transgressed'.[32] While reference to

[29] John of Joinville 1874 pp. 184–6; John of Joinville 1955 p. 109.
[30] John of Joinville 1874 p. 198; John of Joinville 1955 p. 116.
[31] Johansen and Walson 1998; Ortiz and Berger 1998.
[32] *Synodicum Nicosiense* 2001 pp. 100–1, xx.

the use of the rack in the twelfth-century Latin East is rather circumstantial, we can be fairly confident that it was in use during the thirteenth century.

The thirteenth-century laws of the kingdom of Jerusalem and later Cyprus also mention the use of torture in the judicial process. In those laws where it was used, it was typically employed because there were no eye witnesses to critical aspects of the crime. If a slave stole an object from someone and gave it to another free man, and this free man was seen by witnesses talking to the slave, the free man was to be tortured until he agreed to return the possessions to the rightful owner.[33] Another role for torture was to determine the events surrounding an unlicensed burial. If it was discovered that an individual had been buried under a house, rather than in a cemetery, the body was to be exhumed and studied to determine the cause of death. If is was found that the individual had died from suffocation or weapon injuries, the court was obliged to torture those living in the house to find out the events behind the death. Those who admitted during the torture to having committed the murder were then buried alive in the ground, positioned vertically with their heads downwards and feet nearest the surface.[34] Cases of murder sometimes warranted the use of torture by the courts. If a man was accused of murder by relatives of the dead man, then their evidence was not regarded as credible as that of a truly independent witness. The accused man therefore had to undergo three days of torture. If he denied the charges throughout this period of torture, then he was to be put in jail for a year and a day in case any independent witnesses came forward. If no witnesses presented themselves during that time then he would be acquitted. The accused could opt for trial by ordeal during this time in prison and if he passed the test then he was acquitted, although failure led to a conviction for the crime.[35]

Laws such as these demonstrate that by the later years of the Latin East torture had become an acceptable tool for the state to employ even on Christians of Latin stock. However, its use by the courts was restricted to cases where insufficient evidence was available from reliable witnesses. In the first example, the slave was not regarded as a credible witness as he was not a free man, and the circumstantial evidence from witnesses who saw the slave and free man talking together was regarded as sufficiently suspicious to warrant further inquiry. The second, third and fourth cases described were much more serious, in that they referred to murder. In each case, torture was used when there were no witnesses to the alleged crime. Trial

[33] *Assizes of Cyprus* 2002 p. 165.   [34] *Assizes of Cyprus* 2002 p. 209.
[35] *Assizes of Cyprus* 2002 p. 198.

by ordeal was an option that a man accused of murder could request in the absence of sufficient witnesses, to avoid having to languish in prison for a whole year in case any witnesses turned up. However, trial by ordeal was not an option for those who had buried a body under their house. Their fate was to be much worse.

Mutilation was a punishment meted out in some of the crusading armies. In 1190 King Richard I of England laid down a set of laws in order to maintain order in his fleet during the Third Crusade, and these became known as the Oleron laws.[36] A number of the punishments involved mutilation:

Whoever shall slay a man on shipboard, he shall be bound to the dead man and thrown into the sea. If he shall slay him on land, he shall be bound to the dead man and buried in the earth. If any shall be convicted, by means of lawful witnesses, of having drawn out a knife with which to strike another, or shall strike another so as to draw blood, he shall lose his hand. If, also, he shall give a blow with his hand, without shedding blood, he shall be plunged in the sea three times. If any man shall curse his companion, he shall pay him an ounce of silver for every time he has so abused him. A robber who shall be convicted of theft shall have his head cropped after the manner of a champion, and boiling pitch shall be poured on it, and then the feathers of a cushion shall be shaken out upon him, so that he may be known.

Boiling pitch would be expected to cause deep burns to the scalp so that the head would sustain significant scarring. It is likely that much of the hair would never grow back, so this was a highly visible method of mutilating the criminal.

The Frankish courts of the Latin East also employed mutilation against the convicted wrongdoer. Crimes punishable by mutilation ranged from armed assault and rape to medical malpractice. Mutilation had the advantage, from the point of view of a court, of being highly visible and so might have acted as a deterrent to others contemplating such a crime themselves. In many circumstances the area to be mutilated was directly related to the crime so that individuals would have been unable to re-offend even if they had wanted to. If a group of men were jointly accused of stabbing another to death and they were waiting their year in jail for want of witnesses, any one of them could be challenged to trial by combat by any free man. If the free man won the contest, the loser was hanged as the presumed murderer while the other accused were to have their hands amputated and then be expelled from the kingdom.[37] We might expect that the only option left to many after bilateral hand amputation would be a life of begging. Archaeological

[36] Roger of Howden 1853, ii, pp. 140–1; Roger of Howden 1870, iii, p. 36.
[37] *Assises de Jerusalem* 1839 pp. 315–7; *Assizes of Cyprus* 2002 p. 199.

cases of mutilation have been found in a number of medieval skeletons from northern Europe, where a typical punishment would be the removal of a hand or foot, or both.[38] If a man raped a girl in the kingdom of Jerusalem, she was to live out her life in a nunnery at his expense and if the family requested it then the man would also have his genitals cut off.[39] If a medical practitioner was convicted of malpractice so that a free man was maimed or disabled by substandard treatment, then the doctor was to suffer amputation. The Cyprus assizes stated that the whole hand should be amputated while the Jerusalem assizes stated that just the thumb should be removed.[40] In each of these examples it would have been virtually impossible for the same individual to commit such a crime again, since the murderer could not hold a dagger, the rapist had no genitals and the quack doctor could not hold a scalpel.

SUMMARY

It is clear that all sides in the medieval Middle East used torture, whether they were crusader, Muslim or Byzantine. Sometimes this was to extract information from a prisoner but often its use was merely as a grotesque sport for the victor. Techniques described include those borrowed from warfare, those more at home in a butcher's shop or surgeon's operating table, and those specifically designed for the torture chamber. Approaches borrowed from the battlefield included target practice with arrow or lance and amputation of limbs with a sword. Techniques borrowed from surgery or a butcher's shop included dismemberment, pulling of teeth and flaying of the skin. Torture devices mentioned include tight cords which may have caused compartment syndrome, the rack to stretch a prisoner and the bernicles to crush him. Torture was rationalised in the Frankish mind with the decision that it was acceptable to use it on non-Christians, also known as 'pagans'. However, the victim being Christian rarely prevented the use of torture by other Franks if they were angry and powerful enough.

It is only possible to guess at the contemporary perceptions of its use by members of the population. However, the comments of Walter the Chancellor, who refrains from mentioning the most severe forms of torture so that Christians should not use the techniques on each other in Europe, are fascinating. They suggest that he is aware that torture is taking place in Europe and that he personally does not believe that the most unpleasant

---

[38] Brothwell and Møller-Christensen 1963; Mays 1996.
[39] *Assises de Jerusalem* 1839 pp. 150–1; *Assises of Cyprus* 2002 p. 131.
[40] *Assises de Jerusalem* 1839 p. 258; *Assises of Cyprus* 2002 p. 182.

techniques should be used on other Christians. We can only speculate as to whether he would think them acceptable to use on 'pagans', but he may have been so bitter after his ordeal as a captive that his hatred may have enabled him to accept the use of any kind of torture in revenge.

Mutilation was a widely used punishment in the early years of the Frankish states. There are many examples of this form of punishment, both within the framework of the law and by vigilantes. More common forms of mutilation included cutting off the nose, ears or genitals, amputation of a hand or foot or blinding with a hot iron. If such tortures and punishments really were handed out on a regular basis by those in power at the time, then it might be expected that a significant proportion of the population would have suffered disability or disfigurement of some kind.

CHAPTER 5

Injuries and their treatment

Trauma surgery understandably comprised a major part of the surgical workload for practitioners in the Latin East. A significant number of battles, sieges, raids and expeditions took place throughout the 200-year history of the Frankish states. Even discounting the effects of fighting, the Latin East may have been a rough and rowdy place. We hear of 'many sinful as well as pious men, adulterers, murderers, thieves, perjurers and robbers' who set out on the First Crusade in 1096–7.[1] To make things worse, in many areas of Europe convicted criminals facing hanging or amputation could opt for exile in the Holy Land as an alternative punishment. These convicts were sent east by the courts in Europe in the hope that spending time at the Holy Places might reform their characters.[2] However, as Jacques de Vitry noted, 'as they had only changed their climate and not their character, they defiled it [the Holy Land] by numberless crimes'.[3] In 1253 the papal legate Odo of Chateauroux told John of Joinville 'no one knows as well as I do the wicked sins that are committed in Acre'.[4] The legate also noted that Christians who fled Europe to Outremer hoping to find less opportunity to sin discovered there more occasions than at home, and where they expected to be sanctified they were further corrupted.[5] While the region may have been called the Holy Land, not everybody behaved in a holy way.

It might be presumed that the most logical place to look for textual evidence of the treatment of the injured would be medical texts. This approach has been used either on its own[6] or in conjunction with independent evidence for injuries[7] to determine how they might have been treated. One difficulty with this technique is that there are no European surgical texts from the earliest days of the Latin East, and so assessing both early practice and also the evolution of techniques over the decades is problematic.

---

[1] Albert of Aachen bk 1, ch. 2.   [2] Hurnand 1969 pp. 35, 195, 227 n.1.
[3] Jacques of Vitry 1611 p. 1097; Jacques of Vitry 1971 pp. 89–90.
[4] John of Joinville 1874 pp. 334–6; John of Joinville 1955 p. 181.   [5] Innocent IV 1876 p. 220.
[6] Haddad 1986–7; Perrot 1988; Frohberg 1989.   [7] Paterson 1988; Mitchell 1999a.

Clearly not all medieval surgical texts are equally applicable to all events within the entire life span of the Frankish states, and so a late thirteenth-century text has only limited compatibility with an early twelfth-century treatment episode. Furthermore, there has been considerable debate as to how to interpret the content of surgical texts in the medieval period and to what degree it can be assumed that practitioners actually performed the procedures found in these works.[8] Sometimes the wording of a medical text uses practical examples that give the impression that it was written primarily to be used to treat the injured[9] and at other times the inclusion of new techniques suggests that they were practised by the author who recommended their use. However, some texts merely repeat word for word procedures that are found in much earlier works and there may be no evidence that the author even saw such a procedure, let alone performed it himself.

One helpful approach in the study of the treatment of medieval weapon injuries is to use original works on how to maintain health in an army, such as Arnold of Villanova's *Regimen Almarie*,[10] as discussed earlier. The mention of new techniques or information might imply that they were in use at that time rather than merely copied into a text from ancient sources for completeness. Another more rather impartial technique for assessing the actual practice of surgery is to use anecdotal information in non-medical contemporary sources where procedures are referred to. While this would by no means be guaranteed to give evidence for all the surgical procedures that were actually undertaken at that time, with a large enough range of original sources a rough estimate of typical procedures may become apparent. Of course, not all of the surgeon's trauma workload was the treatment of battle casualties. Even in peacetime farmers would have fallen off carts and masons been hit by falling stones, many needing the attention of a *medicus* or *cyrurgicus* if one was available. Some interesting work on such accidents in children has been undertaken using evidence from the miracle cures of saints in medieval England.[11] Typical injuries included lacerations, contusions, fractures, burns and asphyxiation. However, such trauma rarely attracted the attention of most general chroniclers, so that the majority of information regarding the crusades refers to the battlefield.[12]

Evidence for injuries and their surgical treatment in the Frankish states is outlined below with representative examples. The nature of these texts means that care must be taken to use historically plausible accounts and

---

[8] Alvarez-Milan 2000; Savage-Smith 2000.   [9] Paterson 1988.   [10] McVaugh 1992.
[11] Gordon 1991.   [12] Mitchell in press (c).

to avoid taking everything at face value. I hope that the legends and more outrageous stories have been either excluded or highlighted as such, and that those authors known for their active imaginations have been used with appropriate caution. At the siege of Antioch in February 1098 there was a battle between the besieging Franks and the Turks who came to relieve the city. Orderic Vitalis[13] wrote:

Weapons were shattered everywhere and bright sparks flew from brazen helmets. Wound after wound was inflicted and the fields were red with blood. You could see torn entrails, severed heads, headless bodies, corpses everywhere.

While such detail might at first glance seem to suggest Orderic's personal participation in the campaign, this is far from the case. He wrote his chronicle from the comfort of his French monastery several decades after the crusade, used other written accounts as his sources rather than eye witnesses; he himself never even went to the Frankish states. It is probable that this is an example where description of battle scenes was fabricated in a way plausible to the reader to make the story more exciting, as in Greek and Roman epics.[14]

Similarly, the details in the *Canso d'Antioca*[15] describing the wounds sustained in the same battle appear particularly vivid, perhaps at first glance suggesting they were recorded by an eye witness. However, further assessment shows many implausible details in the same passages which arouse significant doubt as to whether they can be authentic descriptions of such injuries. Many named nobles are described giving and receiving wounds in person while fighting hand to hand with named emirs in the opposing army. It is highly unlikely that the leaders in both armies would have actually fought each other in person. It is highly unlikely that knights would have known the name of the emirs they were killing. It is also highly unlikely that the writer of the text (or people he later discussed the battle with) would have been able to see all of these duels even if they had taken place. It seems that this is another example where the vivid descriptions of wounds are probably not sufficiently reliable for us to use in this study. Despite the identification of many such examples as unreliable there are nevertheless many other accounts where the descriptions do appear to be of value in an investigation of weapon injuries and their treatment. However, there will always be grey areas, where some feel a passage to be reliable while others do not. Readers will have to make up their own mind as to how much credence to give to some of these passages. I have highlighted the more

---

[13] *Orderic Vitalis* 1975, V, pp. 80–1.   [14] Salazar 2000.   [15] *Canso d'Antioca* 2003.

controversial authors, such as Usama, in the text as the relevant examples are discussed.

Injuries resulting from trauma will be discussed in this chapter by subdividing them by the mechanism of injury and the part of the body affected. In order to make sense of this we must understand exactly what anatomical knowledge was commonplace at the time of the crusades. This is necessary as knowledge among doctors of the function of different parts of the body varied widely. Medical texts discussing human anatomy date back well before the medieval period.[16] Alexandria in Egypt is known for the human dissections that took place there in Ptolemaic times around 250–300 BCE.[17] Perhaps the most significant single contribution was from Galen in second-century AD Rome, who dissected the pig, ox, dog, bear, barbary ape and other animals.[18] The Roman empire continued in the east as the Byzantine empire, and human dissection is known to have taken place there over the following centuries.[19] Examples come from the fourth to twelfth centuries and were typically the cadavers of condemned criminals. Dissection was undertaken specifically to understand human anatomy in order to treat the sick more successfully. With the rise of medicine in the Islamic world a number of medical texts incorporated anatomical knowledge from Galen and others. While there has been much misunderstanding with regard to the role of human dissection in medieval Islam,[20] there was certainly no prohibition against the dissection of animals to further anatomical understanding. Although Galen was well known in the Middle East by the time of the crusades, some of his anatomical works were not known in Europe until the 1500s.[21]

However, a number of those Arabic texts that had incorporated Galen's discoveries did find their way to Europe and translations of these began to become available from the eleventh century onwards. The most notable works include the *Isagoge* of Hunayn, the *Canon* of Avicenna, the *Liber Pantegni* of al-Majusi and the book of the Almansor by al-Razi.[22] Knowledge of the anatomy of higher mammals advanced significantly in southern Europe from the eleventh to thirteenth centuries with a number of texts which describe how to perform dissection of the pig. Perhaps the earliest is the *Anatomia Porci*,[23] and a number of comparable works were subsequently produced in Italy.[24] One of these, the *Anatomia*

[16] French 1999; Carlino 1999.   [17] Scarborough 1976a; von Staden 1992.
[18] Savage-Smith 1971a; Savage-Smith 1971b; Persaud 1984 pp. 57–69.
[19] Bliquez and Kazhdan 1984; Browning 1985.   [20] Savage-Smith 1995.
[21] Galen 1956 pp. i–xxvi.   [22] Siraisi 1990 pp. 84–7.
[23] *Anatomia Porci Cophonis* 1927; O'Neill 1970.   [24] Corner 1927; Saffron 1975.

Ricardi, was sometimes included in the Articella used to teach medicine in European universities.[25] The production of illustrated Latin translations of anatomical texts from Alexandria appears to have begun by 1150 in southern Europe.[26] Illustrations of human dissection have also been identified in a medical manuscript thought to have originated in thirteenth-century England, perhaps at St Albans.[27] Organs clearly drawn in the female cadaver include the heart and lungs, liver, kidneys, intestines and ovaries. By the late thirteenth century, postmortem examinations were being undertaken in Italy for forensic purposes to help identify cause of death.[28] An interesting parallel is found with the wounding of King Baldwin I of Jerusalem around 1103, described in more detail later in the chapter. Here his doctor asks for permission to give a Saracen prisoner a similar wound and then dissect him to aid in the treatment of the king, but instead a bear was dissected as a compromise.[29] In this example the use of autopsy to investigate a wound occurs at a much earlier date than modern experts in this field would expect, and in consequence is fascinating. Human dissection became more widespread in the teaching of medicine in the fourteenth century (on the cadavers of criminals)[30] and illustrated anatomical works were written by Henri de Mondeville, Mondino dei Luzzi and others.[31]

Another source of anatomical knowledge would have been the procedures undertaken when individuals died away from home and wished their remains to be transported to a specific burial place. This appears to have been a common practice in the twelfth and thirteenth centuries, at least among the nobility of northern Europe. The practice involved either boiling the body to retrieve the bones for transport, or full dissection of the body so that important organs such as the heart were placed in a casket while the eviscerated cadaver was packed with salt or other preservatives for the journey home. This dismemberment is often termed division of the corpse. In many cases is is not entirely clear whether the division was performed by a surgeon or another who possessed skill with a knife, such as a butcher or cook. While the decree of Pope Boniface VIII in 1299 stopped this practice in many parts of Europe, it was still allowed after this date if the death occurred outside Christian lands.[32] Clearly the crusades were a classic example of where nobles would die far from home and there are many examples of this preservation and transport home of Franks, such as those of King Baldwin I of Jerusalem in 1118, Emperor Frederick I of Germany in 1190 and

[25] French 1999 p. 17.   [26] French 1999 p. 22.
[27] MacKinney 1960.   [28] O'Neill 1976; Sinha 1982; Park 1994.
[29] Guibert of Nogent 1996 p. 287; Guibert of Nogent 1997 p. 134.
[30] Alston 1944; Siraisi 1990 pp. 84–7.   [31] MacKinney 1962; Olry 1997.   [32] Brown 1981.

the English earl of Arundel in 1221.[33] This must have given those crusaders performing the preservation a reasonable knowledge of the anatomy of much of the human body. An assessment of the frequency that division of the corpse, autopsy and dissection took place in different parts of medieval Europe has highlighted an interesting finding.[34] It seems that division of the corpse for later burial was mainly practised in northern Europe, and took place throughout the twelfth and thirteenth centuries. Autopsy to diagnose the cause of death mainly took place in Italy, from the late thirteenth and fourteenth centuries. Dissection to aid the teaching of anatomy took place throughout Europe in universities, but was again principally a phenomenon of the late thirteenth century onwards. At the time of the crusades many of those practitioners with an academic medical training would have had a basic knowledge of mammalian anatomy from both texts and dissections of the pig and others may have gained hands on experience of human anatomy either from division of the corpse or forensic autopsy. However, the anatomical knowledge of many of the less well-educated practitioners would probably have been rather limited and none of them appears to have known the correct function of many organs, especially in the thorax and abdomen.[35]

A discussion of the types of weapons and armour used and numbers of casualties in battle enables battlefield injuries described in more reliable accounts to be seen in context. These wounds have been grouped together under crush injuries, blade injuries, penetrating injuries from arrow and lance, burns and head injuries. Cranial trauma is dealt with separately, as the complications and treatment were similar, regardless of the weapon used to cause the injury. Where possible the information is identified as representing either crusader or local medical practice, the latter being performed by either Frankish settlers or those Christian, Jewish or Muslim practitioners indigenous to the region. This may highlight any apparent differences between those from contrasting backgrounds. The evidence is then evaluated in an attempt to ascertain which injuries were most common and which were the most serious. We will also be in a position to determine what kinds of surgical procedures were actually being undertaken at that time in the management of trauma and how closely this resembled the recommended treatments found in contemporary medical texts.

---

[33] Albert of Aachen bk 12, ch. 28; Continuation of William of Tyre 1982, p. 98; Continuation of William of Tyre 1996 p. 88; Matthew Paris [Luard] 1876, III, p. 67.
[34] Park 1995.   [35] French 1978.

NUMBER OF CASUALTIES IN BATTLE

It is possible to make very approximate assessments of the fate of those involved in major battles or sieges based on the information recorded in contemporary chronicles. Sometimes actual figures are given,[36] but it is obvious that such information has to be treated with caution as there is potential for an author to massage the figures up or down to make the engagement sound more impressive for his own side.[37] A more objective approach is to determine the fate of individuals known to have been present at a certain battle. This can be useful when looking at the more important nobles or clergy, who tend to be mentioned by name, but of little help in assessing the fate of the common footsoldier.

The *Itinerarium Peregrinorum et Gesta Regis Ricardi* mentions a number of nobles and clergy by name who joined the siege of Acre which lasted nearly two years, in 1190–1.[38] Nobles and clergy would be expected to share many lifestyle factors, such as reasonable diet and access to medical care, with the major difference being their role on the battlefield. With a few notable exceptions, clergy did not typically play an active military role so it is likely that most deaths in this group were from natural causes, such as infectious disease and malnutrition.[39] Clearly some of these individuals would have died anyway, even if they had stayed back in Europe,[40] and ideally it would be useful to know how many extra died as a result of their participation in the crusade. However, it is difficult to allow for this accurately unless the ages of the clerics and nobles are also available, and the age mix of these individuals remains unknown. This method of calculation will tend to underestimate the true death rates as the fate of many individuals is unknown. To err on the side of caution, these unknowns have been treated as if they survived, to give a minimum death rate. Of the sixty-nine individuals mentioned in the list in the *Itinerarium*, eighteen (26 per cent) died at some stage during the siege while the remaining fifty-one are believed either to have survived or their fate is unknown. Of fifty nobles mentioned, fifteen (30 per cent) of them are thought to have died in the siege. Of nineteen clergy mentioned, three (16 per cent) are thought to have died. Twice the percentage of nobles died in the same period and one plausible explanation is that the higher number was due to injuries on the battlefield.

---

[36] Walter the Chancellor 1896 p. 105; Walter the Chancellor 1999 p. 155; Richard de Templo 1864 p. 7; Richard de Templo 1997 p. 25.

[37] Bachrach 1999.

[38] Richard de Templo 1864 pp. 73–4 and 92–3; Richard de Templo 1997 pp. 82 and 98.

[39] Mitchell in press (b).

[40] Bullough and Campbell 1980; Kunitz 1987; Shahar 1993.

A similar approach has previously been used to look at the situation in the Fifth Crusade to Egypt in 1217–21.[41] However, the method differed slightly as only those whose outcome is known (death or survival) are included. This approach may overestimate the total death rate as a death may have been more likely to have been recorded in a chronicle than survival. Death was a newsworthy fact to note in a chronicle, but a survival would rarely have been so. From a total of 261 named crusaders there is evidence that 89 died at some stage during the campaign (34 per cent). From the upper clergy 9 out of 48 died (19 per cent) while from the feudal aristocracy 35 out of 104 died (33 per cent). This again shows a death rate in the clergy of roughly half that of the knights and figures are surprisingly similar to those derived from the Third Crusade thirty years before. It is possible that the higher total death rate in this later campaign was a result of the expedition lasting longer, but the bias due to the reporting of deaths and survivals in the chronicles may also be to blame. More recent study of deaths in the First Crusade has estimated that about 37 per cent died in the subset under discussion.[42] This analysis again used a slightly different method of calculation. The evidence for the cause of death is not based on the crusader's role (soldier or clergy) but on the information written about the circumstances of his death. This will tend to give a different bias from that resulting from the previous methods described. From a total of 217 named crusaders whose outcome is known, 52 (24 per cent) died in combat, 29 (13 per cent) died from unspecified causes (such as starvation, disease or combat) and 136 (63 per cent) survived. As just discussed for the study of the Fifth Crusade, this approach may overestimate the total death rate as only those with known outcome were included. It will also overestimate the proportion of deaths from disease, as some of those who died from unknown causes are nevertheless thought to have died in battle. As with the other techniques, the information is based on that subset of the crusader army who were sufficiently rich, noble or well known to have been mentioned by name. None of these techniques is perfect, but seen together they all contribute to our understanding of the chance of a typical crusader returning home alive.

These findings suggest that in a long campaign with sieges under difficult conditions, at least 15–20 per cent of the wealthy crusaders might have died from disease and at least a further 15–20 per cent of knights might have died in battle. Thus in these upper echelons of medieval society perhaps

---

[41] Powell 1986 pp. 169–71.   [42] Riley-Smith 2002.

25–40 per cent might have died in a tough expedition lasting two or three years. It is not known what proportion of footsoldiers died from each cause and it might be expected that the figures would be much higher. More would have died from malnutrition as they would have had little money or food supplies in reserve for hard times. Likewise their poor defensive armour may well have resulted in higher casualties in battle.

WEAPONS AND ARMOUR

Some knowledge of the tactics and weapons used in the medieval period, together with the armour employed to protect against injury, helps in the understanding of trauma at this time.[43] Personal weapons known to have been used in the crusades include the sword, dagger, battle-axe, mace, war-flail, war-hammer, lance, spear, arrow and crossbow bolt[44] (Figures 12–14). Siege weapons were able to propel rocks, Greek fire, boiling oil and water and, on occasion, amputated body parts. In defence a typical Frankish knight's protection would have included a coat of chain mail or scale armour, shield and a helmet.[45] The mail typically covered the head, arms, body and thighs in one piece, known as a hauberk. During the twelfth century mail protecting the lower legs, chausses, became more common. Although an effective defence, mail could still be penetrated by lance, cross-bow bolt and arrow and even cut with a heavy blow from a good sword.[46] The mace exploited the flexible nature of mail and crushed the bones and soft tissues underneath without having to penetrate the mail. In consequence, padded cloth (*aketon*) or rigid leather (*cuirasse*) garments could be worn under the mail to dissipate the energy from these blows, so decreasing the resulting damage. The shield was changing from the long pointed 'kite' shape of the Normans to become shorter with a flatter top, easier to use on horseback. Helmets in the twelfth century were evolving from the conical shape with a nasal bar used by the Normans the century before. Their first advance was to become rounded in shape and by the end of the twelfth century the great helm was introduced, which gave protection to the face as well as the skull.

A footman was limited in the amount of defensive equipment he could use. This was partially due to the cost, partially that heavy armour greatly limited mobility and partially a consequence of the intense heat in much of the region. A footsoldier may have worn a helmet, jerkin of padded

---

[43] France 2001.   [44] Nicolle 1988.   [45] Edge and Paddock 1996; Nicolle 1980.
[46] Oakshott 1994; Bradbury 1985.

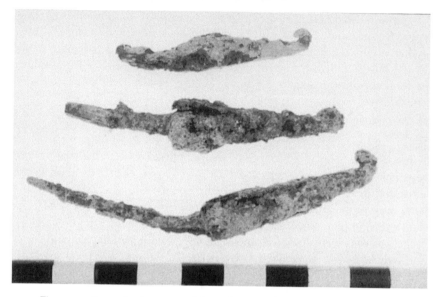

Figure 12.   Arrow heads excavated from the siege of Jacob's Ford castle in 1179
These are of the armour-piercing type, without barbs. Although slightly corroded with
time, it can be seen that the sharp tips (to the right) were deformed by their impact, while
the arrow shafts have long since rotted away.

cloth (*gambeson*) or stiffened leather, possibly some mail and sometimes a
small shield. It was rare to wear protection for the lower legs. A popular
helmet from the end of the twelfth century was the kettle hat (*chapel de fer*).
This was rounded over the skull and had a wide brim, which gave reasonable protection while not impairing the field of vision. Although all this
equipment was available, often the poorest soldiers went into battle with
nothing but a weapon.

In the armies of the Muslim emirs armour obviously varied depending
on the origins of the soldiers. Some came from Asia Minor to the north,
others from Syria and Persia to the east and others still from Egypt and
north Africa to the south.[47] Many Muslim soldiers were well known for
their light armour, which allowed them much greater mobility. Typical
equipment included close quarters weapons such as the sword, dagger, axe
or mace and projectile weapons such as the bow, crossbow and javelin.[48]
The spear was used by both infantry and cavalry, the latter using the

[47] Nicolle 1979.
[48] Richard de Templo 1864 p. 247; Richard de Templo 1997 p. 234; Nicolle 1994.

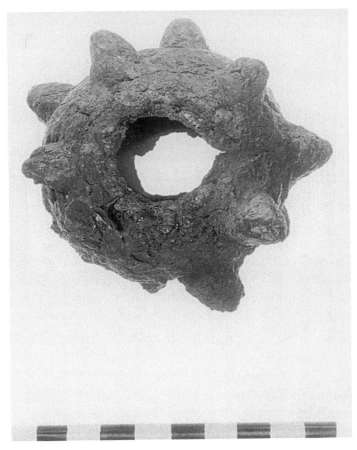

Figure 13. Mace head from Jacob's Ford castle, Galilee (1179)
The central hole was for a wooden handle, which has not survived.

lance as well. Horsemen typically wore conical helmets or a turban and sometimes a combination of the two. Many shields were round or kite-shaped, while infantry had the flat-bottomed shield which could be used to create a defensive wall in battle.[49] These shields could be made from leather, wood or iron. Some cavalry were heavily armoured with mail or lamellar armour to cover the body, arms and legs comparable to the crusader hauberk while others wore just a padded cloth jacket to improve mobility.[50]

[49] Nicolle 1983.   [50] Williams 1978; Nicolle 1999.

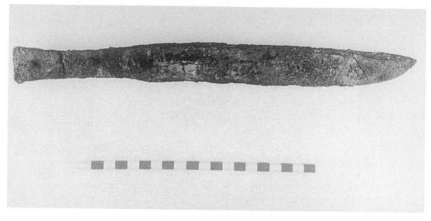

Figure 14.   Dagger from Jacob's Ford castle, Galilee (1179)
The wooden handle to the left has not survived.

While none of this body armour could protect against the projectiles from the massive siege engines[51] used by all sides, it did help considerably in protecting the soldier from blows from hand-held weapons and lighter projectiles such as arrows.

BLADE INJURIES

Wounds from the sword and battle-axe were common, and good archaeological examples have been described from the Frankish settlement of Le Petit Gérin[52] and the castle of Vadum Iacob. The effectiveness of the weapons at close quarters is highlighted in the following examples of injuries from contemporary chronicles. In 1097 the armies of the First Crusade won a battle near Nicaea against Kilij-Arslan, the sultan of Rum. Even at this early stage the practice of decapitation with the sword and use of the severed head as a trophy was widespread. Albert of Aachen wrote that 'the Christians cut off the heads of the dead and wounded and as a sign of victory they brought them back to their tents with them, tied on the girths of their saddles'.[53] When they besieged the city of Nicaea itself these heads were catapulted into the town by the crusaders to frighten and demoralise the defenders. A further use for these heads was when 'a thousand Turks heads were gathered in carts and sacks and loaded on wagons and they took them down to the port which is called Civitot and then they were

[51] Hill 1998.   [52] Mitchell 1997.   [53] Albert of Aachen bk 2, ch. 27.

sent by ship to the emperor of Constantinople'.[54] Again this was meant as a sign of military prowess. Presumably the sight and smell of so many decomposing heads must have had quite an effect when the ship arrived in Constantinople.

In August 1097, shortly after the city of Nicaea was taken by the crusaders, the army came near the town of Antiocheia (west of modern Yalvac). It was here that Duke Godfrey of Bouillon showed off his swordsmanship during an encounter with a wild bear that had attacked a peasant wandering in some woods.

By an unlucky chance, as the beast was escaping the blow of the sword it suddenly drove its curved claws into the duke's tunic, it brought him down to the ground embraced in its forepaws as he fell from his horse and it wasted no time before tearing his throat with its teeth. The duke, therefore, in great distress remembering his many distinguished exploits and lamenting that he who had up to now escaped splendidly from all danger was now indeed to be choked by this bloodthirsty beast in an ignoble death, recovered his strength; he revived in an instant and was on his feet and, seizing the sword which had got entangled with his own legs in the sudden fall from his horse and the struggle with the frenzied wild beast, holding it by the hilt he aimed swiftly at the beast's throat, but mutilated the calf and sinews of his own leg with a serious cut. But nevertheless, although an unstaunchable stream of blood poured forth and was lessening the duke's strength, he did not yield to the hostile brute but persisted most fiercely in defending himself until a man called Husechin, who had heard the great shout of the poor peasant delivered from the bear, and the butcher's violent roaring, rode at speed from the comrades scattered through the forest to assist the duke. He attacked the terrifying wild beast with drawn sword, and together with the duke he pierced its liver and ribs with his blade.

So, with the ferocious beast killed at last, the duke for the first time began to lose heart because of the pain of his wound and the excessive loss of blood; his face turned pale and he threw the whole army into confusion with the wicked news. Everyone rushed together to the place where the brave champion and man of wisdom, head of the pilgrims, was brought wounded. Laying him on a litter, the chiefs of the army brought him down into camp with great lamentation and grief of the men and wailing of the women, summoning the most skilled doctors to heal him.[55]

While Godfrey may have sustained damage to his throat from the bear it sounds as if the worst injury was caused by his own sword after he was pulled from the horse. The laceration appears to have been to one of his calves and the record of heavy bleeding would suggest transection

---

[54] Albert of Aachen bk 2, ch. 28.
[55] Albert of Aachen bk 3, ch. 4; Guibert of Nogent 1996 pp. 285–6, Guibert of Nogent 1997 pp. 133–4.

of an artery, rather than a vein, where bleeding would be less. This is supported by the observation that he turned pale, which is a classic sign of shock due to significant blood loss.[56] While the techniques employed by the doctors are not outlined in Albert of Aachen's chronicle, surgical texts from the medieval period recommend how this kind of injury should be treated. However, it should be remembered that the twelfth-century European surgical texts had yet to be written by this time. One early text that might be helpful is that of Albucasis, who wrote in tenth- to eleventh-century Islamic Spain. Although his text was not translated into Latin until the 1170s, it should have been known to the Eastern Christian doctors who often assisted the crusaders. He describes one interesting technique for stopping arterial bleeding.[57]

Very often there occurs bleeding from an artery which has been cut either by an external wound or in opening an abscess or in cauterising a part of the body and so on, and it is difficult to stem. When this happens to anyone, quickly apply your forefinger to it and closing it properly until the bleeding ceases under your fingers and nothing comes out. Then put in the fire several olive cauteries, small and large, and blow on them to make them very hot. Then take one, small or large according to the size of the wound and the size of the opening of the artery and bring the cautery right down on the artery itself, after promptly removing your finger, and hold the cautery upon it until the bleeding ceases.

This treatment would be expected to be effective as the hot cautery would burn the artery and stop the flow of blood through the middle. This was by no means an easy procedure to perform. All the blood pouring from the vessel would make both instruments and body tissues very slippery to hold and it would often have been difficult to see exactly where to place the cautery as the blood welled up from a deeply positioned artery. Furthermore, time would not have been on the surgeon's side as the duke would have been deteriorating minute by minute. However, from what we hear about the degree of bleeding from his wound we would have expected him to have died from blood loss had the doctors not intervened with a technique such as this. It was January 1098, a full five months later, before we hear that Godfrey had fully recovered from his wound.[58] The duke then continued as one of the prominent leaders of the First Crusade and became the first ruler of Jerusalem after it was conquered in 1099.

Sometimes descriptions of the frantic slaughter after the capture of a town were frighteningly vicious. In consequence, some modern scholars

---

[56] Committee on Trauma 1994 pp. 81–2.   [57] Albucasis 1973 p. 162.
[58] Albert of Aachen bk 3, ch. 58.

do not believe that the details of these accounts should be taken literally, and there is some sense in this. However, a number of these accounts were from eye witnesses, and were often highly graphic. It seems plausible that a significant proportion of the passages written by such witnesses may have been based on the truth, if sometimes embellished. One such eye witness, Raymond of Aguilers,[59] tells us that on taking Jerusalem in July 1099, 'some of the pagans were mercifully beheaded, others pierced by arrows plunged from towers, and yet others, tortured for a long time, were burned to death in searing flames. Piles of heads, hands and feet lay in the houses and streets.' In modern times, letting prisoners go unharmed might be thought of as merciful. The suggestion in this chronicle that mere beheading, without torture, was merciful shows the attitudes of some of the more zealous chroniclers.

There are rare examples of scalping, when a knife was used to remove the hair and scalp from the head as a sign of victory over an opponent. Gervase was in charge of the city of Tiberias in 1108 when he was captured by soldiers from Damascus. As King Baldwin I refused to surrender several cities in return for the knight's life, his captors decided to put him to death. However, Gervase had long white hair which had not been cut for some time and chronicles mention that the scalp was cut off the head, dried and fixed to the top of a spear to remind the Damascenes of the victory and intimidate the Franks in future battles.[60] The practice of scalping in the region had a long history and archaeological cases from the eastern Mediterranean date back as early as the Bronze Age (3,000 BCE).[61]

An attempt to assassinate a Frankish noble with a sword was described by William of Tyre,[62] when in the 1130s

the Count of Jaffa was awaiting passage and lingering in Jerusalem as he was wont to do. One day he happened to be playing dice on a table before the shop of a merchant named Alfanus in the street which is called the Street of the Furriers. The count, intent upon the game, had no thought of danger. Suddenly, before all the bystanders, a knight from Brittany drew his sword in a hostile fashion and stabbed the count again and again . . . The count remained for a while in the kingdom, that his wounds might be cared for and his health restored.

We can only speculate as to exactly how these wounds were healed. It is presumed that the count would have been treated either by a Frankish settler or local practitioner as he was not participating in a crusade at the time of his injury. Albucasis recommended that injuries were cleaned and

[59] Raymond d'Aguilers 1968 p. 127.   [60] Albert of Aachen bk 10, ch. 57.
[61] Ortner 1997.   [62] William of Tyre 1986, II, pp. 654–5; William of Tyre 1943, II, p. 74.

either bandaged or sutured to bring the wound edges together[63] and both these techniques work well for an appropriate wound.[64] By this time the very limited surgical texts available to educated Frankish practitioners had at least been augmented by the Latin translation of al-Majusi at Antioch in 1127.[65] Other treatments such as modification of diet to promote healing, oral medicines and bloodletting were all likely possibilities in the following weeks.

Usama wrote a story in which a Muslim footsoldier attacked some Frankish troops hiding in a cave between Shaizar and al-Ruj.[66] As always, we have to be careful using this author, and certainly this example may well have been embellished for his audience.

Numayr now turned to the man with a sword, intent upon attacking him. But the Frank immediately struck him with the sword on the side of his face and cut through his eyebrow, eyelid, cheek, nose and upper lip, making the whole side of his face hang down upon his chest. Numayr went out of the cave to his companions who bandaged his wound and brought him back during a cold and rainy night. There his face was stitched up and his wound was treated until he was healed and returned to his former condition, with the exception of his eye which was lost for good.

Another very similar injury was described in a Muslim animal dealer who had been fighting the Franks and again a surgeon at Shaizar sewed up the wound to his face and it healed. The man then gained the nickname of 'the gashed one'.[67] While the descriptions of the face hanging downward might seem at first to be exaggerated,[68] the anatomy of much of the forehead, face and cheeks means that if a sufficiently large wound is made then the skin can easily be peeled away from the bones and deeper tissues.[69] If we interpret these tales as true events, these incidents show presumably local surgeons suturing wounds with apparent long-term success.[70] From a modern perspective it might be anticipated that suturing with non-sterile threads would lead to infection and wound breakdown, but this does not appear to have happened here.

It is probable that not everyone would have survived an amputation. The earliest statistics of survival following amputation come from the eighteenth and nineteenth centuries, before the use of antiseptics to kill bacteria. Survival varied greatly between surgeons, the part of the body removed and also on the indications for the treatment. Those with a clean injury appeared to

[63] Albucasis 1973 p. 526–42.   [64] Brunius, Zederfeldt and Ahren 1967.   [65] Burnett 2000.
[66] Usama ibn Munqidh 1929 pp. 106–7.   [67] Usama ibn Munqidh 1929 p. 193.
[68] Nicolle 1993.   [69] McMinn 1994 pp. 453–5.   [70] Hauben 1983.

do better than those who already had gangrene or an abscess. Mortality rates in Paris hospitals during the 1830s averaged 39 per cent for all amputations and rose to 62 per cent of those undergoing thigh amputation. We can only speculate on whether these figures can be compared to the pre-gunpowder Latin East. The time taken to perform an amputation was also an important factor to minimise the pain from the procedure. In the eighteenth and nineteenth centuries it was standard to take less than a minute to remove the unwanted part of the limb and no more than three or four minutes more to stop the bleeding and complete the procedure.[71] The method of amputation described by the eleventh-century author Albucasis[72] is a reasonable example, as by the mid-twelfth century the manuscripts were popular both in the Islamic world and also in Europe. He advised first placing the limb on a block of wood. Ligatures were to be tied round the limb above and below the site of amputation to keep the soft tissues out of the way once they were cut through with the scalpel. After the haemorrhage from the blood vessels was dealt with, the surgeon had to saw through the bone sufficiently high up the leg to ensure that only healthy bone remained. The stump was then bandaged until healed, presuming the patient lived that long. Another time for undergoing amputation was in the course of battle. In May 1191 the forces of King Richard I of England attacked a Muslim supply ship which was sailing to the relief of Acre. The descriptions of the location of wounds corresponds well with the archaeological evidence outlined earlier, such as the battle of Visby.[73] The *Itinerarium Peregrinorum et Gesta Regis Ricardi* recorded how 'the Turks gained boldness from despair and tried with all their strength to resist the attacking sailors, cutting off here a foot, there a hand and even a great many heads'.[74]

Marquis Conrad of Montferrat was assassinated by the Exchange in the city of Tyre on 28 April 1192. Although there were many rumours as to who was responsible, the most likely appears to have been the Islamic Assassin sect.

He had reached the toll-house when two young Assassins, unencumbered by cloaks, rushed up to him at great speed, stretched out the two long knives which they held in their hands and stabbed him this way and that in the stomach, mortally wounding him, before running off at full speed. The marquis at once fell dying from his horse . . . The marquis was already drawing his last breath. Surrounding him, his entourage lifted him gently in their arms and carried him to the palace . . . Then almost at once he died and he was buried at the Hospital.[75]

---

[71] Wangensteen 1967. [72] Albucasis 1973 pp. 562–8. [73] Ingelmark 1939–40.
[74] Richard de Templo 1864 p. 208; Richard de Templo 1997 p. 198.
[75] Richard de Templo 1864 p. 340; Richard de Templo 1997 pp. 306–7.

The marquis appears to have died too quickly for infection from his damaged bowel to have led to peritonitis. A swift death like this from a penetrating injury to the abdomen is most likely to have been caused by uncontrollable blood loss from damaged blood vessels or an organ such as the liver or spleen. The laws of the kingdom of Jerusalem specifically cover the problem of assassination or murder by stabbing. In the *Assises de la Haute Cour* it is stated that the total number of people charged with the murder could not exceed the number of stab wounds.[76] A further refinement of this concept can be seen in the laws of Bologna from 1265, where the total number charged could not exceed the number of stab wounds in fatal parts of the body, as opposed to superficial wounds in less important areas.[77] In some countries or time periods it was doctors who had to assess deceased stab victims[78] but in the kingdom of Jerusalem it could be any free man, and no medical training was required.

At the battle of Mansourah in February 1250 in Egypt, Lord John of Joinville describes[79] some of the facial wounds his comrades received.

There my Lord Hugh of Ecot was wounded by three lance thrusts in the face, my Lord Raoul too . . . My Lord Erard of Siverey was struck by a sword across the face, so that his nose fell over his lip . . . he died of that wound.

After capture by the Egyptian forces in April 1250, John of Joinville[80] tells us,

Lord Raoul of Wanou, who was in my party, had all the muscles at the back of the knees cut through in the battle of Shrove Tuesday and was unable to stand on his feet; and I should tell you that an old Saracen knight, who was in the galley, used to carry him to the latrine hanging from his neck.

Prince Edward of England was in Acre during 1272, where he was attacked by one of the Assassin sect.[81] From the Continuation of Matthew Paris[82] we hear,

the Assassin wounded him twice in the arm and a third time under the armpit. Edward at once hurled the Assassin to the earth with his foot and, wrenching the knife from his hands, slew the villain with it. In wrestling away the knife, however, he wounded himself severely in the hand and as the poison entered and spread in the wounds, they were only cured with great difficulty and by the application of many and various remedies.

---

[76] Kirsch 1969; *Assizes of Cyprus* 2002 p. 199.   [77] Simili 1973.   [78] Amundsen 1979; Simili 1973.
[79] John of Joinville 1874 pp. 122–4: John of Joinville 1955 p. 80.
[80] John of Joinville 1874 p. 176; John of Joinville 1955 p. 105.
[81] *Chronique de Primat* 1894 p. 84; Hayton 1906 p. 228.   [82] Matthew Paris [Giles] 1854, III, p. 379.

The local Chronicle of the Templar of Tyre[83] added that the 'lords assembled and summoned all the doctors and assistants, who sucked the wound and drew out the poison'. It cannot be known for sure if a poison was used on the knife as there is no mention of the symptoms which resulted from it. However, poisons thought to have been in use for arrows and knives in medieval Europe and the Middle East[84] include plant extracts from the white hellebore (*Veratrum album*) and possibly aconitum (*Ranunculaceae sp.*) and henbane (*Hyoscamus niger*). Evidence for the use of aconitum as a poison in the Byzantine period can be found in the case of Emperor John I Tzimisces (ruled 969–976), who appears to have been poisoned by a disgruntled eunuch.[85]

PENETRATING ARROW AND LANCE INJURIES

Both these weapons have effectively the same function, being a wooden shaft with a sharp metal point which could penetrate certain types of armour and pass deep into the body. The tips of some had barbs which made their removal difficult, while others were without barbs. The absence of barbs made the penetration of armour easier and, in the case of the lance, enabled the horseman to use the weapon repeatedly. While the obvious differences between the two are the larger scale of the lance and the fact that the arrow could be used from a distance while the lance was hand held, the injuries caused by both of these weapons would have been similar. They caused a deep, penetrating injury while leaving only a small wound in the skin. As a result it would have been difficult for a surgeon to explore the wound to assess the degree of internal damage without enlarging the wound and perhaps worsening it. If the arrow could not easily be pulled out the way it went in, medical texts recommended pushing it right through so it came out the other side,[86] taking care to cause as little damage as possible to the uninjured tissues. If barbs prevented its immediate removal an alternative approach was to wait a few days for the tissues around the arrow to putrefy and soften, so enabling the arrow to be pulled out. Another potential problem was that it could be very difficult to remove the injured man's armour as the weapon would have effectively nailed it to his body. Sometimes ingenious contraptions were used to remove projectiles such as

---

[83] Templar of Tyre 2000 p. 140.   [84] Bisset 1989.   [85] Lascaratos and Marketos 1998.
[86] Theodorich Borgognoni 1498 p. 112v; Theodorich Borgognoni 1955, I, p. 85.

the crossbow bolt or arrow,[87] including sliding tubes[88] or even a crossbow itself in a supposed case from thirteenth-century Spain.[89] Modern research on arrow wounds has shown that the probability that a particular arrow would cause death was dependent on the type of bow used, the velocity of flight, the design of arrowhead and the part of the body injured.[90] In view of the similarities between the injuries resulting from weapons and lances they are dealt with together here.

On the First Crusade the knight Walter the Penniless was killed in battle near Nicaea in Asia Minor, fighting against Kilij-Arslan, the sultan of Rum. Apparently seven arrows penetrated the metal rings of his hauberk to enter his chest before he died.[91] Many similar examples of arrows piercing the mesh of the hauberk can be found in crusader texts.[92] In the siege of Nicaea itself Baldwin of Ghent died from an arrow through his skull.[93] Presumably a knight of such standing would have been well armed and have a helmet, which would have had to have been pierced by the arrow. Examples such as these go to show how effective a weapon the arrow was as that time. In the siege of Arsuf in 1101 a Christian hostage named Gerard of Avenses was tied to a makeshift cross and set up on the town walls. However, the Frankish army continued to attack with the result that he was inadvertently hit by a number of arrows from the Christians (Albert of Aachen says ten). It was presumed that he had died and he was given up for dead when the siege was unsuccessful and the army left. However, when peace was later made between the Christians and those of Arsuf, Gerard was returned to Jerusalem, 'cured of all his wounds'.[94] It is possible that the arrow wounds were not severe and that he managed to survive them despite languishing in a dungeon. However, if he really was hit by ten arrows when wearing no armour, it would be surprising if he survived. It may be that his wounds were treated by a surgeon in the town so that he could be used for future bargaining or ransom.

The problem of multiple arrow wounds is mentioned in many chronicles and seemed to have been an occupational hazard in large battles. King Richard the Lionheart took part in the fighting around Jaffa in August 1192 while on the Third Crusade. Ambroise[95] tells us how 'his body, his horse, his trappings all were so covered in arrows which the swarthy folk had

[87] Lang 1992; Salazar 1998; Theodorich Borgognoni 1498 p. 112v; Theodorich Borgognoni 1955, I, pp. 85–7.

[88] Paterson 1988.   [89] Burns 1972.   [90] Karger, Sudhues, Kneubuehl and Brinkmann, 1998.

[91] Albert of Aachen bk 1, ch. 21.

[92] Albert of Aachen bk 3, ch. 33; John of Joinville 1874 p. 132; John of Joinville 1955 p. 84.

[93] Albert of Aachen bk 2, ch. 29.   [94] Albert of Aachen bk 7, ch. 2 and 15.

[95] Ambroise 1897 p. 311; Ambroise 1939 p. 151.

rivalled at shooting at him that he resembled a hedgehog'. Not surprisingly he was not in the best of health after the battle and 'King Richard fell ill from the exhaustion of the battle and the stink of the corpses'. He decided that 'he would return to Acre to take medicines and get well'.[96] Lord John of Joinville was injured in the battle of Mansourah in Egypt in 1250[97] when he was

covered with the arrows that missed the men-at-arms. Fortunately I found a Saracen's padded jerkin stuffed with wadding. I turned the open side towards me and made a shield of the jerkin. It served me well for I was wounded by the arrows in only five places, while my horse was in fifteen.

Later that evening[98] we hear,

when I was in bed, where I badly needed to rest the wounds I received during the day, I got no such repose. Before it was properly light there was a shout in our camp, 'to arms, to arms!' . . . I sent to the king for help as neither I nor my knights were able to put on hauberks because of our wounds.

It sounds as if the five arrows had been removed as only the wounds are mentioned at that point.

The possible use of poison on the tips of arrows is demonstrated in this interesting case. Emperor John II of Byzantium was hunting in the Meadow of Mantles near Anavarza, Cilicia, in April 1143. William of Tyre[99] recorded events thus:

suddenly a wild boar which had been started up by the dogs, infuriated by their shrill insistent barking, rushed past the hiding place of the emperor. With marvellous swiftness he seized an arrow but he carelessly stretched the bow too far and wounded himself in the hand with the point of the poisoned arrow. Thus, from so trivial a cause, he received the summons of death. The pain of the wound soon compelled him to leave the woods and return to camp. Physicians were summoned in numbers. He explained the accident to them and did not hesitate to say that he had caused his own death. Full of solicitude for their lord's safety, they applied remedies but the fatal poison had already permeated his system. The means taken did not avail and the venom continued to creep still further to the internal parts, thus effectively preventing all hope of recovery. He was advised that there was only one course of action which might save his life; the injured hand, in which yet all the potent evil was concentrated, might be removed before the poison infected the rest of his body. But the emperor, a man of lofty spirit, although suffering intense agony and

---

[96] Richard de Templo 1864 p. 427; Richard de Templo 1997 p. 370.
[97] John of Joinville 1874 p. 132; John of Joinville 1955 p. 84.
[98] John of Joinville 1874 p. 140; John of Joinville 1955 p. 88.
[99] William of Tyre 1986, II, p. 704; William of Tyre 1943, II, p. 127.

convinced that death was imminent, still steadfastly preserved his imperial majesty and rejected the advice.

The use of arrow poison to increase the effectiveness of the weapon has been employed for thousands of years.[100] Written texts from ancient Greece, the Middle East, India and China all mention it. By the medieval period arrow poison was mainly restricted to hunting animals, although there were laws regarding its use in attempted murder. While several Byzantine chronicles also blame poison on the arrow head, an alternative hypothesis has been proposed for John's death. It is possible that the wound became infected either by bacteria from a dirty arrow head or organisms normally present on the skin.[101] This is because some accounts of the story suggest that he lived for over a week, while most poisons would have killed him much faster.

There are less controversial examples of death following gangrene from an arrow wound. A possible twelfth-century case was that of Shihab-al-Din, who according to Usama was a Muslim from Shaizar. If we believe Usama, Shihab-al-Din was hit by a Frankish arrow in an engagement at the ruined castle of Afamiyah.[102] The arrow hit him in the lower arm and after the skirmish it was removed and bandages applied. However, three days later his arm turned black, he became unconscious and then died. Whether or not we can trust Usama's stories, this description is classic for gangrene. This is a process where bacteria contaminate the wound, spread rapidly through the tissues and can kill in a few days. It is thought that a significant proportion of battle wounds might have developed gangrene in the medieval period. Another potential complication from a penetrating arrow wound is osteomyelitis. In this case infection is in the bone rather than the soft tissues, as is the case with gangrene. A legendary example is that of Robert, duke of Normandy, who was said to have been wounded in the arm by an arrow on the First Crusade. Even though the arrow was removed a sinus developed and the legend states that he went to the doctors at Salerno for treatment.[103] As with most legends there may be an element of truth to the story. Penetrating wounds may lead to a chronic infection in bone if bacteria are introduced into the bone marrow at the time of the injury. This osteomyelitis will lead to chronic discharge of pus via a sinus to the skin and such a problem was described in the legend. Even if this particular example may have been just a story, it is likely to reflect the diseases common at the time.

[100] Bisset 1989.　　[101] Lascaratos and Voros 1998.　　[102] Usama ibn Munqidh 1929 pp. 75–6.
[103] Capparoni 1923 p. 13.

Detail on the impressive penetrating power of the lance can be found in a number of chronicles. On 14 August 1119 Usama fought his first battle with the Franks, and he described attacking a certain knight.[104] If this story from the master of tales can be believed literally,

all of a sudden I saw him spur his horse and as the horse began to wave its tail I knew it was already exhausted. So I rushed on the horseman and struck him with my lance, which pierced him through and projected about a cubit [50 cm] in front of him . . . A few days later a messenger came to summon me before my uncle at a time in which it was not his custom to call me. So I hurried to him and saw that a Frank was in there. My uncle said to me, 'Here is a knight who has come from Afamiyah to see the horseman who struck Philip the knight, for the Franks have all been astounded on account of that blow which pierced two layers of links in the knight's mail hauberk and yet did not kill him.' 'How', I said, 'could he have survived?' The Frankish knight replied, 'The thrust fell upon the skin of his waist.'

It seems that Philip the knight must have been rather overweight so that the lance went through the fat on his waist but did not enter the abdominal cavity. Another vivid demonstration of the penetrating power of the lance comes from the Seventh Crusade to Egypt. Lord Jean de Joinville tells us of a wound at the battle of Mansourah[105] to 'Lord Frederick of Loupey by a lance between the shoulders; the wound was so large that the blood poured out of his body as though from the bung of a cask'. It sounds as though the thoracic aorta was severed by the injury. Clearly with a hole in the largest artery of the body he would not have lived long enough to receive the attention of a surgeon.

The vulnerable areas of a horseman attacked by an infantryman with a spear are highlighted in this passage by Usama.[106] If we can believe this story, a brigand named Zammarrakal infiltrated the camp of the Franks from Antioch to steal what he could during a raid on Shaizar around 1122. After taking a horse, shield and lance he was confronted by a footman. 'As I was making my way out from among their troops a footman pursued me and thrust his lance through my thigh.' He apparently told this story to Usama while sitting on a rock with dried blood covering his leg and foot. The thighs of a man on horseback were closest to the footman, which made an attack on them relatively easy, while it was hard for the rider to protect the legs with a shield which mainly covered the trunk.

The problems facing the doctor attempting to treat a lance injury are shown in the next two passages, which both refer to the same individual and

[104] Usama ibn Munqidh 1929 pp. 68–9.
[105] John of Joinville 1874 p. 124; John of Joinville 1955 p. 80.
[106] Usama ibn Munqidh 1929 pp. 71–2.

may be referring to the same incident. In 1103 King Baldwin I was hunting animals near Caesarea but was ambushed by some Saracen soldiers. While the king's party had swords and hunting bows with them, they were not expecting trouble and were not wearing any body armour nor carrying shields. Albert of Aachen[107] tells us how the king

> was pierced through the thigh and kidneys by the furtive lance of a Saracen hanger-on who was lurking among the branches and thick leaves. At once streams of blood gushed ominously from so cruel a wound of so powerful a king, his face began to grow pale, his spirit and strength to falter, his hand to cease from fighting with his sword, until at length he fell from his horse to the ground as if dead and destroyed, and he was believed to have expired . . . they placed him on a stretcher and took him back to Jerusalem amidst a very great weeping and lamentation of men and women, acquiring very experienced doctors for him, by whose skill and experience their king and strong champion could recover his health after this lethal wound.

The claim that the lance pierced his thigh and abdomen in the region of the kidneys suggests that weapon was used at an angle, pointing either upwards or downwards. If the attack was from a footman then it would be expected that the lance would have been aimed upwards, passing through the thigh and then entering the abdomen. If the attack was from another horseman or from someone hiding in the branches of one of the trees then the lance could have been aimed downwards, so that it passed through the abdomen first and then entered the thigh. In any case, the symptoms which followed suggested that Baldwin lost a significant amount of blood from the injury. He went pale and fell from his horse, which would be expected in significant blood loss as the brain fails to get enough blood, which leads to dizziness and fainting. The suggestion that the king lost consciousness is supported by the information that his companions thought he had died. It would normally take blood loss of about two litres before a fit adult male would lose consciousness from hypovolaemic shock.[108] To lose this much blood so rapidly Baldwin must have suffered a laceration to an artery, large vein or vascular organ such as the liver or spleen. Albert says that the injury was at the site of the kidney but does not specify which side. The liver lies adjacent to the right kidney while the spleen is adjacent to the left kidney and either organ could easily have been damaged.

Interestingly Baldwin survived the trip to Jerusalem so his body must have formed a blood clot at the site of the laceration to the blood vessel,

---

[107] Albert of Aachen bk 9, chs. 21–2.   [108] Committee on Trauma 1994 pp. 80–2.

preventing the loss of a fatal amount of blood. Doctors of a standard to work for a king should have known the basics of anatomy. Although they did not know how the organs worked they would have known that the heart and lungs lay in the chest[109] and that the kidneys were a few centimetres below the lungs, on the back of the abdominal wall below the diaphragm.[110] The anatomy of the kidneys was described in some detail in the works of Galen[111] and al-Majusi,[112] even subtle details such as the right kidney being slightly higher than the left being noted. It is unfortunate that the account does not specify whether these 'experienced doctors' were Europeans who stayed on after the First Crusade or indigenous practitioners.

The incident described by Albert of Aachen may well have been the same injury recounted in the chronicle of Guibert of Nogent.[113] It highlights the difficulties in treating penetrating wounds as the size of the skin wound would usually be far too small to determine exactly which organs had been injured.

He suffered a similarly severe wound in battle, in the course of saving one of his footsoldiers who had supported him bravely. Foresight led the doctor whom he summoned to resist covering the wound with medicinal poultices because he knew that the wound was very deep and while the skin could be made smooth the wound would fester deep within his body. He proposed to conduct a remarkable experiment. He asked the king to order one of the Saracens whom they held prisoner to be wounded in the same place and in the same manner as Baldwin himself had been (for it was forbidden from him to ask for a Christian) and to have him killed thereafter so that he might look more freely into the corpse and determine from the inspection something about the king's own internal wounds. The prince's piety recoiled in horror at this suggestion and he recalled the example of ancient Constantine, declaring that he would not be the cause of death of any man, however insignificant, for such insignificant salvation, when it is ever doubtful. The doctor then said to him, 'if you have decided that no man's life can be spent on your own well being then at least give the order to bring forward a bear, an animal useless except for show, and have it hung up by its front paws, then struck with an iron blade so that I may examine its entrails and I shall be able to measure how far it went in and therefore determine the depth of your own wound.' The king answered him, 'the beast will be brought immediately since it is necessary: consider it a done deed'. Then when the doctor had finished his experiment at the animal's expense he found as we mentioned above, that harm could come to the king if the wound were quickly covered unless the pus was removed and the interior part of the wound would heal.

---

[109] French 1978.   [110] Derenne, Debru, Grassin and Whitelaw 1994.
[111] Scarborough 1976b.   [112] Eknoyan 1994.
[113] Guibert of Nogent 1996 p. 287; Guibert of Nogent 1997 p. 134.

There are a number of unexpected points included in this story. First, it is interesting that Guibert, a Benedictine abbot writing in 1106–9, appears knowledgeable about the problem of pus in wounds. It is not clear whether this was from reading medical texts or perhaps experience in the monastic infirmary. Pus is suggestive of infection and from a modern viewpoint a penetrating wound to the abdomen with a deep collection of pus is likely to lead to chronic fevers, sepsis and potentially death from peritonitis. Guibert and others of his era clearly did not understand the concept of infection as we do but still regularly saw pus in wounds and interpreted this in a way compatible with their own view of disease. Pus was typically thought of as formed from humours altered by putrefaction in the wound.[114] Medieval medical texts varied in their opinion as to whether the formation of pus in the first place was a good ('laudable') or bad thing.[115] However, everyone agreed that once formed it was better out than in and many believed that good pus might clean the wound as it flowed out. The other interesting component of this account is the use of autopsy by European practitioners at such an early date.[116] The initial request was to perform autopsy on a captured prisoner and this was at a time when anatomical dissection does not appear to have been performed in Europe, even on the excommunicated or criminals.[117] The king declined and the alternative was to dissect a bear, one of the animals used by Galen in his own dissections.[118] It is possible that this animal was chosen as it could stand on two legs and therefore perhaps provide a more accurate model for a human wound than dissection of a pig, which was the standard animal in the European anatomical dissection texts of the time.[119]

There does not appear to be any evidence for autopsy in Europe this early, and even human dissection for the purpose of teaching human anatomy is not known at this time in Europe.[120] However, the European evidence for dissection of animals at this early date appears to originate in Italy, especially around Salerno. In consequence, one possibility is that the medical practitioner looking after the king had trained at Salerno and was attempting to make a medical advance by moving on from dissecting animals to humans. However, if it is argued that the choice of a human or a bear would be too novel for a European, then another alternative is that the practitioner was a Byzantine Christian accompanying the king. This should be considered since Galen's texts describing the dissection of bears along with other animals would have been available in the Byzantine world, while they are

---

[114] Theodorich Borgognoni 1498 p. 108r; Theodorich Borgognoni 1955, I, p. 31.
[115] Cope 1958.   [116] Hiestand 1988.   [117] Persaud 1984 pp. 77–88.
[118] Savage-Smith 1971a.   [119] Corner 1927; O'Neill 1970.   [120] Park 1995.

not thought to have been known in Europe at that time. Autopsy was known at exactly this time in Constantinople. A contingent of Scandinavian crusaders under Sigurd Jorsalfar became ill at Constantinople in 1110. Autopsy apparently found that their livers were swollen, and the remaining crusaders were forbidden to drink Greek wine.[121]

HEAD INJURIES

The head was a popular part of the body for an attacker to focus his blows. Examples of fatal and non-fatal blows to the head have been recovered from the Frankish castle of Jacob's Ford, as described earlier. Since the effects and treatment of cranial injuries were similar regardless of the type of weapon used, they are worth discussing as a separate group. Textual evidence for injuries to the head includes those sustained in personal combat from blows with the sword or mace and also from projectiles such as the arrow or rock from a siege engine.[122] The use of a helmet certainly gave some protection but did not completely prevent serious head injury. Penetrating head injuries in the Crimean war and American Civil War were associated with a mortality rate of over 70 per cent.[123] This helps to explain the advice to surgeons found in medieval medical texts recommending caution before agreeing to take on the care of a patient with a head wound.

It was clear that from the start of the crusades those without medical training were aware that some head wounds were treatable while others were incurable. Albert of Aachen[124] wrote of the injury sustained by a knight named Franco, from the town of Maasmechelen in Belgium, once the crusaders had taken the city of Antioch but not the citadel. Soldiers from the besieging Muslim army of Kerbogha injured Franco on the head during an attack on a tower. It was described as a 'very severe and scarcely curable wound', which does suggest awareness that some head wounds were curable while others were fatal whatever was done. This point is borne out in contemporary medical texts from both Europe and the Middle East.[125]

A large number of cases are described in the sources where head wounds resulted in death. There are examples where rocks from a siege engine caused fracture of the skull, and due to the high energy transfer from such wounds the outcome was usually fatal. In the siege of 'Arqah in the First Crusade, Anselm of Ribemont was killed when a rock from the citadel hit his skull.[126] Sword blows were also frequent directed at the head and a firm

---

[121] Hiestand 1989.   [122] Hill 1998.   [123] Rose 1997.   [124] Albert of Aachen bk 4, ch. 35.
[125] Rose 1997.   [126] Albert of Aachen bk 5, ch. 31.

strike with a sharp sword could even cut right through a well-made helmet. The infamous battle of the Field of Blood took place between Antioch and Aleppo in 1119 and the end of battle was brought about by the death of Roger of Salerno, the prince of Antioch, through a blow to the head. Walter the Chancellor was an eye witness present at the battle and mentions the way Roger was killed.[127] Apparently, 'He was struck by a knight's sword through the middle of his nose right into his brain.' Such serious damage to the brain would have caused death instantly.

King Fulk of Jerusalem took part in an ill-fated hunting trip in November 1143, near Acre. William of Tyre[128] tells us,

as they were riding along, the servants who had preceded the train happened to rouse a hare which was lying in a furrow. It fled, followed by the shouts of all. The king, impelled by evil fate, seized his lance and joined the pursuit. In vigorous chase, he began to urge on his horse in that direction. Finally, the steed, driven to reckless speed, stumbled and fell. The king was thrown head foremost to the ground. As he lay there stunned by the pain of the fall, the saddle struck his head and his brains gushed forth from both ears and nostrils. The members of his escort, those in advance and those following him, overcome with horror at the frightful accident, rushed to his aid as he lay on the ground. They found him unconscious, however, unable to speak or understand . . . Tearfully they bore him back to the city, where he lived until the third day, unconscious but still breathing.

The description of material discharging from the nose and ears suggests that the base of the skull was fractured, as this allows cerebrospinal fluid and blood to leak out at these sites. Contemporary medical texts showed awareness that it often took about three days for someone to die after an open skull fracture, if not killed instantly. From a modern perspective it appears that they were referring to the effects of infection. Theodorich wrote one hundred years after this incident,

and most particularly of all, one must be careful that everyone having a wound on the head (especially if there is suspicion of internal injury) keep it from every pollution, because if care is not exercised in head wounds spasm will occur very quickly and when this has happened, according to most evidence, he will die a most bitter death on the third day.[129]

John of Joinville described a case[130] in June 1249 at Damietta in Egypt.

It was that day that my Lord Walter of Autrèche armed himself at all points in his tent and, mounting his horse, with his shield round his neck and his helmet

---

[127] Walter the Chancellor 1896 p. 88; Walter the Chancellor 1999 p. 127.
[128] William of Tyre 1986, II, p. 710; William of Tyre, 1943, II, p. 134.
[129] Theodorich Borgognoni 1498 p. 113v; Theodorich Borgognoni 1955, I, p. 95.
[130] John of Joinville 1874 p. 96; John of Joinville 1955 p. 67.

on his head, ordered the flaps of his tent to be lifted and he spurred his horse towards the Turks. As he rode alone out of his tent, all his people raised a loud cry of 'Chatillon!' But it happened that before he reached the Turks he fell and the horse galloped over his body. The horse, whose housing bore his arms, went over to the enemy; for the greater part of the Saracens were mounted on mares which attracted it to their ranks. Those who saw what happened told us that four Turks attacked Lord Walter as he lay on the ground and as they passed by him they gave him great blows with their maces. The Constable of France, with some of the king's men-at-arms, rescued him and they carried him back to his tent in their arms. When he was brought in he was speechless; some of the physicians and surgeons in the camp came to him and as he did not seem to be in danger of death they bled him in both arms. Very late that evening my Lord Aubert of Narcy told me that we ought to go and see him because we had not yet done so and he was a very brave man and had a fine name. As we went into his tent, his chamberlain met us and asked us to walk gently so as not to wake his master. We found him lying on some rugs of ermine; we went quietly up to him and saw that he was dead.

While Lord Walter clearly received a number of injuries both from his horse and also the mace blows, the description that he was speechless but still conscious suggests that he sustained a significant head injury. Whether his death later that day was from internal bleeding in his abdomen or chest, or whether it was due to cerebral contusions and intracranial haemorrhage, it is not possible to tell.

While many of the serious head wounds described were fatal, there are occasional examples when the wound was survived but left a residual neurological deficit. The Muslim warlord al-Ghazi of Aleppo received a head wound in battle against the combined Christian forces of King David II of Georgia and some Frankish troops in 1121. It took a long time for him to recover and a year later, in 1122, he was still not back to health and was known to be 'afflicted by a kind of paralytic illness'.[131] A possible explanation is that the head injury he sustained in the battle with King David caused damage to the brain which left a long-term neurological deficit. While the functions of the brain are very complex and clearly baffled doctors in the past, doctors did have some appreciation that different areas performed different functions and that injuries to one side of the head might lead to weakness on the other side of the body.[132] The parts of the brain which control movement in the body (the precentral gyri) are located on its surface, just beneath the skull, on the left and right sides of the head.[133] Archaeological research has shown the area of the left precentral gyrus, which controls motor function to the right side of the body, to be the

[131] Walter the Chancellor 1896 p. 114; Walter the Chancellor 1999 p. 171.
[132] Lokhorst 1982.   [133] Fitzgerald 1985 p. 140.

most common site for weapon injuries to the head in the medieval period. In consequence it is not unreasonable to suggest that his head injury could have been responsible for the paralysis noted in the chronicles.

Details of the actual treatment given for a head injury are not found in these sources. However, an indication on how a doctor of the time might have treated al-Ghazi or a crusader who survived the initial injury may be found in the medical texts, where there is broad agreement on management.[134] It is difficult to determine quite how interventionist the surgeons would have been when considering which treatment options to employ, but archaeological evidence for all the approaches described in the medical texts has been found in excavated remains from medieval Europe, as discussed previously. The first decision was whether to take on the care of the patient in the first place. Signs of a poor prognosis included loss of consciousness, seizures, vomiting, fever, discharging pus and inability to speak (note the information on Lord Walter of Autrèche). If none of these were present an assessment was required to see if a fracture had been sustained, or if the injury had just resulted in bruising to the scalp and perhaps concussion. The simplest techniques described involved cleaning the wound and then determining if a fracture of the skull had occurred. Non-invasive tests for a skull vault fracture included palpation of the scalp for any indentations or protruding bone and plucking a taut string with one end held in the teeth as the pitch was believed to be effected by a skull fracture. To detect a base of skull fracture, one option if the patient was conscious was to perform a Valsalva manoeuvre. In this test, attempting to exhale against a closed nose and mouth increases pressure in the airways. This might force air out of any fractures of the skull vault if free air had escaped from the air passages through the skull base fracture. While this test would never be attempted now the phenomenon is occasionally observed in patients, and it does sound a very practical test. A more invasive method was to feel for any fractures with a probe or to cut the scalp with a knife to allow good access and then pour ink into the wound, which would highlight any fractures as dark lines.

Once a fracture was discovered it was the doctor's duty to explore it and remove any sharp bone fragments that might be protruding into the brain and so causing serious damage. This is specifically mentioned in the thirteenth-century legal code of the kingdom of Jerusalem, as described in the *Livre des Assises de la Cour des Bourgeois* (see ch. 8). The passage states

---

[134] Paulus Aegineta 1846, II, p. 430–2; Theodorich Borgognoni 1955, I, pp. 106–24; Hunt 1992 pp. 3–15; Albucasis 1973 pp. 698–710.

that, 'If my servant has a head wound with the bone broken and he doesn't know how to remove the pieces, so that the broken bone pierces the brain so that he dies, reason adjudges that he is legally bound to pay for the servant.' If the injured individual was a free man then the punishment was for the surgeon to be hanged.[135] Similarly the surgeon was obliged to visit the patient daily, as failure to do so was regarded as negligence if the patient subsequently died. The point that this specific law was included among the limited examples of medical negligence in that bill suggests that previous cases may have come to court in the kingdom, and is strongly suggestive that this technique recommended in medical texts was probably employed there. The scalp was shaved and a cross-shaped incision made in the scalp to ensure a clear view of the injury. Depressed or fragmented areas of bone were freed with mallet and chisels, and removed with fingers or forceps. Some texts describe the use of 'non-sinking drills', which had a collar that prevented the drill plunging into the brain once it had penetrated the skull vault.[136] These drills may have been useful in the removal of problematic bone fragments. Rough bone edges were then smoothed off with a rasp, the scalp replaced and the wound dressed with bandages soaked in oil of roses or wine. A comparable example of such cranial surgery is the case of Juan del Frago, who in 1330 had eighteen pieces of broken bone removed by a surgeon in Aragon after an assault, and survived to accuse his attacker.[137] Another case of cranial surgery from early thirteenth-century France was recorded by a medical student watching the operation at the hospital of the Holy Spirit in Montpellier.[138] It does appear that similar operations for skull fractures were taking place in the Latin East too.

CRUSH INJURIES

A crush injury is one in which a blunt force is applied to a part of the body resulting in the crushing of the tissues. This contrasts with sharp injuries from a sword or arrow in a number of ways. The area of tissue damage may be much larger in a crush injury so that it can take a long time to heal. If large areas of muscle are damaged this can lead to renal failure when chemicals from the muscle are released into the blood and damage the kidneys, a process termed rhabdomyolysis. If the damage is severe enough the individual can die. Moreover, it is often difficult to tell early on how much damage has been done, as the tissue may appear intact on initial

---

[135] *Assises de Jerusalem* 1839 p. 258; *Assizes of Cyprus* 2002 p. 181.
[136] Albucasis 1973 pp. 698–710.   [137] McVaugh 1993 p. 160.   [138] Demaitre 1975.

inspection. It is only with time that the damaged tissues swell and become bruised or the patient becomes seriously ill from internal bleeding if an abdominal organ is ruptured, so that the true degree of damage becomes clear. If a limb is crushed then perhaps the most serious complication which may follow is compartment syndrome. This is discussed in more detail in ch. 4.

There are many examples of crush injuries sustained by crusaders either when travelling to the eastern Mediterranean, in battle or on account of natural disasters which intermittently occurred in the Latin East. The overland journey to Jerusalem was notoriously difficult and perhaps the most dangerous section was the mountainous passes in Asia Minor and near Antioch. Near Laodicea (Latakiya) the route of the Second Crusade in 1148 became extremely hazardous. The eye witness Odo of Deuil[139] recounts rather poetically how,

the mountain was steep and rocky and we had to climb along a ridge so lofty that its summit seemed to touch heaven and the stream in the hollow valley below to descend into hell. Here the throng became congested while ascending, pushed forward then crowded closely together, stopped and, taking no thought for the cavalry, clung there instead of going ahead. Sumpter horses slipped from the steep cliffs hurling those whom they struck into the depths of the chasm. Dislodged rocks also caused destruction. Thus when the men had scattered far and wide in order to seek out paths, all feared that they would misstep or that others, in falling, would strike them violently.

Sustaining injuries after falling from a height was not restricted to those on rocky mountain paths. Henry of Champagne, king of Jerusalem, fell from an upper-floor balcony of a building in Acre in 1197. It seems he broke his neck in the fall and died.[140] Sieges were understandably dangerous places to be and there are many accounts of crush injuries during siege warfare. Albert of Aachen noted that at the siege of Nicaea in 1097 on the First Crusade the knight Baldwin Calderun died when his neck was broken by a rock thrown from the walls.[141] Raymond of Aguilers[142] recorded how in November 1098, 'the besieged of Ma'arrat-an-Nu'man hurled stones from catapults, darts, fire, hives of bees and lime on our men who had sapped their walls'. On the Fourth Crusade to Constantinople there was a skirmish outside the city walls in 1203. Geoffrey of Villehardouin[143] recalls, 'in their

---

[139] Odo of Deuil 1948 pp. 116–17.
[140] Roger of Wendover 1886, I, p. 266; Roger of Wendover 1994, II, p. 164.
[141] Albert of Aachen bk 2, ch. 29.
[142] Raymond d'Aguilers 1969 p. 97; Raymond d'Aguilers 1968 p. 78.
[143] Geoffrey of Villehardouin 1938 p. 168; Geoffrey of Villehardouin 1963 p. 69.

pursuit of the Greeks they followed so close to the gate that men on the walls threw great heavy stones down on top of them . . . During this fight Guillaume de Champlitte's arm was broken by a stone.'

Once the armies had reached the flatter land by the coast the terrain posed less of a threat than the rowdy mob of crusaders. There are a number of versions in the chronicles explaining how Peter Bartholomew died in 1099. He claimed he had found the Holy Lance, which pierced Jesus's side after his crucifixion, in the floor of the church of St Peter in Antioch shortly after the crusaders had taken the city. Some believed his story while other thought he had made it all up. He agreed to undergo trial by ordeal which took place on 8 April 1099 at 'Arqah, when he had to walk between two rows of burning wood which apparently gave out such searing heat that no one could get close to it once it was lit. Those who did not believe Peter took his death after the ordeal as proof that he had been lying. Those who supported him said his survival of the ordeal in the short term proved his innocence and explained his later death as accidental crushing from the crowd. Certainly death from the crush in medieval crowds affected by religious fervour, especially in the proximity of relics, is well known.[144] Raymond of Aguilers,[145] who believed Peter, wrote,

As he emerged, Peter waved to the crowd, raised the lance and screamed out, 'God help us.' Whereupon the crowd seized him, seized him I say, and pulled him along the ground. Almost everyone from the mob pushed and shoved thinking Peter was nearby and hoping to touch him or snatch a piece of his clothing. The mob made three or four gashes on his legs in the tussle and cracked his backbone . . . After Peter's wounds were bound up, he rested.

He lasted until 20 April[146] when 'Peter Bartholomew, debilitated by illness resulting from his crushing blows and wounds . . . on the hour set by God, died peacefully'. Clearly he received some kind of medical care for his injuries, whether they were burns, lacerations or fractures, but there is no detail of who dressed his wounds.

Trial by ordeal was a common technique right across Europe from 800 to 1200.[147] It was used in cases from simple theft and sexual offences to murder and heresy. Ordeal was usually employed when no other mode of proof was available, such as witnesses. There were many variations in the type of ordeal used. Some involved holding the skin next to something that would normally burn it, as happened with Peter Bartholomew, and the individual was vindicated if no burn occurred. Usually candles, boiling

[144] Dickson 2000.   [145] Raymond d'Aguilers 1969 pp. 120–2; Raymond d'Aguilers 1968 p. 102.
[146] Raymond d'Aguilers 1969 pp. 128–9; Raymond d'Aguilers 1968 p. 108.   [147] Bartlett 1986.

water, hot iron, ploughshares or axe were used. Other versions of ordeal included trial by water, by the cross (where two contenders stood with their arms out like a cross and the first one to tire was deemed the wrongdoer) or by combat.

Trial by combat was described in the Frankish laws of the principality of Antioch as the method to determine guilt in cases of murder.[148] Usama wrote two interesting stories about about the Frankish use of ordeals to determine innocence and guilt. They are clearly included by him for their amusement value, but it is not so clear whether they are true events that were recorded for their comic aspects, or fabricated stories used to stereotype the Franks. One was a tale of trial by combat between two Franks in Nablus. It seems that one man was accused of acting as guide to a Muslim raid on a nearby Christian village and was made to fight the local blacksmith, both armed with a club and a shield. The blacksmith, used to wielding a hammer all day, beat the suspect to death and the body was then hung.[149] A further story about trial by water was described. Here the son of a Frankish father and local mother was suspected of murdering Franks when he had the chance, as he had become a Muslim. He was lowered on a rope into a barrel of water and since he floated he was convicted of his crime and blinded.[150] Blinding was sometimes preferred to capital punishment as it gave opportunity for later repentance and spiritual salvation.[151] Regardless of how literally we take these tales, they do confirm the use of trial by ordeal by the Franks or else Usama's Muslim audience would not have understood them. In the context of the legal evidence for such ordeals, the accounts may have some truth to them.

There are some examples that describe how large numbers of people were crushed to death when the mass of a crowd tried to enter a confined space. Typically it was those near the front who died as a result of pushing from the back of the crowd. When the crusaders stormed Jerusalem in July 1099 the army was so keen to enter the city through the few narrow open gates and sections of breached wall that some were crushed under the stampede.[152] Once in the city many locals tried to hide from the crusaders in the royal cistern, a large water storage facility filled from rain falling on nearby roofs. There were many openings in the vaulted roof which could be used as wells from above, but it was possible to fall down these. 'As many Christians as Saracens fell headlong in the flight and blind rush and were not only in danger of drowning but also died of broken necks and limbs or

[148] *Assises d'Antioch* 1876 p. 62. [149] Usama ibn Munqidh 1929 pp. 167–8.
[150] Usama ibn Munqidh 1929 pp. 168–9. [151] Bruce 1941. [152] Albert of Aachen bk 6, ch. 21.

ruptured entrails.' When Godfrey of Bouillon defeated the Egyptian army near Ascalon in Autumn 1099 many of the vanquished ran towards the city. There was not room for the thousands of people to get through the gates in such a hurry and many died in the crush.[153] In 1107 panic spread through Frankish forces near Jaffa who were planning to engage a larger force of Muslim troops from Ascalon. As they fled back to the city those on horseback apparently rode over and trampled many of the footsoldiers in their race to get to the gates before the pursuing Ascalonites cut them down.[154]

Sometimes it was an accident due to faulty crusader engineering that led to crush injuries. The method of undermining the walls of a besieged castle is described well at the siege of Nicaea in 1097. After constructing a protective covering they began:

hollowing out the earth under the foundations of the tower with mattocks and sharpest iron, until [the master of the siegework] could construct beams, posts and other enormous oak timbers in that same excavation under the foundation, on which the walls would be supported after the earth had been taken away so that they would not suddenly fall down on top of those still digging. Now once a great excavation had been made, both wide and long, on the instruction of the master-craftsman, everyone in the army, small and great, gathered twigs, stalks and sticks and dry reeds, pieces of tow and all sorts of kindling and heaped it between the posts and beams and the splendid timbers, everywhere where the excavation was occupied by these pieces of wood. After this, fire was put in by the master of the siegework, it was encouraged by a great breath until, roaring and racing in different directions, the unconquerable flame grew stronger and stronger and it reduced the posts, the beams and all the wood that had been put underneath to ashes. When these things had been reduced to embers and there was no prop for the foundations either of earth or of wood, the building of that very ancient tower fell flat in a moment in the middle of the night and it made such a noise that it was taken for a crash of thunder by all the people who were awoken from their sleep.[155]

The anonymous Syriac chronicle described the fate of Joscelyn of Edessa in 1131, when this technique did not go to plan. Joscelyn,

who was advancing in years but did not rest from fighting, gathered an army to destroy a castle named Tell 'Arran, between Aleppo and Mabbiy where dwelt robbers who wasted the country continually. He dug tunnels under it to make breaches in it, went down to see them for himself and a breach fell on him and buried him. When they dug him out he was at his last gasp so they carried him back to Tell Bashir, for his body was crushed and he was very ill.

---

[153] Albert of Aachen bk 6, ch. 49.   [154] Albert of Aachen bk 10, ch. 13.
[155] Albert of Aachen bk 2, ch. 36.

William of Tyre[156] adds, 'His people rescued him with much difficulty and he was found to be suffering from many fractures. For a long time he had been ill from his injuries.' Presumably his doctors would have been treating the fractures during his protracted recovery.

Battle was not the only time when crush injuries occurred and a terrifying cause of such injuries was the earthquake. The Frankish states lay on the Dead Sea transform fault system, which is a continuation of the Great African Rift.[157] Movement of the western Sinai tectonic plate relative to the eastern Arabian plate results in earthquakes in the eastern Mediterranean to this day. There is evidence for thirteen or fourteen earthquakes during the 200-year existence of the Frankish states and several more were felt in Frankish lands but did no damage as the epicentre was elsewhere.[158] As an eye witness Walter the Chancellor recorded in his chronicle,[159]

In the 1115th year from the incarnation of Our Lord Jesus Christ, on the eve of the feast of St Andrew the Apostle and in the silence of the dead of night, when human frailty was accustomed more suitably and more sweetly to sleep, there was an immense and terrible earthquake in Antioch and its region. And as a matter of fact, in that same unexpected earthquake men were horribly knocked around and they felt, saw and heard the collapse of walls, towers and different buildings deeply threatening to themselves and others; some thought to escape by running away, some to slide down the walls, certain men gave themselves up and threw themselves down from high houses. More, indeed, were caught piecemeal in their sleep by the collapse, in such a way that even if a part of the wall remained intact they were nowhere to be seen. Others indeed were terrified; they abandoned their homes, scorned their wealth, left everything and behaved as if demented in the streets and squares of the town. They stretched out their hands towards the heavens because of their manifold fear and powerlessness and cried tearfully without ceasing in different languages, 'Spare us, Lord, spare your people'.

Another serious earthquake which caused many crush injuries occured in the year 1170:[160]

In June of the following summer, that is in the seventh year of King Amaury, a great and terrible earthquake, more violent than any other within the memory of men now living, occurred in the orient. Strongly fortified cities dating from very early times were completely demolished. The inhabitants, caught in the ruins of their homes, were crushed to death and only a few survived. Not a spot in the entire country was left untouched by loss of property and domestic tragedy.

---

[156] William of Tyre 1986, II, p. 634; William of Tyre 1943, II, p. 51.
[157] Girder 1990.   [158] Amiran, Arieh and Turcolte 1994; Poirier and Taher 1980.
[159] Walter the Chancellor 1896 p. 63; Walter the Chancellor 1999 pp. 80–1.
[160] William of Tyre 1986, II, pp. 934–5; William of Tyre 1943, II, p. 370.

Other crush injuries were sustained during recreational activities. In 1159 Emperor Manuel I of Byzantium visited King Baldwin III of Jerusalem at Antioch after giving his niece Theodora to marry Baldwin. William of Tyre[161] tells us,

they were riding through the forest, as hunters do in the pursuit of that sport, when on the solemn day of the Ascension of our Lord, an accident befell them. The king, borne along on his fleet horse, was riding over rough ground covered with low-growing shrubs and brambles, when he was flung headlong to the ground from his horse and suffered a fractured arm. As soon as the emperor learned of the accident, he took upon himself, with the most gracious sympathy, the office of surgeon; he knelt down by the king and attentively administered to him, as if he himself were merely an ordinary person. Meanwhile, his nobles and kinsmen were dumb with wonder and dismay. That the emperor, regardless of his imperial majesty, should lay aside his august dignity and show himself so devoted and friendly to the king appeared to all unseemly. When, on account of this accident, they returned to Antioch, he visited the king daily, himself renewing the poultices and healing ointments and then carefully replacing the bandages.

A number of other occasions are known when Emperor Manuel personally treated patients, in contrast to the emperor's more socially accepted role merely as official protector of the hospitals and other charitable institutions in the Byzantine empire.[162] The treatment of a fractured long bone such as this involved firm longitudinal traction followed by manipulation to return the bone fragments back to their original position relative to each other. This position was then held by bandaging and splints or plaster, employing a technique that maintained the position for the weeks it might take for the bones to heal. Sometimes plasters were made from flour and egg white, while others recommended splints made from parallel wooden sticks.[163] The laws of the kingdoms of Jerusalem and Cyprus also discussed when a surgeon treating such a fracture could be regarded as negligent.[164] The *Livre des Assises de la Cour des Bourgeois* state that:

If a doctor treated a servant, male or female, for a broken arm or leg and said that he would cure it completely and would be the case if he had acted properly and he made a solemn covenant but then broke it and acted badly, applying useless plasters which left men forever crippled, reason judges that the doctor is liable to take the servant and pay his master what he cost . . . If he crippled a Christian man or woman, reason adjudges that he should lose his right thumb.

[161] William of Tyre 1986, II, p. 848; William of Tyre 1943, II, p. 280.
[162] Lascaratos and Voras 1996.
[163] Paulus Aegineta 1846, II, p. 427–60; Albucasis 1973 pp. 676–83; Theodorich Borgognoni 1498 pp. 118v–119r; Theodorich Borgognoni, I, 1955 p. 161.
[164] *Assises de Jerusalem* 1839 p. 258; *Assizes de Cyprus* 2002 pp. 181–2.

Clearly it was expected that a surgeon should have been able to straighten
long bone fractures and hold them in reasonable alignment with bandages,
plasters or splints until they healed.

BURNS

Burns appear to have been a surprisingly common cause of injury among
the crusaders and the heat may have come from a number of very different sources. The possibility of trial by fire to determine guilt of a crime
has already been discussed.[165] Many buildings were highly flammable, the
conditions hot and dry for much of the year and fires were a real problem. Sometimes forest fires were responsible for burns and these could be
natural or started deliberately. In 1101 a group of around one thousand
soldiers travelling across Asia Minor to the Holy Land were trapped by
Turks near Kastamonu. On account of the rugged terrain the Turks were
unable to attack the crusaders directly. In consequence they 'lit a big fire
from branches of the bushes and dry plant material and filled the valley all
around, and the thousand men were consumed by it'.[166]

As well as the possibility of being caught in a burning building or forest
fire, a common weapon used in siege operations in the Middle East at that
time was Greek fire. This appears to have been developed by the Byzantines
in the seventh century AD and was in widespread use by the time of the First
Crusade. It was used by all the major armies and was quickly incorporated
into the arsenal of the crusader forces, who found out how to make it from
local Christians. Different sources described slightly different constituents
in making Greek fire,[167] from naphtha, olive oil and lime which were then
distilled, to other versions such as tar, resin, sulphur and animal fat which
were heated together. Whatever combination of combustible materials were
used, the mixture was typically placed in a pottery container, and hurled
at the enemy. The pot then broke on impact, allowing the contents to
spill out and burn the soldiers or siege engines which were the target. Some
combinations had to be lit just before use, while others ignited on impact.[168]
The fear of Greek fire arose from the inability to extinguish the flames with
water – alternative liquids had to be used. Vinegar was found to be the most
successful fire extinguisher and the large amount of wine that accompanied
armies in the medieval period should have provided a reasonable source
of this.

[165] Raymond d'Aguilers 1969 pp. 120–2; Raymond d'Aguilers 1968 p. 102; Bartlett 1986 pp. 2,
      16 and 48.
[166] Albert of Aachen bk 8, ch. 12.   [167] Bradbury 1994 pp. 277–8.   [168] Bradbury 1979.

As early as the siege of Nicaea on the First Crusade in 1097 the defenders used Greek fire against the attacking siege engines. We hear that they 'mixed together grease, oil and pitch with tow and strongly burning torches and poured the mixture from the walls and it burnt up completely the apparatus of the battering ram and the wicker frameworks'.[169] It is possible that some of the men working the ram would have suffered burns as well. The use of vinegar is highlighted in a number of passages. During the siege of Jerusalem in July 1099 the Saracen defenders covered a tree trunk with 'tow soaked and anointed with pitch, wax and oil and all kinds of things for kindling fire'. They then lit it and lowered it down on a chain to burn up a crusader siege engine. However, the

native fellow-Christians had explained to the Christians how this fire, which could not be put out by using water, could only be extinguished with vinegar. So vinegar which had fortunately been placed in wineskins inside the engine was thrown onto the trunk and poured out and in this way the great fire was put out.[170]

It is not clear why vinegar should be more effective at extinguishing the Greek fire than water. However, armed with this information on how to protect themselves, it might be expected that fewer crusaders would have suffered burns during sieges than had they continued to use water, which was apparently ineffective.

In the siege of Arsuf in 1099–1100 by Godfrey of Bouillon, Greek fire was used by the defenders to burn a crusader siege tower. Unfortunately the fire took hold quickly and many soldiers in the tower were unable to escape and were burnt under falling timbers.

More than fifty warriors, appointed by the duke and other leaders, were now overtaken everywhere by the invading flames and they suffered destruction along with that same machine. Some had broken backs and necks, others legs half cut off, hips or arms, certain had burst intestines from the unbearable weight of timbers; having no strength for freeing themselves, they were reduced to ember and ash along with the timbers.[171]

In the unsuccessful siege of Tyre by King Baldwin I in spring 1112, Greek fire was again used with great effect by the Muslim defenders. The Franks had erected two tall wooden siege towers which allowed them to fire downwards at the men defending the city walls. Large wooden rings were constructed by the defenders and coated with pitch, sulphur, wax and fat mixed with tow. Once it was lit the ring was thrown from the walls onto the tower in an

[169] Albert of Aachen bk 2, ch. 33.   [170] Albert of Aachen bk 6, ch. 18.
[171] Albert of Aachen bk 7, ch. 3.

attempt to burn it down. 'Unbearable flames surrounded it on all sides and burnt it with a great and unquenchable fire, along with a great part of the men, who tried to shake off and put out the fire and were completely unable to escape.'[172] A good campfire tale was that about Emir Husam al-Din 'Abu' I-Haija' al-Samin. The story went that he sustained nasty burns when he was knocked from his horse while carrying a jar of Greek fire to burn down a Frankish siege tower in the siege of Acre in 1190. The *Itinerarium Peregrinorum et Gesta Regis Ricardi* states that 'the flask in which he was carrying the Greek fire was broken by the fall and the inextinguishable liquid set alight the Turk's genitals'.[173] Clearly an emir would be unlikely to be loaded down with a heavy vessel of dangerous chemicals, and the very fact that it was his genitals that were burnt does suggest this example was probably a fictional one. However, it does highlight the use of Greek fire in battle, as such tales would have needed to be plausible or else no one would have found them amusing.

Passages on burns in the medical texts are generally very similar and recommend an approach distinct from that used for other wounds.[174] Texts point out the need to prevent blister formation and so early treatment was directed towards this aim. The burn was to be prevented from drying out and was anointed with cooling medications. It could be placed in a bowl of vinegar or covered with wet compresses of vinegar, oil of roses or a number of herb extracts. Alternatives were ointments made from combinations of egg, rose oil, vinegar, opium and a range of herbs, covered with a dressing. Once blisters had developed then different drugs were used. Three ointments described by Theodorich Borgognoni were frankincense, mastic and elder bark mixed with oil and wax; egg white, camphor, ceruse with oil of roses and wax; thistle root with pork fat and wax.

DISCUSSION

The evidence gathered has formed a significant source of textual information on weapon injuries and their treatment in the Latin East. This allows a number of conclusions to be drawn regarding the experiences of soldiers who fought in the twelfth and thirteenth centuries. Attempts at objectively assessing the mortality in three crusading armies have given surprisingly similar results. In the upper echelons of the crusader armies at least

---

[172] Albert of Aachen bk 12, ch. 6.
[173] Richard de Templo 1864 p. 105; Richard de Templo 1997 p. 109.
[174] Paulus Aegineta 1846, II, pp. 42–5; Theodorich Borgognoni 1498 pp. 137v–138r; Theodorich Borgognoni 1960, II, pp. 135–6.

25–35 per cent seem to have died in tough expeditions lasting two or three years. About half of the deaths were the consequence of injuries and half due to malnutrition and infectious disease. A considerably higher proportion of footsoldiers would have been expected to die on account of their limited armour and reserves of food.

The most common injuries in pitched battles were from arrows and crossbow bolts. In the course of just a single engagement it is common to hear how many individuals suffered multiple arrow injuries, to the point where soldiers resembled hedgehogs. Arrows often rained down in showers that made it very difficult for soldiers to avoid them. While their armour gave some protection, the sharp tips were able to penetrate the links of chain mail and cause penetrating injuries. The jerkin of padded cloth (*gambeson*) was a useful protective garment against the arrow, as John of Joinville discovered at Mansourah on the Seventh Crusade.

While the sword and mace were certainly very effective, the lance used on horseback appears to have been the most formidable and lethal of weapons. The closed ranks of the heavy Frankish cavalry were extremely effective in the early years of the twelfth century[175] and when such charges failed in later times it was often because the opposing army opened a path for them to ride through, to avoid meeting the attack. The reason that the lance was so effective was that it still had the penetrating tip, as did the arrow, but carried with it much more energy. It was heavier than these airborne projectiles but still moved at speed with the momentum gathered by the cavalryman on horseback. It was common to hear of the lance penetrating body armour and on occasions coming right out the other side of the target. When this penetrating power was combined with the ability to guide the weapon up to the last minute, unlike the arrow, then a higher proportion of injuries might be expected to be in mortal areas of the body. It is common to read of survival after even multiple arrow wounds, but extremely rare after lance wounds. The sword and mace were still invaluable in close quarters fighting when the horse was able to move little, but at a gallop the lance was a deadly weapon.

The evidence for the practice of surgery in armies of both crusaders and Frankish settlers provides a range of fascinating information. In many cases the textual record shows that doctors were called to an injured person and treatment given, but frustratingly little detail of the management may be included. In these situations we can only make educated guesses as to what procedures or medication were employed based on the recommendations

---

[175] Bennett 1992.

in medical texts of the time. However, a good range of examples were also found where details of the treatment were recorded. This information tells us what treatments were actually being used to treat the injured. No longer are we obliged to guess whether the techniques recorded by the highly educated medical authors wrote in their books was always put into practice. The bandaging of wounds, burns and fractures along with the application of poultices is mentioned on many occasions throughout the texts. Bandaging was a simple technique to learn and may well have been applied by the common soldier as well as medical practitioners such as barbers and surgeons.

It is not known whether there was a formalised network of battlefield orderlies, as today, or if new soldiers just learnt the basics of wound care from their more experienced comrades. In the absence of evidence for the former option it seems possible that the latter may well have been the case. Poultices were applied to the injured, although no details of their composition were included in the relevant passages. Interestingly, there was contradictory advice in medical texts as to whether poultices should be used on fresh weapon injuries. Theodorich Borgognoni recommended wine or vinegar to wash the wound followed by bandaging, without a poultice. However, he did advise the use of a poultice in abscesses and to make pus appear in old wounds 'which the effect of air had already changed'.[176] Arnold of Villanova writing at the end of the crusades recommended that a powder from certain herbs be applied topically to weapon injuries once they had bean cleaned,[177] so he appears to have been an advocate of the poultice even in fresh wounds. Burns were treated differently from weapon injuries in the medical texts, which differentiated between burns with and without blistering. Although the topical use of wine on wounds is described by both European and Middle Eastern medical authors[178] there are no actual examples of this technique identified in the anecdotal descriptions. Frankish laws refer to the correct management of long bone fractures with plasters and show that those surgeons who crippled people by their inability to manage fractures properly were punished, in some cases by amputation of their thumb.

Likewise, standards were set for the management of skull fractures. Those surgeons who were unable to safely remove dangerous pieces of bone were hanged if their bungling resulted in the death of a freeman. It is interesting that the surgeon was expected to get this operation right. A number of the laws suggest that it was acceptable to fail to cure a patient, as in the

---

[176] Theodorich Borgognoni 1498 p. 106v; Theodorich Borgognoni 1955, I, p. 13.
[177] McVaugh 1992.
[178] Avicenna 1930 p. 520; Theodorich Borgognoni 1498 p. 110r; Theodorich Borgognoni 1955, I, p. 54.

case of measles or ulcers, so long as accepted techniques were employed.[179] The point that skull fracture was not included in this bracket suggests that the operation was normally performed without killing the patient. If everyone with this injury died then head injuries would most likely have been included in the no fault category, along with measles and ulcers. This suggestion is supported by the evidence of healing in many excavated cases of trepanation from Europe. As operating around the brain was clearly going to have some element of risk, this might imply that the advice on careful selection of patients prior to surgery was generally performed. A patient with no brain damage prior to surgery would be expected to have recovered much better post-operatively than someone comatose even before the surgeon arrived.

The removal of arrows was clearly common in the army. There are frequent references to soldiers hit by a number of arrows and by the next day the injuries were referred to merely as wounds. It might be presumed that basic attempts to remove the arrows would be made by the soldier himself or his colleagues and that only those that were difficult to remove would have been sent to the barber or surgeon; but there is no firm evidence for this in the sources. Medical texts describe a number of techniques to assist the extraction of an arrow, which was often difficult on account of the barbs, but unfortunately no details of the techniques employed were mentioned in the battlefield descriptions.

Bloodletting may have been used in only a limited way in the management of trauma, as many of the injured had already lost significant amounts of blood. However, crush injuries where no overt blood loss had occurred were managed with bloodletting, as in the case of Lord Walter of Autrèche. Texts on the use of bloodletting did advise that phlebotomy from a part of the body distant (termed revulsion) from a source of significant blood loss could actually stop the bleeding by diverting the blood elsewhere.[180] Balancing this, weakness was regarded as a significant contraindication to the use of bloodletting[181] and this reason is often cited in crusader chronicles for not performing bloodletting on a sick patient. It may have been a more common treatment in the weeks of recovery following injury rather than on the battlefield itself.

There was also a fascinating case of early twelfth-century medical experimentation when King Baldwin I sustained a penetrating injury. The doctor called to treat the king was clearly not sure exactly what organs might have

---

[179] *Assises de Jérusalem* 1839 p. 262.
[180] Brain 1986 pp. 13–14; Theodorich Borgognoni 1498 p. 110v; Theodorich Borgognoni 1955, 1, pp. 61–2.
[181] Voigts and McVaugh 1984 pp. 56–7.

been damaged and hoped to dissect a Muslim prisoner, given a similar wound, so that he could understand the injury better. In the end a dancing bear was dissected instead and the king did survive. It is not known if he then underwent an operation at the hands of the doctor or if supportive treatment such as wound care, dietary modification and oral medication was used.

Another more surprising aspect was the apparent use of poison on weapons at that time. The accusation that someone died from poisoning was common in the era of the crusades, especially if there was any suspicion as to the cause of death or if enemies had much to gain.[182] It is easy to dismiss all these claims as fanciful since none of those in Frankish sources gives any symptoms to suggest poisoning with a particular substance. However, doctors clearly thought that poisons were used on the battlefield and Arnold of Villanova mentions how to treat them in his *Regimen Almarie*.[183] What is more interesting is that Emperor John of Byzantium may have wounded himself while on a hunting trip with an arrow that was deliberately dipped in poison, although gangrene has also been suggested as an alternative diagnosis. His doctors even offered to amputate his hand in an attempt to save him, so they clearly knew how effective such poisons could be. With evidence such as this, it is possible that some of the descriptions of attacks where arrows or knives were claimed by chroniclers to have been dipped in poison may have been correct.

The evidence for the practice of surgery in Muslim armies is again interesting. On a number of occasions texts mention the use of sutures by indigenous surgeons to bring together the edges of wounds. Although it is presumed that the materials used would not have been sterile, when long-term outcomes are given they often suggest that the wound healed satisfactorily. It could be argued that a bad infection would have killed the patient and so only those who healed well would be alive for any comment on long-term healing. However, the evidence does suggest that this technique may have been reasonably standard practice and had some success in certain parts of the body.

With all these examples of surgery it would be ideal if comparison could be made between treatment practised by European-trained crusaders and the techniques of the indigenous practitioners who had trained in the eastern Mediterranean. It is a commonly held belief today that the Franks

---

[182] William of Tyre 1943, II, p. 117; Continuation of William of Tyre 1871 p. 51; Continuation of William of Tyre 1996 p. 44; Tritton and Gibb 1933.
[183] McVaugh 1992.

were of poor standard compared with the indigenous practitioners. However, the evidence for such an assumption is extremely flimsy, and is discussed in some detail in the later chapter on the exchange of medical knowledge with the crusades. The definitive approach to allow comparison between European and indigenous practitioners might be to look at the success and failure rates of each group, but this is not possible using textual sources as such information was just not recorded. An archaeological approach may be possible in the future, where injuries on human skeletal remains from Frankish cemeteries can be compared with those of comparable socioecconomic status from non-Frankish areas. If the tibial fractures healed straight in one group and angulated in the other this might suggest variation in the ability to treat such fractures. However, even this approach may be limited by the presence of the indigenous practitioners who were treating the Latin population. Another line of inquiry would be to assess multiple, detailed textual examples where practitioners from each group were treating similar injuries, and this would highlight the similarities and differences in their approach. Unfortunately such data are not yet available. In many of the cases described above the origin of the treating practitioner is unknown, and modern educated guesses may be incorrect. Furthermore I have been unable to identify examples where members of each group are treating the same type of injury, where sufficient details are given to enable meaningful comparison. Certainly an approximate assessment of the general type of procedures and techniques can be made and used to compare the two groups. By this final criterion there is little evidence to suggest that typical practice by crusaders, Frankish settlers or indigenous Christians, Jews and Muslims was dramatically different.

Having discussed what is found in these descriptions, it may be worth considering what is not found. The absence of certain treatments from the record can be interpreted in a number of ways. Perhaps the first reaction might be that if a treatment is not mentioned in these sources then it might not have been practised at that time. In some examples this may have in fact been the case, but alternative reasons should also be considered. It is possible that some procedures were so common that no one bothered writing the details down in a chronicle. This is a plausible argument as to why there is an absence of reference to the use of cautery in the treatment of trauma. This is presumed to have been popular among Islamic doctors on account of the large sections discussing the technique by Albucasis[184] and to a lesser

---

[184] Albucasis 1973.

degree Avicenna,[185] but it was also included in European texts.[186] Using hot iron was thought useful in trauma cases with bleeding and gangrene, so it is surprising that no examples of its use have been identified. However, cautery was mentioned in Frankish laws with regard to elective procedures such as treatment of haemorrhoids,[187] so it may well be that the technique was used after all.

Another theory to explain the absence of certain techniques is that the chroniclers may not have seen the more complicated operations being performed. These might well have taken place in the privacy of a battlefield tent, so that the only information the chroniclers could write was that treatment was given and the individual either died or recovered. This reason must be considered when it is noted that there were no examples of surgical treatment of abdominal injuries with a description of damaged intestines, and this was well known to have been a very grave injury. It is not known if the surgeons would attempt to suture the intestines as described in medical texts,[188] or if the patient was merely left to die from peritonitis without any attempt at surgical intervention. However, there are some examples of attempts to treat such wounds in medieval Europe.[189] Unlike an elective operation on the abdomen, the surgeon would surely not be blamed if the patient died after surgery for such an injury as patients were known to invariably die in any case if left untreated. While we do have examples of abdominal injuries undergoing treatment, such as King Baldwin I after the bear was dissected, the lack of detail subsequent to this suggests that the eye witnesses who gave the rest of the story to the chronicler were kept out of the tent where the treatment took place.

This approach has demonstrated a wide range of treatments used in the management of weapon injuries resulting from medieval battles. The interaction between weapons, armour and injuries has been explored, the mortality in crusader armies estimated and the most common and most lethal weapon injuries discussed. The evidence for the practice of surgery has been compared with techniques recommended in the medical texts of the time. It seems that treatment for common weapon injuries was similar to the approach advocated in the medical texts. However, evidence

---

[185] Avicenna 1930 p. 525.
[186] Theodorich Borgognoni 1498 p. 127v; Theodorich Borgognoni 1960, II, p. 36.
[187] *Assises de Jérusalem* 1839 p. 262; *Assizes of Cyprus* 2002 p. 184.
[188] Albucasis 1973 pp. 536–50; Theodorich Borgognoni 1498 p. 118r; Theodorich Borgognoni 1955, I, p. 154.
[189] Lang 1992.

for complicated and dangerous procedures such as chest and abdominal surgery is not found in the non-medical sources used here. Whether it is simply the result of chance that such procedures were not recorded, whether such procedures were just not performed in public view for the chroniclers to watch or whether this really suggests that such operations were not undertaken at all is open to discussion. It may well have been a mixture of all these.

CHAPTER 6

The practice of elective surgery and bloodletting

Having considered the evidence for the urgent use of surgery in the management of trauma, it is interesting to consider those procedures that took place in the elective setting. Elective surgery refers to planned operations for chronic conditions, in contrast to the treatment of emergencies. Medieval surgical texts from Europe[1] and the Islamic world[2] mention a wide range of procedures but some recent research has questioned just how many operations were really performed. It has been suggested that many of the procedures described in these manuscripts were no longer in use by the medieval period and that their inclusion by copying details from older texts was for prestige value or completeness rather than in the expectation that surgeons would put them into practice.[3] This is further compounded by the fact that the profusion of surgical instruments recovered from excavations of classical Greek and Roman sites[4] is not mirrored in medieval settlements. While this is believed to represent a trend away from the burial of practitioners with their equipment towards the handing on of such expensive instruments to others, it does take away a very useful source of evidence regarding the practice of medieval surgery. Those instruments that have been recovered seem to have been lost accidentally by their owners or sometimes found in the ruins of fire-damaged houses.[5] While the total number is relatively small, medieval surgical instruments have been recovered from Europe, the Byzantine empire and Islamic world, and include scalpels, forceps, hooks, probes, scissors, saws, cautery irons and phlebotomes for bloodletting.[6]

It is generally agreed that, outside the context of trauma, surgery was often the last option to be employed to treat disease.[7] Once diet, drugs,

---

[1] Murray-Jones 1994; Siraisi 1994b; McVaugh 2000.
[2] Nabri 1983; Azmi 1984; Haddad 1986–7.   [3] Alvarez-Milan 2000; Savage-Smith 2000.
[4] Milne 1907; Jackson 1988 pp. 112–94; Bliquez 1993; Kunzl 1996; Rimon 1996; Kunzl 1999.
[5] Stephan 1993; Møller-Christensen 1938 pp. 167–80.
[6] Bliquez 1984; Hamarneh and Awad 1977; Bliquez 1999.   [7] McVaugh 1993 p. 158.

bloodletting and perhaps baths had been utilised the patient had to decide if the symptoms were sufficiently severe to warrant an operation. Interestingly, there is good textual evidence for certain elective surgical procedures in medieval Europe, including operations for hernias, bladder stones and cataracts.[8] In order to assess the degree to which elective surgery was undertaken in the Latin East a range of non-medical textual sources have been studied. Once such evidence has been identified then comparison of the available details with techniques included in contemporary medical texts can highlight any contrasts between theory and practice in this population.[9]

One notable example of surgical practice involved large numbers of individuals with a complication of malnutrition. The patients were soldiers participating in the Seventh Crusade and the location was Egypt. King Louis IX of France led the crusade and took the coastal port of Damietta. By the beginning of 1250 he had advanced to the town of Mansourah in the Nile delta where between February and April the army became trapped between canals. The soldiers became reliant on supplementing their diet by fishing from the canals hemming them in, which were clogged with the dead of both sides. At this point large numbers of the army became sick and for want of a better explanation they blamed the illness on the fish. John of Joinville developed the symptoms himself[10] and wrote

The only fish we had to eat in the camp for the whole of Lent were eels, which, being greedy creatures, feed on the dead. On account of this evil circumstance and because of the unhealthy climate – for not a drop of rain ever falls in Egypt – a disease spread through the army of such a sort that the flesh on our legs dried up and the skin became covered with black spots and turned a brown earthy colour like an old boot. With those who had the disease the flesh on the gums developed gangrene and no one who fell victim to it could hope to recover, but was sure to die. An infallible sign of death was bleeding from the nose . . . I fell victim to the sickness that had stricken the army and it affected my mouth and legs . . . The sickness that had stricken the army now began to increase to such an alarming extent and so many people suffered from mortification of the gums that the barber surgeons had to remove the gangrenous flesh before they could either chew their food or swallow it. It was pitiful to hear around the camp the cries of those whose dead flesh was being cut away; it was just like the cry of a woman in labour.

After his capture by Muslim forces, Joinville writes, 'Then one of the Saracen knights told our rescuer to bid us take comfort for he would give me something to drink that would cure me within two days. And this, I may say, he did.'

[8] De Moulin 1971; Park 1998; McVaugh 1998a; McVaugh 2001.
[9] Mitchell, 2004 (a).   [10] John of Joinville 1874 p. 166; John of Joinville 1963 pp. 237–44.

It is interesting that as a secular writer Joinville does not blame the illness on sinful activities in the army, as the priests and bishops often did on crusades, but tried to explain it with logical, natural theories. He thought it might have been the result of eating the eels which had been feeding on decomposing human bodies and it is perfectly reasonable to propose that disease would follow from drinking contaminated water and eating fish from such a polluted source. As it happens we can identify the disease and explain its cause and show that the eels were not to blame. However, this does highlight the sensible attitudes to the cause of disease held by many lay people in the thirteenth century. The most likely explanation for the symptoms described by de Joinville is that he and many others in the army had developed scurvy. This is a condition resulting from the lack of vitamin C (ascorbic acid), normally obtained by the consumption of fresh fruit and vegetables. Symptoms include progressive weakness with loss of weight, and by the terminal stages, swollen spongy gums with fungating masses projecting beyond the biting surface of the teeth, which themselves may loosen and fall out. Purple spots are seen on the feet and ankles as a result of bleeding from blood vessels and this is followed by large spontaneous bruising all over the body, especially on the legs. There is almost always some infection of the gums and where this occurs the breath has an offensive smell.[11] Stress and exertion increase the rate at which vitamin C is used up by the body[12] and so sieges or harried, underfed armies, particularly after long sea voyages, are likely to provide cases of scurvy.

This account gives interesting information regarding the practice of surgery by the barbers in the camp. The excision of the superfluous tissue forming on the gums is a procedure which was described well before the crusades by authors such as Albucasis.[13] The fact that screams were heard around the camp during the operations on the gums suggests that neither analgesia nor anaesthesia was being used. The use of opium and other drugs (such as dwale or the soporific sponge) to make surgery less horrific for the patient is described in medieval medical manuscripts[14] and this is discussed in detail later in the chapter. However, it seems clear that little or no use of such drugs was made on this occasion. If they had been used then these battle-hardened soldiers would surely not have been screaming in pain the way they did. There are several possible explanations for this. One option is that that pain-killing drugs were reserved for major operations and a quick trim of the gums would not have been classed as major.

[11] Passmore and Eastwood 1986 p. 325.   [12] Norris 1983.
[13] Habib Khan and Riaz Ali Perwaz 1980.   [14] Olivieri 1968; Voigts and McVaugh 1992.

Another alternative is that with such large numbers of sick to treat, the barbers were overwhelmed with work. They would not have had the time to give the drugs to each soldier and wait for him to become drowsy before performing each operation. Another interpretation is that the procedure was specifically described as being performed by barbers, rather than more formally trained surgeons, and so they may not have known how to use pain-killing drugs, or even been able to afford to buy them in the first place. It is also possible that after months of battle the doctors may have treated so many injured that they had run out of most of their drugs and so had no pain-killers left.

An attempt to treat mental illness using surgery to the scalp is found in the twelfth-century work of Usama. If we accept the story as a true event, the surgeon was an unnamed Frank from Europe and the operation took place at the Frankish castle at al-Munaytirah, now in Lebanon.[15]

He examined the woman and said, 'This is a woman in whose head there is a devil which has possessed her. Shave off her hair.' Accordingly they shaved it off and the woman began once more to eat her ordinary diet – garlic and mustard. Her imbecility took a turn for the worse. The doctor then said, 'The devil has penetrated through her head.' He therefore took a razor, made a deep cruciform incision in it, peeled off the skin at the middle of the incision until the bone of the skull was exposed and rubbed it with salt.

A number of medical texts of the period discuss mental illness along with the various treatment options for patients.[16] The term phrenitis was used to describe an acute mental disturbance associated with fever and was thought to be caused by an excess of yellow bile. Melancholia was a chronic condition associated with anxiety, sadness and delusions, due to an excess of black bile. Mania was associated with excitement and wild behaviour, arising from an excess of yellow bile. Incubus referred to recurrent nightmares, while love-sickness caused sleeplessness and sadness. Possession was only described by some authors and was applied to those patients who believed themselves to be under the control of higher powers (either good or bad) and some of whom made predictions about the future.

It has been shown that in early medieval Europe it was rare to attribute mental illness to sin, witchcraft or sorcery.[17] However, possession was actually a quite common reason given in non-medical texts, with thirty-one out of fifty-seven cases recorded in one study of eleven pre-crusader chronicles.[18] While most contemporary medical authors interpreted mental illness in the

---

[15] Usama ibn Munqidh 1929 p. 162; Conrad 1999.   [16] Jackson 1972.
[17] Neugebauer 1979.   [18] Kroll and Bachrach 1984.

context of humoural imbalance, the Frankish doctor mentioned here gives the explanation of a devil in the woman's head. It is possible that this doctor had diagnosed the woman in the account as suffering from possession. However, alternative explanations include his blaming a devil as a way of explaining the illness to the observers in a way they would understand, or this was perhaps a poorly educated practitioner who genuinely believed that devils were the cause of mental illness. Typical treatments for mental illness in the medical texts were chosen in the hope that they would redress humoural imbalance. This involved the modification of diet, the use of drugs either orally or topically to the head, bloodletting to veins of the scalp or elsewhere and therapeutic baths. Shaving the head or trimming the hair very short was thought to help the head breathe freely. Cupping and scarification of the head were also treatment options. The fact that hardly any of these techniques were employed in the case from Usama would fit with the doctor's explanation that it was not humoural imbalance but a devil causing the illness. Once shaving the head to help it breathe had failed, it is possible that cutting into the scalp was undertaken in an attempt to flush out the devil. While skull trepanation was described in the treatment of epilepsy[19] and the use of a cruciform incision in the scalp was well described in medical texts to give access to skull fractures[20] such a treatment for mental illness does not appear to have been described widely in the texts. However, as with many of Usama's stories it is not clear how reliable this particular tale is, especially as he admits that he did not witness the events himself.

Osteomyelitis is infection in the bone and bone marrow. This can result from a fracture with a wound in the overlying skin or alternatively bacteria causing the infection can be carried to the bone via the blood from other sites of infection in the body, such as a dental abscess or urine infection. It was a common problem in the medieval period due to the chronic course of the disease and the difficulty in its cure. Cases have been recovered from excavation at the crusader period settlement of Le Petit Gérin involving bones of the spine and forearm.[21] Usama wrote of the successful surgical treatment of one of the Frankish royal court, under King Fulk (1131–42), who had osteomyelitis. As always with this author, we have to take care in interpretation, but the description does seem plausible enough.

[19] Corner 1937.
[20] Paulus Aegineta 1846, II, p. 431–4; Theodorich Borgognoni 1498 p. 115r; Theodorich Borgognoni 1955, I, p. 119.
[21] Mitchell 1994; Mitchell 1997.

The king of the Franks had for treasurer a knight named Bernard who (may Allah's curse be upon him) was one of the most accursed and wicked among the Franks. A horse kicked him in the leg, which was subsequently infected and which opened in fourteen different places. Every time one of these cuts would close in one place, another would open in another place. All this happened while I was praying for his perdition. Then came to him a Frankish doctor and removed from the leg all the ointments which were on it and began to wash it with very strong vinegar. By this treatment all the cuts were healed and the man became well again.[22]

It sounds as if Bernard sustained an open fracture to either the tibia (shin) or femur (thigh) of the leg when the horse kicked him. This is believed to have been a common injury in times when the horse was the major form of transport. The broken bone in itself should have healed satisfactorily given that Bernard was of high status and would have been treated by reasonable doctors, presumably realigning the bone and holding it in a splint until healed. However, we are also told that numerous ulcers formed on the leg around the injury and these were extremely difficult to heal. This suggests that at the original injury to the leg the skin was broken by the kick and infection took hold at the site of the break in the bone – osteomyelitis. Kicks from farm animals are notorious for causing this as there is often animal excrement on their hooves.[23] Once the infection takes hold pus is formed deep in the bone as the immune system of the body tries to kill the bacteria. The pus drains to the skin via a sinus and bursts through it to form an ulcer. The multiple openings on various parts of the leg are classic indicators for osteomyelitis, as is the observation that when one ulcer heals another opens. This is because the pus has to drain out from the bone and if one sinus closes then a new path must form to allow the pus out.

Interestingly the treatment found to be successful was vinegar. This has proven antiseptic qualities capable of killing a range of bacteria.[24] Unlike the ointments applied to Bernard's leg by previous doctors, the vinegar could be used to wash not only the skin ulcers but also the deep infection in the bone. By inserting the vinegar in one sinus the antiseptic liquid could flush through the diseased part of the bone and wash out again through the other holes. While this approach would be unlikely to kill every bacterium in the bone, it might well have suppressed the infection sufficiently to allow the body to kill off the remaining organisms or at least minimise the amount of pus produced so that the ulcers could heal for a while.

---

[22] Usama ibn Munqidh 1929 pp. 162–3.   [23] Tsukayama and Gustilo 1996.
[24] Kass and Sossen 1959; Phillips, Fernandez and Gundara 1963.

he nor Albucasis nor Paulus Aegineta makes any mention of complications of haemorrhoid surgery such as anal stenosis from overzealous cautery. The fact that this complication is included in the medical negligence legal collection shows that such surgery was taking place in the Frankish states. Perhaps more interestingly, this evidence demonstrates that whether or not the procedure cured the complaint (and it might well have helped), the citizens expected that the operation would not leave them worse off than before the surgery.

Ascites (dropsy) was a term used to describe the distension of the abdomen by a large collection of fluid in the peritoneal cavity. Causes of ascites include liver disease, heart failure, tuberculosis and metastatic cancer.[36] The legal code of the *Livre des Assises de la Cour des Bourgeois*[37] discusses some of the complications that can result from the surgical procedure of tapping the fluid to make the patient more comfortable.

If I had a servant, male or female, with dropsy possessing an enlarged belly and a doctor is contracted to cure and this doctor taps the belly where the illness is and then doesn't know how to let the water out that was inside, but lets all the fluid come out at the first or second occasion and the patient is so weakened that he loses his breath and dies, reason judges and commands that the doctor should replace the servant.

If all the fluid is tapped at one session then as it re-forms in the abdomen insufficient fluid is left in the blood vessels, which can lead to shock and death. Theodorich described the procedure in some detail.[38]

You should perforate the skin and peritoneum as well, from three fingers below the umbilicus . . . After having made the perforation, introduce a bronze or silver tube so that the water may be evacuated by itself. Take care not to let it drain for any length of time, since perhaps by reason of release of the animal spirit the patient may die or he may suffer fainting and approach death. But drain it according to the amount of the patient's strength and then withdraw the tube and stop up the hole.

The procedure, along with the risks of excessive drainage, had been mentioned by Paulus Aegineta back in the seventh century and again by Albucasis in the tenth.[39] Albucasis advised using a tube with a ring on its outer end, presumably to prevent its being lost inside the patient. Despite warnings in the medical texts it appears that some doctors of the time were

[36] Burkitt *et al.* 1996 p. 178.
[37] *Assises de Jérusalem* 1839 pp. 260–1; *Assizes of Cyprus* 2002 p. 184.
[38] Theodorich Borgognoni 1498 p. 133v; Theodorich Borgognoni 1960, II, p. 94.
[39] Paulus Aegineta 1846, II, pp. 337–40; Albucasis 1973 pp. 382–6.

still draining too much ascitic fluid from the abdomen and ending up in the Frankish courts.

The simple procedure of bloodletting was widely practised from classical times to the nineteenth century.[40] Up to the twelfth century most bloodletting appears to have been performed by *medici*, medical practitioners who might undertake all aspects of treatment. Medical subspecialisation became more common in the twelfth century so that bloodletting was undertaken by barbers or bloodletters. There is little archaeological evidence of bloodletting as it is difficult to distinguish bloodletting bowls at excavation from those used for meals, and medieval phlebotomes have only been recovered from a few sites.[41] Interestingly, the medieval infirmary at Soutra in Scotland has excavated pits into which the blood may have been poured. The authors have proposed this function on account of the darker colour of the soil and positive tests for blood products.[42] However, the findings have not been reproduced at other sites using this technique and therefore the approach of testing the soil remains contentious, given the potential for false positive results.

The reason bloodletting was such a widely used treatment was that it was thought to remove bad blood and redress any imbalance in the bodily humours,[43] believed to be responsible for so many kinds of disease. For the same reasons, phlebotomy was also used to correct such imbalance early, before any symptoms of disease became apparent. In consequence the technique was used not only to treat established disease but also prophylactically to maintain health. A number of sources demonstrate the practice of bloodletting in the medieval period. It is described in some of the large medical texts[44] but others take it for granted that everyone knew how to perform the procedure and merely mentioned the best veins to open for each disease. A number of specialised bloodletting manuals were also written, often in the vernacular for the better educated barbers who could read.[45] Other sources include sections of works on preventative medicine such as the regimen of health (*Regimen Sanitatis*), which discuss bloodletting amongst the various methods required to ensure that an individual avoided becoming unwell.[46] *Hisba* manuals from the eastern Mediterranean

---

[40] Seigworth 1980; James 1983; Gil-Sotres 1994; Kuriyama 1995; Kerridge and Lowe 1995.
[41] Thompson 1942 pp. 76–83; Kirkup 1981; Hamarneh and Awad 1977; Bliquez 1999.
[42] Moffat and Fulton 1988 pp. 14–30.   [43] Brain 1986 pp. 122–34.
[44] Albucasis 1973.   [45] Voigts and McVaugh 1984.   [46] *Regimen Sanitatis Salerni* 1953 pp. 83–92.

also included sections on bloodletting, such as the twelfth-century Arabic manual written by a Syrian named al-Shayzari.[47] Albucasis summarises the procedure well.[48]

The blood vessels in the body which it is customary to open are thirty in number. There are sixteen of them in the head . . . in the arm and hand there are five . . . three veins in the leg and foot . . . The three veins that are opened in the elbow are the veins which universal custom has used for bloodletting. There are two ways of venesecting these, either by piercing with a broad myrtle-leaf scalpel or a rather fine olivary; or by cutting with a knife-edged scalpel . . . The venesector should sit on a cushion raised above the cushion of him whose vein is to be opened. Then let him stretch out his arm and let the venesector chafe it two or three times with his hand; then he should bind a bandage round it by means of thongs twisted two or three times. The ligature should be moderately tight, for any other sort of ligature, be it too tight or too loose, will hinder the flow of blood. After putting on the tourniquet, the patient about to be venesected should chafe his own hands together until the veins swell up and become obvious. Then the venesector should wipe over his knife with a little olive oil, preferably old. Then he should place the forefinger of his left hand on the vessel itself below the place where he wishes to cut, lightly, so that the vein does not slip away and elude the stroke . . . then he should apply the knife . . . Now in each case you should extract blood in proportion to the person's strength and to the prevailing colour of the blood.

There were four factors of principal concern to ensure the safe practice of phlebotomy.[49] The first was custom, meaning that those unaccustomed to venesection should not be bled. The second was the strength of the patient, which meant that bloodletting should not be performed in hot weather or during a new moon as people were thought to be weaker at this time. The third was time, since in cold seasons the blood was more viscous so that good blood was lost rather than bad blood, which was the point of the procedure. The fourth was age, as children were not treated in this way, and nor were old men unless they were plethoric. The amount of blood removed depended on the strength and age of the patient. Galen even went as far as to state that recommending a specific volume to let was rash, as it would need to be different for every patient on every occasion.[50] While a few practitioners advocated bleeding until the patient was on the verge of unconsciousness, most preferred the technique of apoforesis, when repeated letting of smaller volumes allowed the patient to recover between visits while still giving the intended eventual outcome. A number of complications of bloodletting were also recognised. Disease might be allowed into the veins from the

---

[47] 'Abd al-Rahman 1999 pp. 108–13.   [48] Albucasis 1973 pp. 624–46.
[49] Voigts and McVaugh 1984.   [50] Brain 1986 p. 53.

outside, such as when an abscess was overlying the vein that was opened. Laceration of an artery, as opposed to a vein, might lead to a haematoma (large blood clot), arteriovenous fistula or even death from exsanguination. Bleeding patients with intermittent fever too early after its onset might weaken them and worsen their condition. In order to help a patient recover from the procedure it was common to give either strengthening electuaries or foods afterwards, and those prone to fainting could be given such an electuary beforehand too.[51] With this basic knowledge of bloodletting it is interesting to look at the evidence for its use in the Latin East.

The institutional use of bloodletting is best demonstrated by the examples of the major military orders and these show strong parallels with monastic practice in Europe.[52] In the Order of the Temple information on bloodletting can be found in the Retrais of the Infirmarer Brother, statutes dating from 1165.[53] It was the infirmarer who give permission for members of the order to undergo bloodletting. Once they had undergone the procedure, 'healthy brothers, when they are bled, should eat only three times' of the special food in the infirmary. It is presumed that the special diet there was to help them recover their strength. The need to specify that only three meals were allowed may suggest that some people tried to eat there for a longer period. This would not have been too surprising as the infirmary diet offered more variety and the wine was of better quality than that drunk by the healthy brothers.[54] The Teutonic Order also practised bloodletting. The procedure was referred to indirectly as the rule specifies certain days of the year when the procedure was forbidden,[55] presumably to avoid the risk of illness developing if it was performed in the wrong season or with the moon in the wrong phase.

The practice is described in the Order of St John, both in its statutes but also in the chronicles of pilgrims who were patients in their hospital. The anonymous cleric who wrote of his experiences in the hospital of St John in Jerusalem in the 1180s mentioned the bloodletting that took place.[56] As the doctors performed their twice-daily ward rounds, one of the sergeants who accompanied him made a note of those who required bloodletting. The *minutores* who performed the phlebotomy were paid a regular salary by the hospital to bleed the patients there. Statutes of the order showed that knights, sergeants and clergy in the Order of St John also underwent bloodletting, as well as the patients in the hospital. The procedure was performed both for prophylaxis against ill health and also

[51] Voigts and McVaugh 1984.   [52] Gougaud 1924.
[53] *Rule of the Templars* 1886 pp. 138–41; *Rule of the Templars* 1992 p. 65.
[54] Riley-Smith 1967 p. 259.   [55] *Die Statuten* 1890 p. 165.   [56] Kedar 1998.

to treat established disease. In the *Esgarts* (judgments) of the order in 1239 it is recorded that, 'if any brother have himself bled without leave, unless it be in case of illness . . . let him undergo seven days' penance'.[57] The need for such punishments suggests that undergoing bloodletting was an attractive prospect and this might been the case as those who were bled received the tastier diet of the infirmary, just like the Templars. The *Usances* (customs of the Hospital) of the same year also include information on the prophylactic use of phlebotomy as, 'in the house of the Hospital it is customary that the brethren should be bled on Saturdays'.[58] Having all the planned bloodletting on the same day may have helped the monastic life run smoothly, as the bloodletter could be pre-booked for the use of the infirmary and the kitchens plan for the extra meals required to help those bled to regain their strength.

Having considered the evidence for the practice of bloodletting members of Frankish institutions, there are also plenty of examples where it was applied to named individuals. Just as today, not everyone was happy with the idea of voluntarily losing blood. The events noted in the twelfth century by Usama[59] might have been applicable wherever venesection took place.

There used to visit us in Shayzar a man from Aleppo who was meritorious and learned . . . In case he got sick, the physician would prescribe bloodletting and every time the bloodletter came, Salim's colour would change and he would shiver; and when the bloodletter applied the knife, he would faint and remain unconscious until the cut was bandaged, upon which he would return to consciousness.

Clearly this was the kind of patient that medieval texts advised should have been given strengthening electuaries before and after the procedure.[60] King Richard I of England also underwent bloodletting. Saphadin had come to discuss a truce between Sultan Saladin and King Richard on 7 November 1191, between Yazur and as-Safiriya. However, we are told that 'the king did not wish to talk with him that day because he had just been bled'.[61] This suggests that sufficient blood had been removed to make him feel weak or at least not at his best to bargain with a foreign dignitary. On this occasion there is no reference in the texts to his being ill, so this may be an example of prophylactic phlebotomy. In 1241, Earl Richard of Cornwall returned from crusade and visited Emperor Frederick of Germany on the way home. Matthew Paris[62] noted how 'the emperor also ordered him to

[57] *Cartulaire Général* 1894–1906, II, p. 546, cart. 2213 stat. 78.
[58] *Cartulaire Général* 1894–1906, II, p. 548–61, cart. 2213, stat. 105.
[59] Usama ibn Munqidh 1929 p. 175.   [60] Voigts and McVaugh 1984.
[61] Richard de Templo 1864 p. 296; Richard de Templo 1997 p. 273.
[62] Matthew Paris [Luard] 1877, IV, p. 147; Matthew Paris [Giles] 1852, I, p. 369.

be gently and mildly treated with blood letting, baths and divers medicinal fomentations to restore his strength after the dangers of the sea'. John of Joinville described the bloodletting of Lord Walter of Autrèche after his fatal wounding in 1249 at Damietta.[63] 'Some of the doctors and surgeons in the camp came to him and as he did not seem to be in danger of death they bled him in both arms.'

Bloodletting was also included among those treatments covered by the medical negligence clauses of the *Livre des Assises de la Cour des Bourgeois*.[64]

If my servant should be ill with fever so that he has great heat within his body and the doctor bleeds him before the due time and removes too much blood so that, both by the weakness of the fever that he has so disturbed and by the bleeding, the fever climbed into the head of the patient, he relapsed and died, reason commands to judge that the doctor is held liable in law and by the Assize to pay compensation to the value of the servant . . . If a doctor has treated a free man or woman, reason judges and commands the doctor be hung.

This legal passage mentions two of the complications of bloodletting, namely bleeding too early in a febrile illness and excessive bleeding (exsanguination) leading to death. It does not bother to include less serious complications such as the haematoma or arteriovenous fistula, as these were not life threatening. This highlights the complicated nature of medieval bloodletting, the detailed structure of rules that had been developed for its use and the profound effect of its misuse as perceived by contemporary medical and legal minds.

A number of authors have investigated bloodletting from a modern scientific viewpoint. Bloodletting would have made perfect sense to the medieval practitioner as the therapeutic removal of blood perceived to be of bad quality was logical in the context of the humoural theory. However, modern scientists have also wondered what effect the procedure may have had upon the patient and the practitioner's perception of the disease. Some have considered what kind of information might be gained by inspecting the blood collected in the bowl held under the arm.[65] While it might be expected that all blood would look dark red and form a clot in the bowl, a number of conditions could modify this process. Those diseases associated with systemic inflammation, such as infections, result in the production of special proteins in the blood. These cause the red blood cells to clump together and precipitate out at the bottom of the blood sample, leaving

[63] John of Joinville 1874 p. 96; John of Joinville 1955 p. 67.
[64] *Assises de Jerusalem* 1839 p. 260; *Assizes of Cyprus* 2002 p. 183.
[65] Macfarlane 1962; Ell 1984; Cameron 1993 pp. 159–68.

straw coloured liquid at the top. Such a process is the basis of a standard clinical test for inflammation, the erythrocyte sedimentation rate (ESR). If this were noted in the sample in a bloodletting bowl then it may have conveyed information to the practitioner on the health of the patient, showing that all was not well.

Another area of investigation has been the effect of bloodletting on the health of patients. It has been suggested that venesection might in fact have had beneficial effect upon health.[66] In the 1970s it was realised that one of the methods employed by the body to fight infection was to take free iron out of the blood and store it away from the invading organisms where they could not access it to grow and multiply, known as 'nutritional immunity'.[67] The loss of iron in red blood cells removed from the body during venesection results in a state of iron deficiency, with a corresponding low level of free iron in the blood. In consequence it has been suggested that venesection during an infection helps the body in the task of ensuring that serum iron levels are reduced to starve the microorganisms.[68] However, more recent work has shown that the effect of 'nutritional immunity' was overstated and that the concept was also simplistic.[69] While it is agreed that iron is crucial for the growth of bacteria, many species of bacteria have developed effective methods to extract iron from blood proteins regardless of the free iron concentration in the serum.[70] The notable exception to this is malaria, which is more dependent on the free iron concentration. Furthermore, iron deficiency actually impairs the ability of the body to fight infection with white blood cells, which along with antibodies make up the two principal defence mechanisms of the body. Metanalysis of the large number of clinical studies undertaken over the years has failed to show any concrete evidence that iron deficiency anaemia protects against infectious disease.[71] At the most there may be a slight tendency for iron deficiency to worsen bacterial infections in non-malarious areas, but it may possibly give some protection against malaria in endemic areas. However, such arguments would have been of no consequence to medieval practitioners for whom the beneficial effects of bloodletting would have gone without question.

ANAESTHESIA DURING OPERATIONS

It is common to find sections in medieval surgical texts describing the use of plant extracts to relieve pain or sedate the patient prior to an operation.

---

[66] Brain 1979.   [67] Weinberg 1974.   [68] Brain 1979.   [69] Oppenheimer 2001.
[70] Bullen, Griffiths, Rogers and Ward 2000.   [71] Oppenheimer 2001.

However, the use of such drugs is rarely mentioned in the non-medical sources and it is unclear why. It is possible that they were used so commonly that no one bothered mentioning them when describing an operation, but an alternative is that they were hardly ever used at all. William of Tyre mentioned opium in his chronicle covering the Latin East during the twelfth century.[72] While describing the Nile flood plain at Phium in Egypt, he noted that, 'the best opium found anywhere grows there and is called by doctors Theban'. Clearly opium was known in the Frankish states and the quality of the product from various regions appears to have been a topic worthy of discussion. Perhaps more importantly, the reference was not to the recreational use of the drug, as medical practitioners were specifically mentioned. This clearly suggests that opium was a drug found useful by doctors in the Latin East, even if we remain ignorant of how widely it was used.

A number of plants with sedative and analgesic effects are mentioned by authors working in the eastern Mediterranean at the time of the crusades. The thirteenth-century Jacobite medical author Gregorius Barhebraeus lived much of his life in the principality of Antioch and the county of Edessa. One of his works was an abridged version of the *Book of Simple Drugs* by Muhammad al-Ghafiqi, who had died by 1165 in Cordoba, Spain. Barhebraeus' text left out the Greek terms for plants as Greek was not widely spoken in the Levant and omitted those plants only found in Spain and not in the eastern Mediterranean.[73] This suggests that those plants he did include were found either growing or at least for sale in the Levant. Henbane (*Hyoscyamus sp.*) is included in the text as a sedative,[74] which might suggest its use at that time. Similarly, Moses Maimonides wrote his *Glossary of Drug Names* in Cairo and mentions such sedative plants as henbane, hemlock, poppy and poppy syrup, deadly nightshade and mandragora root.[75]

Since there is reasonable evidence for the medicinal use of opium in Frankish sources and suggestive evidence for a range of other sedative and analgesic drugs, it is interesting to consider how they may have been used by medical practitioners of the time. Opium has a long history in the eastern Mediterranean, being in use as early as the Bronze Age.[76] Sometimes opium was described in medieval medical texts for use alone but often it was in

[72] William of Tyre 1986, II, p. 897; William of Tyre 1943, II, p. 330.
[73] Barhebraeus 1932b, I, pp. 35–7.   [74] Barhebraeus 1932b, II, pp. 340–3.
[75] Moses Maimonides 1979.   [76] Merrillees 1962; Kritikos and Papadaki 1967.

combination with others.[77] In the eleventh century Avicenna wrote in his *Canon of Medicine,*

the most powerful of the stupefacients is opium. Less powerful are seeds and root-bark of mandrake, poppy, hemlock, white and black hyoscyamus, deadly nightshade, lettuce seed.[78]

If it is desirable to procure a deeply unconscious state, so as to enable the pain to be borne which is involved in painful applications to a member, place darnel-water into the wine or administer fumitory, opium, hyoscyamus (half-dram dose of each) nutmeg, crude aloes wood (four grains of each). Add this to the wine and take as much as is necessary for the purpose. Or boil black hyoscyamus in water, with mandragora bark until it becomes red. Add this to the wine.[79]

This technique of infusing wine with medicinal plants was to become very popular in medieval Europe, with Arnold of Villanova writing his *Liber de Vinis* devoted to the subject around 1310.[80] A popular analgesic infusion in medieval England was known as dwale.[81]

While some versions of this prescription were taken orally in wine others used the soporific sponge, a technique described in European manuscripts from the ninth century.[82] In this form a similar range of plants were boiled in a cauldron and concentrated onto a sponge. Theodorich Borgognoni included a standard prescription for this in his *Cyrurgia*:

The composition of a saviour to be made by a surgeon, according to Master Hugo, is as follows: take of opium and the juice of unripe mulberry, hyoscyamus, the juice of spurge flax, the juice of leaves of mandragora, juice of ivy, juice of climbing ivy, of lettuce seed and of the seed of lapathum which has hard round berries and of the shrub hemlock, one ounce of each. Mix these altogether in a brazen vessel then put into it a new sponge. Boil all together out under the sun until all is consumed and cooked down onto the sponge. As often as there is need, you may put this sponge into hot water for an hour and apply it to the nostrils until the subject falls asleep. Then the surgery may be performed and when it is completed, in order to wake him up, soak another sponge in vinegar and pass it frequently under his nostrils.[83]

It was noted in the same manuscripts that advocated their use that overzeal-ous application of the sponge could kill the patient. In his section on head injuries, Theodorich warns against using the sponge before operating as some of the patients never woke up afterwards, 'since it is impossible to

---

[77] Ellis 1946; Robinson 1947 pp. 3–26; Demirhan 1980; Carter 1996.
[78] Avicenna 1930 pp. 526–7.   [79] Avicenna 1930 p. 413.   [80] Arnold of Villanova 1943.
[81] Voigts and McVaugh 1992; Carter 1999.
[82] Baur 1927; Deffarge 1928; Corner 1937; Keys 1963 p. 7; Olivieri 1968.
[83] Theodorich Borgognoni 1498 p. 146r; Theodorich Borgognoni 1960, II, pp. 212–13.

apportion the medication accurately in accordance with the condition of the wounded'.[84] The risk of this happening would have been higher in head injuries as suppression of the drive to breathe is a common complication of a serious head injury and the action of these sedative drugs would further exacerbate the problem. The warnings of such complications are further evidence to suggest that the treatment may have been in use after all.

One question often asked of medieval prescriptions is whether they made the patient better, or even had any effect on the patient at all. The list of plants mentioned in the prescriptions of Avicenna and Theodorich do contain a range of active compounds and many are still used today in medicine in their refined forms.[85] The opium poppy (*Papaver somniferum*) has the strongest medicinal effects of all the poppy family. Juice was collected by cutting or scarifying the unripe capsule of the poppy. Alkaloid extracts from the poppy include morphine and codeine,[86] both well known today for their analgesic (pain killing) and sedative effects. Other members of the poppy family such as *P. bracteatum* are indigenous to the Middle East and also contain opiates such as thebaine, which has a milder analgesic but stronger narcotic effect.[87] Side effects of these compounds include vomiting and with a high dose suppression of the drive to breathe, which can be fatal. Black and white henbane (*Hyoscyamus niger* and *H. albus*) contains the alkaloids hyoscyamine and hyoscine.[88] Deadly nightshade (*Atropa belladonna*) contains hyoscyamine and atropine,[89] while mandrake (*Mandragora officinarum*) contains atropine but also hyoscine and scopoletin.[90] Fumitory (*Fumaria officinalis*) contains protopine.[91] These anticholinergic compounds share a number of characteristics as they compete with the body's chemical transmitters at nerve endings.[92] When used together they would cause blurred vision, dry secretions, relax smooth muscle, cause amnesia and at low dose sedate the patient. Hyoscine is an anti-emetic and its action of preventing vomiting would be particularly useful when opiates, well known for triggering vomiting, were also in use. Protopine also kills bacteria which might theoretically enable better wound healing after an operation. Hemlock (*Conium maculatum*) contains a number of active alkaloids based on coniine.[93] These block spinal reflexes and cause muscle paralysis at the right dose, although with too high a dose death

[84] Theodorich Borgognoni 1498 p. 115r; Theodorich Borgognoni 1955, 1, p. 118.
[85] Juvin and Desmonts 2000.   [86] Evans 1996 pp. 368–73; Bruneton 1999 pp. 926–48.
[87] Kettenes-Van Den Bosch, Salemink and Khan 1981.
[88] Evans 1996 pp. 351–4; Bruneton 1999 pp. 811–22.
[89] Evans 1996 pp. 354–7; Bruneton 1999 pp. 811–22.
[90] Evans 1996 p. 358; Bruneton 1999 pp. 811–22.   [91] Evans 1996 p. 493.
[92] Rang and Dale 1987 pp. 122–3.   [93] Bourman and Sanghvi 1963; Daugherty 1995.

from paralysis of the respiratory muscles could follow. Preventing a patient from moving a limb would make most operations much easier to perform and for this reason muscle relaxants are commonly used in anaesthetics today. Lettuce (*Lactuca sativa*) contains a mild sedative in its seeds.[94] Wine is a central nervous system (CNS) stimulant at low doses, but acts as a CNS depressant at higher levels, explaining the heavy sleep of a drunkard. Spurge flax would have been one of the many species of *Euphorbia* that grew in the medieval Mediterranean region. Several of the hundreds of species of spurge in the world have been analysed for their medicinal components, but little is known of the pharmacognosy of the species indigenous to the Mediterranean. For example *E. hirta*, native to Australia, has been shown to contain compounds which act as a sedative and anxiolytic.[95] *E. acaulis*, native to India, contains extracts with anti-inflammatory properties which might lead to decreased pain after a surgical procedure.[96] Since the genus is well known for the medicinal actions of its sap it is quite possible that whichever species of *Euphorbia* was meant by Theodorich would also have contributed to the pharmacological activity of the treatment.

While it is convincing that the alkaloids contained in these plants would have significant effects on anyone who absorbed them there are still a number of factors that remain problematic. It is unknown quite how well these compounds would have been extracted by medieval pharmaceutical techniques to be suspended in the wine or concentrated on the sponge. Similarly, we have no idea how effective soaking such an impregnated sponge in water and holding it under a patient's nose while the vapours were inhaled would have been as a method to get those compounds into the body. An experiment using the soporific sponge prescription on rats found that some became sedated but none fell asleep.[97] However, a nineteenth-century scientific paper did describe its successful use in five human patients undergoing surgery.[98] It is likely that drinking wine in which these plant extracts had been infused would have been much more effective than waving a hot sponge under the nose. The absorption of a solution of these drugs in the gut will be much better than the alternative route relying on vapours condensing on the nasal mucosa. Whichever way we interpret the data on the effectiveness of these methods of administration of the drugs, we do know that if enough of the alkaloids were absorbed at the right dose by the patient then such a cocktail would have had a range of effects that should have made any operation less of an ordeal for the patient and easier for the surgeon too.

[94] Evans 1996 p. 493. [95] Lanhers *et al.* 1990. [96] Singh *et al.* 1984.
[97] Infusino, O'Neill and Calmes 1989. [98] Dauriol 1847.

SUMMARY

There are markedly fewer examples of elective surgical procedures in Frankish sources than is the case for the treatment of trauma and this is exactly what might be expected. When a soldier suffered a serious wound he would be aware that his life hung in the balance and might be more prepared to undergo surgery than if suffering from a chronic condition that would otherwise be unlikely to kill him that day. However, when seen from the opposite point of view it is perhaps surprising that there is as much evidence for elective surgery as has been found. With recent views suggesting that very little surgery was undertaken by the medieval period despite the inclusion of procedures in medical texts, the evidence presented here does confirm that certain surgical procedures were being undertaken after all. By avoiding medical texts we can be more confident that the evidence discussed is a genuine, if approximate, indicator of surgical activity in the Latin East. There are examples of excision of overgrown gum tissue in scurvy, cranial surgery for mental illness, operative and non-operative treatment of osteomyelitis, cautery to haemorrhoids and draining ascitic fluid from the abdomen. While any operation has its associated risks, what is notable is that all of these procedures were relatively safe. There are no examples of surgery to the contents of the chest or abdomen, where the likelihood of patient survival would have been much less. The presence of practical medical negligence legislation covering a number of complications of such surgical procedures not only suggests that these basic operations were being performed but also that the Frankish authorities expected them to be performed to a reasonable standard.

Bloodletting has been shown to be an activity that pervaded all aspects of crusader life. It was used therapeutically to treat the sick and prophylactically to keep them healthy. The statutes of all the major military orders included clauses that regulated when and how the regular bloodletting should be performed. This was to ensure that the activity did not disrupt monastic life any more than was necessary and also that it was not abused by those who wanted the benefits of the tastier infirmary diet after the procedure. A number of named individuals who underwent phlebotomy have been considered and the activity was seen to interrupt even diplomatic negotiations at the highest level. The complications of its inappropriate use were also covered in the medical negligence clauses of the *Livre des Assises de la Cour des Bourgeois*. These show that it was believed possible to kill a patient by venesection at the wrong time in a disease or by removing more blood than the patient could tolerate, and that a doctor or barber could be hanged if convicted of the murder of a free person in this way. Modern scientific research into whether iron deficiency, such as might result from bloodletting, would have protected people against infectious diseases remains controversial. At present there is no conclusive evidence that would indicate that bloodletting would have been protective in this way.

The use of drugs to alleviate pain and cause sedation during surgical procedures is also considered. There is reasonable evidence for the use of opium by medical practitioners in the Frankish states and suggestive evidence for a number of other plants for this purpose. Scientific assessment of the alkaloids in plants included in the common prescriptions indicates that in theory such treatments may well have been effective in giving pain relief and sedation if they could be administered to the patient in an efficient way. The side effects of these plants, now often regarded as poisons, mean that the risk of death from inadvertent overdose would have been significant. Medieval texts describe how the plant extracts were either dissolved in liquids such as wine or concentrated on a sponge. It seems likely that the technique employing wine would have been a more effective method of administration than the sponge. Quite how widely these analgesics were used remains unknown.

CHAPTER 7

Exchange of medical knowledge with the crusades

An obvious question asked about the crusades is the effect they may have had on the participant countries in the longer term. There are many different aspects to this including the possible effect on military tactics, torture techniques, art, religion, architecture, judicial legislation, culinary styles, recreational activities such as steam baths and even population demographics from the loss of so many men.[1] From a medical point of view one of the most intriguing topics is whether the migration of peoples resulted in the spread of diseases.[2] Another logical question is whether the interaction between medical practitioners from different ethnic groups in the Frankish states led to significant transfer of medical knowledge between them. At a superficial level great changes in medicine were taking place in Europe at the time of the crusades. Universities sprang up in the major cities, many new medical texts were written (especially in surgery), huge numbers of *hospitalia* and *leprosaria* were established, while the functions of the non-specialised *medicus* were divided between physicians, surgeons, barbers and apothecaries. Whether these changes were in some way a direct result of the crusades or whether the timing was just coincidental remains a matter for debate. In order to assess the level of exchange in medical knowledge that may have taken place the evidence for a number of these issues requires analysis. This interaction can be divided into the theoretical concepts believed to explain the causes of disease and the practical skills needed at the bedside to actually treat a patient. It might be assumed that one group with a lower level of knowledge or ability would learn the most from interaction with another group with greater knowledge, although clearly some form of two-way exchange is to be expected.

---

[1] Goss and Bornstein 1986.
[2] Mitchell 1999b; Mitchell 2002; Mitchell and Stern 2000.

THEORETICAL MEDICAL KNOWLEDGE AND ACADEMIA

For many years it has been believed that the academic interaction between Europe and Islam was primarily in Spain and Italy and that the Latin East was a cultural desert in the academic sense.[3] The medieval period was one in which much of the the the literature of the classical world was being rediscovered in Europe through translations into Latin of Arabic versions of the original Greek and Latin texts.[4] While the translation of medical texts does not appear to have been as systematic and prolific as at Toledo in Castile and at the court of Frederick II Hohenstaufen in Sicily,[5] there is still a good deal of evidence for such activity in the Frankish states.

Medical texts used in the Latin East may have originated in the Byzantine empire, Islamic world or back in Europe, depending on the cultural and religious background of the reader. Such texts may have been translated and transcribed at established centres of learning such as Antioch, purchased for money, received as gifts, transferred from Europe with the medicomilitary orders or captured in battle. A possible example of capture in battle is when the armies of the First Crusade routed the forces of Kerbogha at Antioch in 1099. They left almost everything in their tents as the Muslim troops fled. When the crusaders looted the camp, 'they found countless volumes in that same camp of the gentiles, in which were written the sacrilegious rites of the Saracens, Turks and all the other races and wicked charms of prophets and soothsayers with detestable writings'.[6] Clearly the vast majority of the army could not read the languages of the Middle East and they could only guess at what was written in the books. However, it is quite plausible that doctors in an army the size of Kerbogha's might have taken medical books with them, just as the religious might have taken books of prayer and religious philosophy. It is also plausible that these books might have subsequently been kept in the city of Antioch and contributed to the collection of manuscripts used for the translation which took place there over the next two centuries. Similarly, Usama's library of over 4,000 books was captured in 1145 when his ship was driven ashore near Acre.[7] As it is known that Usama practised medicine himself[8] it is reasonable to assume that some of these books would have been medical texts. Another example is the Arabic book acquired by the astrologer Vincent de Beauvais. He accompanied King Louis IX of France on the crusade to Egypt in 1248–50 and found the astrological treatise in Damietta.[9] There is also evidence that

---

[3] Woodings 1971; D'Alverny 1982; Getz 1998 p. 39. [4] Burnett 1997. [5] Burnett 1994.
[6] Albert of Aachen bk 4, ch. 56. [7] Beddie 1933. [8] Usama ibn Munqidh 1929 p. 163.
[9] Wickersheimer 1929 p. 196.

the military orders owned books originating from Europe and these were presumably bought or received as gifts rather than captured. It is known that the Order of the Temple in Aragon owned a copy of the *Cyrurgia* of Theodorich Borgognoni,[10] which may theoretically have been for use in the order's infirmary. This particular text was in the local vernacular, rather than Latin, so presumably for use specifically in Aragon. Unfortunately no comparable lists from other regions survive, but it is possible that the military orders may have acquired European medical works on trauma and other relevant topics for use in their infirmaries in the Frankish states. While it is known that many of the soldiers in the military orders were poorly literate[11] the medical practitioners employed to treat the sick would have been able to read and write.

The crusaders did not need to establish any translation centres themselves as they inherited a number that were already there, the most notable being at Antioch and Tripoli. A number of European scholars even went east to make the most of the opportunity of access to the manuscripts that consequently became available. Adelard of Bath (born c.1080) was an Englishman who wrote and translated scientific and philosophical works in the early twelfth century.[12] Adelard went to Antioch around 1114 to use the manuscripts there and a number of the Arabic translations he made in his lifetime may have resulted from this visit. Perhaps the most important of these translators from a medical perspective was Stephen of Pisa. Stephen travelled to Antioch in the early twelfth century and started work on the manuscripts there. He was a treasurer at the Benedictine monastery of St Paul in the city and had a house in the Pisan quarter between 1126 and 1130.[13] He began work on the late tenth-century text by al-Majusi,[14] the 'Complete Book of the Medical Art' (*kitab kamil as-sina'a at-tibbiya*, also known as *kitab al-malaki*). The title of his translation was *Regalis dispositio* (the royal arrangement) and a number of the chapters specifically state that they were written in 1127 in Antioch. Some mention the help of the scribes Alduinus and Pancus too.[15] The work was comprised of two parts, the *theorica* and the *practica*, with ten books in each.[16] The *theorica* and part of the *practica* had previously been translated by Constantinus Africanus in the eleventh century under the title *Pantegni*, but this was acknowledged to be a poor translation and parts of the original were omitted.[17] Stephen also added an alphabetical catalogue in Greek, Arabic and Latin of those *materia medica* found in Dioscorides and these were later referred to as 'Stephen's synonyms'.[18] The

[10] *Viage Literario* 1806, v, pp. 200–2; Forey 1998. [11] Forey 1998.
[12] Cochrane 1994 pp. 32–40. [13] Hunt 1950. [14] Fisher 1996. [15] Burnett 2000.
[16] Haskins 1960 pp. 131–3. [17] Burnett and Jacquart 1994. [18] Sarton 1931, II (2), p. 236.

Regalis dispositio reached Europe and was copied both in its entirety and also as extracts in medical compendia.[19] Stephen is also believed to have translated the *Almagest* (a work by Ptolemy on astronomy) from Arabic into Latin, and is also likely to be the author of another astronomical work entitled the *Liber Mamonis*.[20] The importance of astronomy to the practice of medieval medicine has been stressed previously. Another scholar from Frankish Antioch was Theodore, a Jacobite Christian born in the 1190s. He studied languages, philosophy, mathematics, astrology and medicine in Antioch, Mosul and Baghdad. He translated medical extracts from Averroes and the pseudo-Aristotelian *Secret of Secrets* (*Sirr al-asrar*) from Arabic to Latin.[21] Theodore of Antioch spent the last years of his life working in the court of Emperor Frederick II of Germany and died by 1250.[22]

Away from Antioch there is further evidence for academia in medicine. Philip of Tripoli continued the work of Theodore of Antioch and translated the entire pseudo-Aristotelian text as *De secretis secretorum* around 1243.[23] Philip dedicated it to Guido de Vere of Valencia who appears in at least one manuscript as bishop of Tripoli. Several clerics with the name Philip are known from the early thirteenth century. One suggestion[24] is that he was a clerk of Foligno who received a canonry at Tripoli in 1227 in recognition of his services to the patriarch and church of Antioch.[25] In 1247 this same Philip was at Lyons with the pope as representative of the patriarch of Jerusalem and was referred to in terms of his 'knowledge of letters',[26] which would be an appropriate accolade for a recognised translator.

Acre has recently been identified as a centre where Arabic-speaking Europeans studied medical texts.[27] One manuscript of particular interest is that of *The Hundred Books on the Medical Art*, by the Eastern Christian physician Ab Sahl al-Mas h. He is believed to be the teacher of Avicenna, and the text must have been written before 1010 as he died that year. However, a copy of the manuscript dating from 1196 has been found, which was written in a surprisingly clear form of Arabic as if to be read by a foreigner. This manuscript has numerous Latin annotations in the margins, in a style thought to be of an Italian or possibly French hand. The notes translate the names of foods, and notes on fevers, spasms and tremors, vomiting and diarrhoea, pleurisy, the pulse, urine and so on. Study of the manuscript has led to the conclusion that these annotations were probably added in

---

[19] Burnett and Jacquart 1994 pp. 329–20.
[20] Burnett 2000.   [21] Sarton 1931, II (2), p. 492.
[22] Kedar and Kohlberg 1995; Sarton 1931, II (2), p. 492.   [23] Sarton 1931, II (2), p. 563.
[24] Haskins 1960 pp. 137–40.   [25] *Les Registres de Grégoire* 1896, I, p. 59, docs. 118–19.
[26] *Les Registres d'Innocent IV* 1884, I, p. 473, doc. 3138.   [27] Savage-Smith in press.

crusader Acre between 1196 and 1291.[28] However, the annotation of this manuscript in other known Frankish translation centres such as Antioch or Tripoli are also possibilities. Other general collections of books are known outside Tripoli and Antioch which demonstrate scholarly activities at other centres. For example, a list thought to date from the late twelfth or early thirteenth centuries refers to books in the possession of the church of Nazareth and bishop of Sidon, although exactly where the volumes were stored is not clear.[29]

When we think of the medieval translation of medical texts, we often think of transfer from Arabic to Latin. However, this was by no means the only translating going on at that time. There was a strong tradition of translating and copying of medical and religious manuscripts in the Christian communities in the medieval eastern Mediterranean.[30] One good example is Gregorius Barhebraeus, the Jacobite cleric and medical practitioner. He lived part of his life in Frankish Antioch and Tripoli, but also spent many years outside the Frankish states in cities to the east. He is known to have translated a medical treatise on simple remedies by al-Ghafiki from Arabic to Syriac, and his Syriac translation of the Qanun of Ibn Sina was ongoing at the time of his death.[31] Clearly some believed it was important to make these Arabic works available in local languages such as Syriac, to increase the number who could read them.

Having considered the translation of medical texts it is worth mentioning some of the new works thought to have been written in the Latin East and its close ally Armenia. The *Ars Probatissima Oculorum* was the work of Benvenutus Grapheus Hierosolimitanus, a Christian oculist who lived in the second half of the thirteenth century. It is believed that he spent his life in a number of countries around the Mediterranean, including Italy, North Africa and the Latin East. Along with his name (Jerusalemite), there are a number of references in his book as well as more subtle evidence that has led his biographers to believe he did spend time in the Frankish states.[32] Exactly how many of his ideas originated in Latin Europe and how much in the eastern and southern Mediterranean countries is hard to determine. However, he does provide yet another potential source of the spread of medical knowledge between regions. In the nearby Christian state of Armenia, which was closely allied to Antioch, Mekhitar of Her wrote the medical treatise 'Consolation in case of fever' in 1184.[33]

[28] Savage-Smith in press.   [29] Beddie 1933.   [30] Hunt 1997–8.
[31] Barhebraeus 1932b; *Geschichte der Christlichen* 1947, II, pp. 272–81; Barhebraeus 1872; Segal 1971.
[32] Kedar 1995.   [33] Sarton 1931, II (2), p. 70.

The *Sortes Regis Amalrici* was a Latin text describing a method of predicting the future based on the lunar calendar, that has been linked with the kingdom of Jerusalem.[34] This divinatory text is of particular interest from the medical viewpoint as it may have been written by the *medicus* of King Amalric of Jerusalem (ruled 1163–74). We hear how, 'a certain doctor of the most unconquered and kind Amaury established this work of twenty-eight questions concerning fates'. Some sections refer to Arabic terminology but these show that whoever did perform the translations was not very proficient at Arabic, as a number of bad errors are included that make it rather difficult to use the predictor. It is theoretically possible that the text originated in its entirety in France and was attributed to the kingdom of Jerusalem to make it more exotic and intriguing. However, it is also possible that at least part of the work did come from Jerusalem but that subsequent modifications or poor copying back in Europe may have led to a number of mistakes and cultural adaptations prior to the final form of the text preserved today.[35]

A number of medical works were written back in Europe by those who went on crusade. Some directly refer to the treatment of cases in the east, such as that of Gilbertus Anglicus. In his *Compendium Medicine* master Gilbert mentioned his treatment of the diseased eyes of the son of a Frankish noble.[36] Other are known to have accompanied crusading armies and been responsible for surgical works with large sections on the management of wounds. Theodorich Borgognoni (c.1160–1257) wrote his *Chirurgia* based on the teachings of his mentor, Hugo of Lucca.[37] Hugo was a master *medicus* contracted to the army of Bologna who participated in the Fifth Crusade to Egypt in 1219–21. While Theodorich's text makes no specific mention of any techniques Hugo may have learnt or developed while treating the wounded on this crusade, some authors have proposed that it was this military experience that gives the book such a practical tone.[38]

Several academic works were written on the topic of how to stay healthy on a crusade, usually presented to leaders planning to go east. Similar works had been composed in the east before the period of the crusades. Qusta Ibn Luqua was a Christian practitioner working in Baghdad who wrote a medical regimen in the ninth century for pilgrims travelling to Mecca. This covered topics varying from sensible eating to improving the quality of drinking water, and from diseases caused by dust to the treatment of dracunculiasis worms.[39] The best-known medieval European text on such

---

[34] Burnett 1998–9.   [35] Burnett 1998–9.   [36] Gilbertus Anglicus 1510.
[37] Theodorich Borgognoni 1498 p. 110r; Theodorich Borgognoni 1955, I, pp. 54, 112.
[38] Edwards 1976.   [39] Qusta Ibn Luqua 1992.

a topic was by Adam of Cremona. He wrote a treatise on the hygiene of an army or large body of pilgrims for Emperor Frederich II around 1227.[40] It was entitled *Regimen iter agentium vel peregrinatium* and divided into three parts. The first covered diet and sleep, camping, exercise, delousing, bathing, bloodletting and cupping and seasickness. The second discussed fatigue and rest together with care of the feet, while the third was on soldiers' morale and the religious purpose of a crusade. The Italian doctor Guido de Vigevano wrote a comparable work for King Philippe VI of France in 1335. The title of *Texaurus regis Franciae acquisitionis Terrae Sanctae de ultra mare necnon sanitatis corporis* specifically shows the proposed use on a crusade. It included advice on how an 'ageing' crusader such as the forty-two-year-old king might stay healthy on the expedition.[41] It seems that without the impetus of the crusades, such works on how an army might stay healthy on such a pilgrimage would probably never have been written in Europe in the form that they were.

While Arabic surgical texts such as that by Albucasis were being translated into Latin and also vernacular European languages,[42] a significant number of surgical texts were being written in Europe at the time of the crusades. There are works by Roger of Frugard, Rolando of Parma, Bruno Longoburgo, Gilbertus Anglicus, Guglielmo da Saliceto, Theodorich Borgognoni, Lanfranco of Milan and Arnau de Vilanova.[43] It is obvious that many sections are copied from older Arabic manuscripts (which themselves often copied classical authors), but the very fact that new surgical works were written at all does show a desire to improve on these translated works. This continued evolution of the medical text requires three sources of information. The first is the work of previous authors, the second is debate and discussion with colleagues and the third is practical experience of employing such techniques. Without these sources of ideas the passages tend to be regurgitated in a static way, but with them the texts evolve and change over time. The crusades can easily be shown to have contributed to all of these sources.

However, what is not so clear is how to determine which academic centres were most important in the transfer of medical knowledge between cultures around the medieval Mediterranean. Plausible arguments include those that translated texts for the first time, those who translated the largest number of manuscripts, or even those whose texts were regarded as core works for use in the university setting. It is known that Spain and Italy

[40] Adam of Cremona 1913; Sarton 1931, II (2), p. 653.
[41] Wickersheimer 1951; Leopold 2000 pp. 42–3.   [42] Trotter 1999.
[43] Agrimi 1994; McVaugh 1994; Siraisi 1994b; McVaugh 1998b.

possessed centres where translations of medical manuscripts from Arabic into Latin were made.[44] It has been suggested that it was the translations from these centres that were responsible for the evolution of medieval medicine that took place in Europe at that time and that the Latin East was unimportant in this respect.[45] If interpretation was this simple then it might be expected that such knowledge would have had a major impact in Spain and Italy. However, research on thirteenth-century Castile has shown that the translations at Toledo in the twelfth century had very little effect at all on medicine in that country.[46] Evidence such as this shows just how difficult it is to determine which centres of translation had the most profound effects and which were irrelevant. What is not clear is whether the timing of this evolution in Europe was a coincidence, or whether the situation of the crusades was in some way associated with or even the trigger for these new texts. If it is no coincidence, then the phenomenon of the crusades should be thought of as playing a more important role in the context of the evolution of medical academia in the medieval period than previous work has given them credit for.

PATIENT MANAGEMENT

Having considered the effect of the crusades on medical academia, it is just as important to assess the potential exchange of knowledge with regard to practical patient management. It has been stated by many authors that the hands-on abilities of Frankish medical practitioners was poor compared with those in neighbouring Muslim and Byzantine lands.[47] Typically, three are sources quoted as evidence for this view: the writings of Usama, Frankish medical licensing legislation and a passage from William of Tyre. A balanced examination of these passages should demonstrate whether this concept of the ignorant crusader or Frankish clinician is reasonable or unjustified.

Usama described an incident where a local Christian doctor named Thabit was asked to treat two sick people at a Frankish castle.[48] He described how both of the patients appeared to improve with his treatment until a European doctor arrived and took over. Both the patients then died,

---

[44] Garcia-Ballester 1987; McVaugh 1993 pp. 49–64.   [45] Woodings 1971; D'Alverny 1982.
[46] Garcia-Ballester 1987.
[47] Munro and Haagensen 1933; Woodings 1971; Ell 1996; Dolev and Knoller 2001.
[48] Usama ibn Munqidh 1929 p. 162.

allegedly from his drastic surgical management. The story has to be treated with some caution, but is certainly worth giving in detail.

The Lord of al-Munaytirah wrote to my uncle asking him to dispatch a physician to treat certain sick persons among his people. My uncle sent him a Christian called Thabit. Thabit was absent just ten days when he returned. So we said to him, 'How quickly you have healed your patients!' He said, 'They brought me before a knight in whose leg an abscess had grown and a woman afflicted with imbecility. To the knight I applied a small poultice until the abscess opened and became well and the woman I put on a diet and made her humour wet.

At this point an unnamed Frankish doctor arrived, who took over the care of both patients. The knight underwent amputation of the leg and the woman underwent surgery to her scalp, and both soon died. It has long been suggested that this passage shows that the abilities of Frankish doctors from Europe was inferior to the local, non-European practitioners.[49]

However, recent reassessment has shown that this passage fits a classic style of Islamic writing for the period, where extreme examples that apparently contradict each other (didactic dichotomy) were used when describing a topic.[50] As most authors omit the examples of exceptionally good outcomes following treatment by Frankish doctors which follow this passage, the result is the impression that Europeans were much worse than their Middle Eastern counterparts. In fact there is very little evidence to support that theory. Interestingly, the sultan of Egypt at the time of the crusade of 1249 of King Louis IX also had a leg amputated for an abscess.[51] Despite the fact that al-Salih Ayyub never went near a Frankish physician, he died the day after the operation. Clearly death after amputation for infection was not uncommon and not restricted to those treated by Latin doctors. In just the same way, Usama wrote of a number of good and poor treatments prescribed by local doctors and again these are rarely used as evidence. The problems arising from the medical writings of Usama have recently been reconsidered in the context of Islamic literary styles of the medieval period.[52] It appears that this technique of providing extreme examples to embellish a text was in common usage at that time in almost all topics that received literary attention. It seems that Usama has been misunderstood, and the stories accepted at face value by those medical historians who were not experts in Islamic literature. Even despite this, the selective use of some stories to support a theory while conveniently omitting others

---

[49] Munro and Haagensen 1933; Woodings 1971; Hillenbrand 1999 pp. 352–4.
[50] Conrad 1999.   [51] Klein-Franke 1986.   [52] Conrad 1999.

that do not support the argument has encouraged the belief that European doctors were of inferior quality to their local Christian, Jewish and Islamic counterparts. When assessed as a whole, the evidence in Usama's chronicle does not actually support such an assumption.

The legal collection the *Livre des Assises de la Cour des Bourgeois* includes two sections on expected standards of medical care in the Latin East.[53] These describe how doctors who came from Europe had to undergo examination by local doctors and the bishop before a licence was given that allowed the visitor to practise medicine in any particular town (see ch. 8). This has been interpreted by some to suggest that European doctors were of such poor quality at that time that the examinations were required to ensure that such quacks and charlatans did not move east and kill or maim all the inhabitants.

> The standard of military surgery remained at an abysmally low level during the ensuing centuries of the Middle Ages. Physicians who accompanied the crusaders were usually so incompetent or inexperienced in tropical diseases that they were forced to undergo examinations before being allowed to practise in Jerusalem.[54]

However, a balanced assessment of the legislation shows that such an interpretation is a little rash. The passage referred not just to Europeans but also doctors from neighbouring Muslim states as well. It seems more likely that the examination was to assess the knowledge of doctors not known to the town authorities, to ensure that quacks did not harm the population. There was no exemption for any practitioner who came from elsewhere, regardless of the region. In consequence there is no evidence from this text that doctors from Europe were believed by the Frankish authorities to be any worse than those from Egypt, Syria or Persia. In fact it was these very regions that introduced such examinations to improve practice in the first place,[55] with the Franks subsequently adopting the idea too.

William of Tyre also wrote a passage that is frequently quoted, often in an inappropriately selective manner.[56] He says, 'our eastern princes, through the influence of their women, scorn the medicines and practice of our Latin physicians and believe only in the Jews, Samaritans, Syrians and Saracens'. At face value, this might easily be taken to imply that crusaders felt that local doctors were better than those from Europe, and so avoided Frankish practitioners, and many have stated as much.[57] However, if the

---

[53] Amundsen 1974; Kirsch 1969.   [54] Adamson 1982.   [55] Karmi 1979.
[56] William of Tyre 1986, ii, p. 859–60; William of Tyre 1943, ii, p. 292.
[57] Munro and Haagensen 1933; Woodings 1971.

whole passage is read then interpretation is rather different. William gave an example of how he believed King Baldwin III was killed by the poor treatment of a local Syrian doctor named Barac. He then follows with the words quoted above and continues, 'Most recklessly they put themselves under the care of such practitioners and trust their lives to people who are ignorant of the science of medicine.' Clearly William had a low opinion of many of the Eastern practitioners working in the Frankish states at that time.

It should be remembered that William was not from Europe, but was born and brought up in the Latin East, although he did receive some of his education in Europe. We might expect him to give a more impartial opinion than the zealous clerics from Europe or Islamic chroniclers such as Usama, who looked down on crusaders as uncultured invaders. This apparent use of Eastern clinicians by Franks may not necessarily have indicated that they were actually any better. Isaac Israeli in his 'Fifty Admonitions to Physicians' wrote in ninth-century Egypt how, 'if a physician but comes from a distant land and speaks in a foreign tongue, not understood, the multitude will think him enlightened and gather unto him and take counsel from him'.[58] With this concept in mind it is possible that the crusaders sought out local doctors in the early years for their novelty value, regardless of their abilities. Indeed, it could be argued that the views of important statesmen such as Archbishop William regarding local doctors may have been relevant to the introduction of medical licensing within the Frankish states. If we believe William's statements, it could easily be argued that licensing was introduced to ensure that local doctors were up to the standard of Europeans, rather than the other way round, as is usually assumed. While I am not suggesting that European practitioners were in fact any better than their Eastern counterparts, I hope that this has highlighted the fact that many of the preconceptions regarding medical practitioners in the Latin East are based on very poor evidence. Ibn Jumayr' was a physician in the court of Salah al-Din in the late twelfth century and wrote a medical treatise on the revival of the art of medicine. He complained bitterly regarding the poor standard of many practitioners in Egypt, most of whom were only interested in making as much money as possible. He was concerned by 'the state of ruin into which it [i.e. medicine] had fallen at this time, and also about the ignorance and incompetence dominant among most of its practitioners and adherents'.[59] Clearly practitioners in the Islamic world were of varying ability and the widely held presumption that all were of

[58] Bar-Sela and Hoff 1962. [59] Ibn Jumayr' 1983 p. 6.

a higher standard of ability than the Frankish newcomers is no longer defensible.

Having clarified some of the past misconceptions, a fresh look at other evidence is highly illuminating. A study of the treatment of casualties on the First Crusade from 1097–9 has assessed the textual evidence for the standard of medical practice of those doctors accompanying the army. Such an approach has the potential to provide a baseline level of knowledge and skills that allows comparison with Eastern practices at that time. It also enables any changes in expected standards of medical practice to be compared over time, so that possible influence from local practitioners can be accounted for. The study concluded that medical practice in the armies of the First Crusade was comparable with Byzantine and Islamic practice, both in terms of practical treatment and also the theory behind the origins of disease, such as the outbreak of epidemics. It was largely devoid of talismans and charms and medical care appears to have been predominantly based upon practical and logical concepts, albeit logical by medieval standards. This suggests that European practitioners probably had much less to learn from their Eastern colleagues than is typically assumed.[60] Similarly, the evidence outlined in the chapter on trauma and its treatment earlier in this book failed to identify significant differences between the practice of a typical crusading practitioner from Europe, the Frankish settler or indigenous Christians, Jews or Muslims with regard to trauma.

Clearly there was interaction between European and local medical practitioners and many records imply this. European and local practitioners were examined and given licences by the same assessment panel in each town (see ch. 8). The Order of St John had variations to the oath taken by the doctors it employed in their hospitals so that non-Christians did not have to swear by the saints, showing that it was not just Christians who treated the sick there.[61] Unfortunately there is much less direct evidence for the transfer of medical knowledge as a result of this interaction. Without such examples, it is difficult to show whether the changes in the approach to medicine in the medieval period were a consequence of the Latin East or perhaps interaction between the cultures in Spain or Italy. There are a few examples of this direct transfer, however. Usama wrote of an artisan from Shaizar who travelled to Frankish Antioch with his son. If we choose to believe this story, the lad apparently suffered from scrofula, which is tuberculosis of the lymph nodes of the neck and armpits. A Frankish man told

[60] Edgington 1994.   [61] Edgington 1998b

the artisan how to treat his son using topical poultices based on vinegar, oil, fat, lead and herbs and it seems it was effective. The father presumably later told Usama about this, as Usama claimed that he tried it out in his own practice. 'I myself treated with this medicine many who were afflicted with such disease and the treatment was successful.'[62] Clearly this treatment was not known to Usama and other medical practitioners in the area, or he would not have bothered writing about it. The claim that Usama himself then used the technique on patients confirms to some degree that the exchange of medical knowledge was a two-way phenomenon.

It has been suggested that the Frankish medicomilitary orders were responsible for the rise of medical treatment in hospitals of the Latin west.[63] Before the time of the crusades medical care was principally given either in the patient's home by a medical practitioner employed to treat them, or in some cases at the local monastery. While large numbers of *hospitalia* were founded in Europe in the twelfth century, they were not for the medical treatment of the acutely sick but the religious salvation of the poor and infirm. The institutional care provided by the Order of St John and the Teutonic Order in the Levant certainly did evolve from the European-style *hospitale* into institutions that hired doctors and treated disease of the body as well as the soul. Evidence from dietary regulations in the statutes of these orders suggests Eastern influence upon some aspects of medical practice within them. It seems that the evolution in their function was a consequence of interaction with local Eastern practitioners, as many of the advances followed the practices in Eastern institutions such as the Islamic *bimaristan* and the Byzantine *nosokomeion*. These medicomilitary orders established houses in Europe and while the evidence is rather scanty, some of their *hospitalia* do appear to have cared for the sick and employed doctors by the thirteenth century. However, there is no evidence as yet identified that show any European institutions in the twelfth and early thirteenth centuries on the scale of the infirmaries of the principal houses in the East. Interestingly, in the thirteenth century a number of other *hospitalia* in France, Italy and Germany started to employ medical practitioners and it has been suggested that some incorporated medical statutes of the Order of St John into their own rule.[64] By the fourteenth century the hospitals of Europe began to increase in their inpatient capacity, most notably in Italy,[65] and start to show even more similarities with the famous hospital of St John. Bearing in mind the evidence such as borrowing of Eastern Frankish infirmary statutes by developing *hospitalia* in Europe,

---

[62] Usama ibn Munqidh 1929 p. 163.   [63] Miller 1978.   [64] Miller 1978.   [65] Henderson 1989.

it seems likely that Frankish military orders were a significant trigger to the evolution of the hospital in western Europe. This may have resulted both from the experiences of crusaders in the infirmaries of the Frankish states and perhaps also those who interacted with the European branches of these orders.

CONCLUSION

Having assessed the evidence available to date for the possible spread of knowledge between groups at both an academic and also a practical level there still remains a fundamental difficulty. It can never be known how medicine in the medieval period would have evolved without the effects of the crusades. It could be argued that the translation of works into Latin in Italy and Spain would have resulted in just the same level of knowledge in the medical texts available for use in universities of the thirteenth and fourteenth centuries. The presence of Jewish and Muslim doctors in Spain and Sicily would have encouraged the exchange of practical expertise to the Latin communities of Europe. Likewise, the battles raging across Europe in the twelfth and thirteenth centuries would have provided ample experience for surgeons to refine their techniques in the treatment of wounds.

From the other perspective, it can be stated that at an academic level medical and scientific manuscripts were translated into Latin at Frankish centres such as Antioch and Tripoli. We do know that there was interaction between doctors from differing ethnic groups, although the degree to which each accepted new ideas from the others is not at all clear. The incredible carnage seen on a regular basis as armies massacred each other over the 200-year life of the Frankish states would certainly have given a large number of doctors experience that they might well not have gained if they had stayed at home. Some of these doctors went on to write medical works and we must presume that the experienced they gained in the East must have affected what they wrote. The medicomilitary orders of St John, St Lazarus and the Teutonic Knights did set up hospitals and other medical establishments in Europe and, while it appears to vary just how comparable these were in function to the hospitals in the Latin East, some definitely were providing medical treatment by the early thirteenth century.

I think it is fair to suggest that the crusades were probably not the pivotal factor in triggering the evolution in medicine seen in the medieval period. It is also safe to say that quantifying any change that may have resulted from the crusades is extremely difficult. However, the crusades do appear to have played a part in moulding the direction this evolution took in Europe and were probably influential in the rate at which this change took place. While the explosion in the number of surgical texts written in thirteenth-century Italy is tantalisingly circumstantial, there is little direct evidence to attribute this to the need to treat the injured in the eastern Mediterranean. Overall, it seems that any effects of the crusades were most likely to have been seen in the practical treatment of the patient, especially the injured, and that academic university life was only enriched in a limited way by the translations from the Latin East.

CHAPTER 8

Frankish medical legislation

A range of legal documents have survived which help us to understand the legal process in the Latin East. The earliest legislation of the Latin East is that of the council of Nablus in 1120.[1] The canons of the council were ecclesiastical in nature and did not cover medical practice, but they did mention a number of punishments, including mutilation and execution, that are seen in the better-known thirteenth-century legal codes. A number of thirteenth-century commentaries on the laws of the kingdom of Jerusalem, the kingdom of Cyprus and the principality of Antioch have survived, even though the original laws of these states have not. It is possible that any written records were lost, or alternatively they may have been handed down orally, rather than as a formal written tradition. The legislation of the kingdom of Cyprus claimed to be modelled on that of the kingdom of Jerusalem and continued to be used up until the sixteenth century, well after the fall of the mainland Latin East.[2] One consequence of having to rely on these commentaries for our evidence is that we do not know exactly when the original laws came into force, although they clearly must predate the writing of the commentaries.

The earliest dated commentary is known as the *Livre au Roi*, which was part of the *Assises de la Haute-Cour* of the kingdom of Jerusalem and was written before 1205. Another early commentary, which is roughly contemporary to the *Livre au Roi*, comes from the principality of Antioch, and is known as the *Assises d'Antioch*.[3] The principal legal commentary which contains sections on medical negligence and licensing in the kingdom of Jerusalem is found in the *Assises de la Cour des Bourgeois* and was probably written around 1240–4. Study of this commentary suggests that the original laws of the kingdom were probably based on Roman customary law brought over from Europe, modified by the customary law of northern

---

[1] Kedar 1999.   [2] *Assizes of Cyprus* 2002.   [3] *Assises d'Antioch* 1876.

France and Italy as well as by local Syrian Christian legal traditions.[4] The author of the commentary was a lay burgess who worked in judicial administration in the courts at Acre. Consequently, we can only wonder quite how comparable this text was with the decisions of the other burgess courts in the Latin East. The author was not highly educated or legally trained, but seems to have acquired his knowledge as a law practitioner.[5] While much legislation of the Latin East is thought to have been influenced by European law, it is interesting that the sections discussing medicine were probably not.[6] In consequence it is likely that it was local Syrian customary practice that formed the basis for the regulations. This is suggested by a number of factors, including reference to the role of the *mathessep*.[7] The *mathessep* was a Frankish version of the Islamic *muhtasib* who was responsible for ensuring quality and fairness among craftsmen, businessmen and medical practitioners.[8] A recent edition of the *Livre au Roi* is now available,[9] and an edition of the commentary on the Court of the Burgesses for use in Cyprus has also just been published.[10] However, the two editions of the commentary on the Court of the Burgesses at Acre are both over one hundred and fifty years old.[11] The edition by Beugnot appears to have been based on a seventeenth-century copy of a fifteenth-century manuscript, and consequently includes a number of errors.[12] The edition by Kausler is based directly on a fourteenth-century copy of the manuscript, and is therefore believed to be much closer to the original text as used by jurists in Acre in the thirteenth century.[13] In consequence, the Kausler edition has been used here for the medical negligence sections and the Beugnot edition for those extra chapters not edited by Kausler. This provides a useful starting point from which to explore the legal control of medicine in the Latin East. An English translation of the Kausler edition, by Vivian Nutton, follows the discussion of its contents below.

FRANKISH COURTS

Courts in the Latin East were divided into two by the social status of those who used them. The nobles settled their disputes in the High Court (*Haute-Cour*) while the freemen used the Court of the Burgesses (*Cour des Bourgeois*).[14] There were perhaps thirty to forty burgess courts in all.[15] In

---

[4] Grandclaude 1923 pp. 50–70; Prawer 1980 p. 390.   [5] Prawer 1951; Prawer 1980 p. 366.
[6] Prawer 1980 p. 368: Amundsen 1974.   [7] *Assises de Jérusalem* 1843 pp. 236–44.
[8] Prawer 1972b, p. 147; Conrad 1999.   [9] *Livre au Roi* 1995.   [10] *Assises of Cyprus* 2002.
[11] *Assises de Jérusalem* 1839; *Assises de Jérusalem* 1843.   [12] Grandclaude 1926; Coureas 2002 p. 22.
[13] Coureas 2002 p. 22.   [14] Edbury 1997 pp. 155–62.   [15] Prawer 1980 p. 263.

the kingdom of Jerusalem the courts were convened in such cities as Acre, Caesarea, Jerusalem and Tyre. Each of these burgess courts was autonomous and unfortunately we do not have a copy of the *Assises* of any of them. The activities of the court were presided over by the viscount, who was a man chosen by the local lord. In the case of Acre, a city of the royal domain, the viscount was appointed by the king. Twelve jurors were appointed by the lord from among the Latin population of Christian freemen. Eleven of these jurors passed verdict and sentence while one acted as counsel for the defendant.[16]

From a medical perspective, one particularly interesting point is the way in which the court coped with those who claimed to be unable to attend their court hearing because of ill health. This is discussed in the legal commentary by John of Ibelin, the count of Jaffa (died 1266) included in the *Assises de la Haute-Cour*.[17] If someone excused themselves citing sickness, then doctors were sent by the court to assess the medical fitness of the patient. If the sick man claimed to be injured then a *cyrurgicus* would examine his wound and determine whether it was sufficiently serious to prevent his attendance before the judge. Similarly, if someone had other forms of illness a *physicus* would examine the pulse and urine and determine whether the man was genuinely unwell or faking illness to avoid appearing in court. He would then report back to the court with his opinion as to the validity of the excuse.

MEDICAL LICENSING

The licensing of medical practitioners in the Frankish states is an item of particular interest to be found in the medical legislation. This was not a practice found in Europe prior to the crusades, while it was widespread in the Islamic world by the eleventh century. In consequence it appears that licensing was adopted by the Frankish settlers from local customs, although some previous assessments of the *Assises* have failed to consider this option and looked only to Europe for precedents.[18] It could also be argued that this Frankish adoption and adaptation of Islamic legislation then led to the introduction of medical licensing in medieval Europe, although possible alternative routes for this transfer from Islam include the multicultural kingdom of Sicily under Roger II of Salerno. The difficulty in accurately dating the original clauses incorporated into the *Assises de*

---

[16] *Assises de Jérusalem* 1843 pp. 236–8; Kirsch 1969.
[17] *Assises de Jérusalem* 1841 pp. 338–40; Brittain 1966.   [18] Brittain 1966; Amundsen 1974.

Jerusalem means that this debate will probably remain unresolved. The Frankish regulations state that all doctors arriving in a town had to undergo examination before they could practise there. For some reason the licence did not allow practice anywhere in the Frankish states, just in the town that issued it. All practitioners were required to undergo examination regardless of their religious, cultural or geographical origins. The examiners were the most respected local doctors under the supervision of the bishop, who gave successful candidates a letter confirming their right to practise. Those who failed were beaten out of town if they treated patients without a licence, even if they were never guilty of malpractice.

Medieval Islamic *hisba* manuals are very enlightening with regard to the standards of medical practice expected in Islamic states. Since Frankish licensing appears to have adopted Islamic procedure to a large extent (including the *mathessep*), it is possible that the Franks may have used a version of the relevant sections of such *hisba* manuals themselves. These manuals included great detail on the theoretical knowledge and practical skills expected for safe practice by physicians, surgeons, ophthalmologists, bonesetters, bloodletters and pharmacists. This assessment was required as the Islamic world did not issue practitioners with a certificate or degree on completion of their medical training, so it could be difficult to determine how competent any individual was.[19] Some *hisba* manuals outline the range of equipment and instruments that those in each profession should own to allow them to treat their patients adequately. The twelfth-century manual of al-Shayzari required that surgeons possessed at least one set of lancets, scalpels, a saw, dressings and ointments. Ophthalmologists were to own hooks, scalpels, a scour and eye ointments. Bloodletters were to carry lancets, oil for the skin, string to tie around the arm and musk to revive a patient who fainted. Physicians were to possess cautery irons, pincers, syringes, tweezers, probes and gynaecological instruments.[20]

Often a specific medical text was referred to in the *hisba* manuals as the standard by which to assess practitioners. The *Ten Treatises on the Eye* by Hunayn was a typical text used in the examination of ophthalmologists, the musculoskeletal section of Paul of Aegina for bonesetters, *The Trial of the Physician* by Hunayn for physicians, Galen and Albucasis on wounds for surgeons.[21] A number of medical texts were specifically written on how to examine doctors, including works by al-Razi, Galen and Hunayn.[22] It has been stated that medical licensing in the kingdom of Jerusalem was of poor

---

[19] Leiser 1983.   [20] 'Abd al-Rahman 1999.
[21] Karmi 1979; Levey 1963; 'Abd al-Rahman 1999 pp. 116–17.   [22] Iskandar 1962; Karmi 1979.

quality compared with the Islamic *hisba* system, based on the argument that
the local bishop was responsible for assessing the applicant.[23] However, it
was not just the bishop but also a panel of respected local doctors who performed the examination. In any case, a significant proportion of *physici* from
Europe were also clergy and so there was a reasonable chance that a Latin
bishop would have some knowledge of medicine himself. No evidence has
yet come to light that might suggest that the standards required to obtain
a licence in Frankish towns were any different from those in neighbouring Islamic areas. Certainly the details in the medical negligence clauses
discussed below do suggest that a high standard of medical knowledge was
expected.

Medical licensing in Europe began in the twelfth century but only started
to become widespread in the thirteenth and fourteenth centuries. It was
once thought that King Roger II of Sicily gave the masters of Salerno the
right to license medical practitioners from 1127, but this document was
subsequently identified as a forgery dating from the fifteenth century.[24]
However, the Assises collection of Roger II dated to 1140 did briefly state
that doctors were required to undergo examination before they were given
a licence that entitled them to practise in the kingdom of Sicily.[25] By the
1220s universities such as Bologna were granting degrees to those students
who successfully completed their course of studies in medicine and this
was another form of evidence available to demonstrate medical skill. The
legislation of Emperor Frederick II Hohenstaufen in 1231 was based on the
previous laws of Roger II and confirmed the use of medical licensing in
Italy by that time.[26] These statutes give much more detail than those of
Roger II and show that the licences were given by the government, not by
each town. This was in contrast to the situation in the Latin East, where a
licence was only valid in the town where it was issued. Under Frederick II
doctors were required to have written proof that they had undergone the
required number of years of study as well as demonstrating adequate knowledge in an examination. Those who practised without a licence were to be
imprisoned for a year and have their belongings confiscated.[27] This was
much harsher than the penalty in the Latin East, where the offending
doctor was merely beaten out of town. A large number of the licences from
Naples have now been identified and edited.[28]

In France comparable legislation was also introduced around this time.
While the university in Paris was issuing degrees to successful students from

[23] Kirsch 1969.   [24] Kristeller 1945.
[25] *Liber Augustalis* 1854 pp. 149–50; *Liber Augustalis* 1971 pp. 130–1.
[26] Hartung 1934; Sigerist 1935.
[27] *Liber Augustalis* 1854 pp. 149–50; *Liber Augustalis* 1971 pp. 130–1.   [28] *Fonti per la Storia* 1962.

around 1220, the problem remained as to how to regulate those practitioners who had trained via apprenticeship rather than via the academic route. From the 1250s the city provost formed a panel of respected surgeons and these men examined those who wished to practise surgery in the city.[29] The successful surgeons were issued with a licence, but the difficulties in enforcing such legislation meant that illicit practice in the city continued for some time. In Spain it was only at the end of the thirteenth century that good evidence for licensing in the Christian kingdoms has come to light. This is despite the proximity to the Islamic kingdom of Granada, which would have followed the *hisba* system. In the crown of Aragon the first evidence so far identified for medical licensing with the examination of physicians and surgeons dates from 1289. In this law King Alfons III extended to doctors the same licensing procedure already in place for other professionals such as lawyers. The examinations were to be performed in each town and the text implies that the assessment panel would be local doctors and town councillors. By the fourteenth century the examination involved the applicant reading a passage from an appropriate medical text chosen by the examiners, with subsequent discussion of the text providing the required evidence of the applicant's knowledge and experience. The procedure was the same for practitioners of any religion, whether they were Christian, Jewish or Muslim.[30]

MEDICAL NEGLIGENCE

In Frankish towns a medical practitioner who had obtained a licence was still required to maintain satisfactory standards in his work. In the kingdom of Jerusalem it seems that this would have been the responsibility of the *mathessep*. The master sergeant in this post assisted the viscount of the court and commanded a company of armed men who supported him in his role. The earliest legal commentary to mention the *mathessep* is a fourteenth-century text from Cyprus accompanying the *Assises*, known as the *Abrégé*.[31] However, there is evidence that the post was in existence well before this, both on the mainland and in Cyprus itself. A report of 1243 from the bailiff of the Venetian quarter in Tyre to the doge of Venice mentions the 'matesep' of Tyre.[32] Interestingly, it explains how the Venetians were unhappy that this *mathessep* imposed the same rules for the Venetians as the rest of the city, despite their protected status there. The matter was resolved by the Venetians creating their own *mathessep* with jurisdiction over just

[29] Bullough 1958; Jacquart 1994; O'Boyle 1994.
[30] Garcia-Ballester 1989; McVaugh 1993 pp. 69–72, 95–103.
[31] *Assises de Jérusalem* 1843 pp. 236–44.   [32] Marsilio Zorzi 1991 p. 140; Glick 1971.

their own quarter, a man named John of Palermo. Another 'mataseb' is mentioned in 1301 and 1302 in Famagusta, in Cyprus. One document mentions the building he used as his base, while the other mentions his name as Laurencius de Pas.[33] The likelihood that the *mathessep* was a Frankish version of the Islamic *muhtasib*[34] suggests that this was another example of how the crusaders adopted some of the good ideas in practice in the eastern Mediterranean on their arrival. Exactly the same process occurred in Spain. The Islamic post of *muhtasib* was modified by the Christians of Castile to become the *almotacen* in the twelfth century and when King James I of Aragon conquered Valencia in 1238 the *muhtasib* became the Christian *mustaçaf*.[35]

The *muhtasib* is known to have been present in cities of the Islamic world at least by the ninth century and by the eleventh century a number of manuals were available.[36] The *muhtasib* was responsible for ensuring high standards in all aspects of public life, known as *hisba*.[37] This included commercial transactions in the marketplace, workplace health and safety, moral and religious purity, also included in his remit was medical practice. In consequence it was not merely sufficient for a medical practitioner to prove that he knew how to practise safely, which was tested when he obtained a licence, but also that he was trustworthy enough to treat appropriately. For example, the constituents of medicines were tested to ensure they contained the drugs stated and were not diluted or substituted with worthless plants, while the weights used in the pharmacy to ensure that the correct amount was given to the patient were also checked. It seems that the medical negligence legislation from the kingdom of Jerusalem was a way of both Latinising and supporting the Islamic *muhtasib* function, by placing it within a Frankish legal framework, backed by the state.

Medical negligence is often presumed to have been commonplace in the ancient and medieval world, although research has shown that this was by no means always the case. In classical Greece a medical practitioner could in theory be charged with murder if he was believed to have killed his patient, but there was no specific medical legislation to cover negligence.[38] In the Roman empire codices such as the *Lex Aquilia* demonstrate that there were facilities for redress for the victims of malpractice, but the law was ill defined and did not give the patient much protection. For example, there was no penalty in Roman law for the negligent killing of a freeman by a medical

---

[33] Lamberto de Sambuceto [Pavoni] 1982, p. 42, doc. 33; Lamberto de Sambuceto [Pavoni] 1987 p. 79, doc. 57.
[34] Conrad 1999.   [35] Glick 1971; Vernia 1988.
[36] 'Abd al-Rahman 1999; Karmi 1979; Vernia 1988.   [37] Levey 1963.   [38] Amundsen 1977.

practitioner.[39] The only mention of medical negligence in the seventh-century Visigoth medical regulations refers to the cash compensation to be paid if a patient lost too much blood during phlebotomy.[40] There is a fair amount of evidence for court cases in Europe from the end of the thirteenth century century and later[41] and there is even evidence for malpractice insurance for high risk cases.[42] However, twelfth- and early thirteenth-century Europe has left little record in this respect. The contrast between the seventh- and fourteenth-century evidence suggests that it was exactly at this time that medical negligence legislation appears to have evolved so dramatically in Europe. It would be interesting to know exactly what counted as negligence and what was done about it if a practitioner was found guilty. This point highlights just how important the Frankish regulations are for modern research, while also explaining the difficulty in finding appropriate comparisons for comment.

It has been suggested that the medical negligence clauses in the *Assises de Jerusalem* were a version of the *Lex Aquilia*.[43] However, this very early Roman legal code was really about damage to property, and reference to medical negligence was restricted to slaves on account of their financial value.[44] The Frankish code does cover the loss of value of a disabled slave, but it also covers many other areas too. While I can see that these two texts share some aspects in common, the similarities are rather basic. Not only is the information defining negligence very much more specific in the Frankish commentary, but a completely new emphasis is added. In the *Lex Aquilia* the purpose was to compensate the owner for the loss of value of his slave, while the Frankish code adds the concept of actually punishing a medical practitioner for poor standards of treatment, regardless of any financial loss caused. The practitioner could be beaten and humiliated around his home town, he could be banished from the town, he could suffer amputation of his right thumb, or even be hanged. This is so different from the financial aims of the *Lex Aquilia* that any link between the two must be seen as rather distant. Frankish perspectives of right and wrong in this context seem more comparable with modern attitudes to medical negligence than Roman ones. Clearly, early legal codes mentioning medical negligence would have been known to medieval legal experts, and would often have influenced medieval legislation. However, if the Frankish text did indeed have its origins in the *Lex Aquilia*, then a considerable degree of evolution had occurred prior to the writing of the Jerusalem code.

---

[39] Amundsen 1973.   [40] Amundsen 1971.
[41] Cosman 1972; Post 1972; Cosman 1973; Shatzmiller 1989.
[42] Cosman 1982.   [43] Prawer 1980 p. 370.   [44] Amundsen 1973

In the *Assises de Jerusalem* the medical negligence clauses follow a standard pattern. Each example starts with the nature of the disease, continues with the agreement between the doctor and whoever is paying the bill, goes on to mention the potential poor outcomes of treatment and concludes with the punishment appropriate for each example. Medical treatments described vary from oral medications and enemas to bloodletting. Surgical treatments included cranial surgery for fracture, cautery for haemorrhoids, drainage of peritoneal fluid for ascites (dropsy), wound care with poultices, and the manipulation and splinting of fractures (Figure 15). The complications mentioned are sometimes not described in medical texts of the era, suggesting that the examples were based on actual cases heard previously in the court. For example, the complication of anal stenosis from cautery of haemorrhoids is not mentioned in Paulus Aegineta, Albucasis or Theodorich Borgognoni.[45] Archaeological evidence suggests that some of these procedures may have been undertaken successfully in areas where doctors were available. A number of tibial fractures were identified from the excavation of crusaders and Frankish settlers from the city of Caesarea[46] and all had healed straight, not at an angle indicating negligence.

It is interesting that certain diseases were exempt from accusations of negligence, with the examples mentioned in the regulations including measles and dry ulcers. These exceptions may have been introduced as they were conditions that medieval treatments would have found difficult to cure. The low success rate is also suggested by the fact that the fee was dependent on success of treatment. Comparisons can be found in neighbouring regions such as Egypt. One example from the Cairo Geniza documents is a case where a doctor named 'Makarim ibn Ishaq was to be paid for operating on a girl's eye if her sight recovered, but would not be liable for any consequences should the procedure not go well.[47] Other factors that precluded a conviction of negligence were if the doctor was unable to visit his patient on account of his own illness or capture by Saracens. Similarly, if the patient undertook a lifestyle against the advice of the doctor, perhaps eating the wrong food or engaging in sexual activity, then this precluded a conviction regardless of whether the doctor also performed substandard treatment. The evidence required to lead to a conviction could come from a number of sources. The most important were eye witnesses, either the patient if still alive or his or her relatives or friends who were present at each consultation. More than one witness was required as the doctor could not

---

[45] Paulus Aegineta, 1846, II, p. 403; Albucasis 1973 p. 512; Theodorich Borgognoni 1498 p. 135r–v; Theodorich Borgognoni 1960, II, pp. 111–14.
[46] Smith 1999.   [47] Baker 1996.

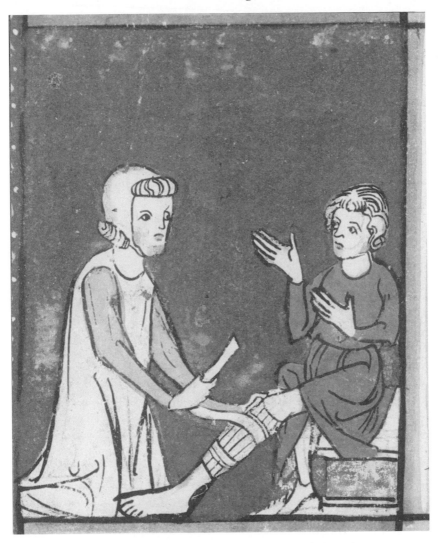

Figure 15. Application of a splint for an injury to the lower leg
This illustration from a thirteenth-century European medical text also demonstrates
the attire of a Frankish practitioner.
British Library MS Sloane 1977 fol. 9r. *Livres de Cyrurgie* (middle left image). Illustrations
preceding the surgical text of Roger of Parma. By permission of the British Library.

be convicted on the unsupported word of one accuser. Interestingly, the patient could claim that 'because the doctor had given him such things he felt strongly in his body that he would die' (see Professor Nutton's translation below) and this could be accepted as evidence of substandard practice by the doctor. The medieval Islamic *hisba* manuals describe how the family of a patient who died was able to go to the chief doctor in the town for an assessment of the treatment of their deceased relative. The chief doctor would look at copies of the prescriptions written during the illness and give judgment as to whether he felt the doctor treated the patient appropriately or was guilty of negligence.[48] However, there is no mention of the use of any such written prescriptions in the Frankish regulations.

The punishment suffered by a guilty doctor varied markedly depending on the circumstances. In general the fundamental facts of importance were whether the patient died or merely suffered disability due to the treatment, and secondly whether the patient was a slave or free member of the population. If the patient was a slave then the negligent doctor had to pay the owner the value of the slave if he or she died, or the drop in the slave's value if disabled. However, if the patient were free then the doctor suffered mutilation if the patient suffered disability and was hanged if the patient died. To add further insult to the process, as well as act as a warning to others, the condemned man would be beaten through the town for all to see, holding his urine flask in his hand so that everyone knew he was a doctor. The choice of mutilation was removal of the right thumb, rather than castration, nasal excision or blinding, which were also common punishments of the time. It is presumed that removing the thumb would prevent continued medical practice, as it would have been very difficult to perform any therapeutic procedures unless the doctor happened to be left handed.

While the cases of medical negligence recorded in the *Assises* are likely to have taken place over a number of years, it is not known whether they date from over the entire existence of the kingdom or just the last decades prior to 1240. One consequence of this is that it is difficult to know exactly how views changed over time in the way we might if each case was dated. One possible approach for future research might be to identify dated examples in historical records of the treatment of those diseases covered in the statutes and compare how closely practice followed the legal advice.[49] If the early cases showed marked contrasts followed by later convergence between

[48] Levey 1963.   [49] See Amundsen 1974 n. 24.

historical cases and the legislation, then it might suggest that the legislation may have been introduced around the time of the later historical case.

SUMMARY

Medical licensing in the Latin East appears to have been adopted from the local *hisba* system that was in force when the Franks arrival. The Frankish *mathessep* was the individual appointed by the court to ensure satisfactory standards for a range of craftsmen and professions, presumably including the medical profession. While we know for sure that licensing was standard practice by the 1240s, the evidence as to exactly when it was adopted is lacking. In consequence it remains unknown whether the practice in the kingdom of Jerusalem predated the regulations of Roger II of Sicily in 1140. Whether or not the crusaders were the first Europeans to adopt medical licensing, by the mid-thirteenth century the Franks in the kingdom of Jerusalem certainly possessed a complex system of medical regulations to assess medical practice and accusations of medical negligence. These were based on case law and the observation that some of the complications were not included in contemporary medical texts suggests that they were summaries of previous cases that had been to court, not merely details extracted from these books. The information given on procedures and unacceptable complications demonstrates that a surprisingly high standard of theoretical knowledge and practical skills was expected of medical practitioners of the time. Physicians had to bleed their febrile patients on the correct day for each illness and give the appropriate strength purgatives for their condition, while surgeons were required to remove bone fragments from skull fractures without damaging the brain and to treat broken long bones in plaster without leaving the bones to heal malaligned. None of these activities would have been easy even for experienced, well-trained practitioners. This suggests that charlatans, con men and bogus doctors would have experienced great difficulty if they tried to bluff their way through such a system to obtain a licence.

Frankish Medical Licensing and Negligence Regulations from the Livre des Assises de la Cour des Bourgeois

Translated by Vivian Nutton

From a fourteenth-century manuscript in E. H. Kausler (ed.),
Les Livres des Assises et des Usages dou Reaume de Jerusalem sive Leges et Instituta Regni Hierosolymitani. Stuttgart: Adolf Krabbe 1839, I, docs. CCXXXI and CCXXXIII.

CH. 231. THE LAW REGULATING SURGERY

Here you will have the account of all doctors, usually of wounds, who medicate or cut an injured person other than one should and hence the injured person dies, what right one has of that doctor.

If it happens that I accidentally injure my servant, man or woman, or someone else injures them and I bring in a doctor and that doctor contracts with me for a fixed sum and tells me on the third day after seeing the wound that he will cure it without fail; and it happens that he cuts it badly or cuts for something that should not be cut and then he dies; or if he should have cut the wound along the lips or along the swelling and he makes a cross cut, so that he dies; reason judges and commands us to judge that that doctor must pay for the servant, male or female, the value on the day he was injured or the price for which he was bought, for this is the law and reasoning of the Assise. And the court should order the doctor to leave the town where he effected that bad treatment.

Likewise, if my servant had a wound in a hot place or in a place to which hot things are appropriately applied, like the brain or the nerves or on joints which are of a cold nature, and he always applies cold things and the slave dies, reason judges and commands us to judge that he is obliged to pay for that slave, man or woman, for that is right and reasonable.

Likewise, if my servant had a swelling in a dangerous place and it required emollients to soften, break down and remove the problem and the doctor

Professor Vivian Nutton is at the Wellcome Trust Centre for the History of Medicine at UCL, University of London.

applies heating and dry things so that the problem gets worse and he dies, reason judges that he is by law responsible for compensation.

Likewise, if my servant has a head wound with the bone broken and he doesn't know how to remove the pieces, so that the broken bone pierces the brain so that he dies, reason adjudges that he is legally bound to pay for the servant.

Likewise, if my servant had a wound in the head or in the upper arm or in any dangerous place and the doctor was one or two days without treating it, or he used so many heating substances with the result that the top of the arm or thigh became infected, or the wound putrefied, or because he could not stay to treat him daily and the man dies, reason judges and commands that the doctor must repay me as much as the servant cost, for that is the law and judgment by the Assise of Jerusalem.

Likewise, if the doctor can show in court, with good guarantee, that he whom he treated lay with a woman or drank wine or ate some bad food that he had forbidden him, or did anything other than he should, reason judges and commands to judge that even if the doctor should still have treated him differently from what he should have done, he is not held liable to pay compensation, for the most expert argument is that he died from doing what was forbidden him, not through a poor doctor, and that is the reason and judgement of the Assise. But if a doctor had not stopped him from eating or drinking, or touching a woman and he did so, or ate or drank when he ought not and he dies, reason adjudges that the doctor is rightly held to pay compensation since the doctor is rightly liable, on seeing the sick, to tell him what to eat and what not; and if he does not and an accident happens that is the doctor's responsibility.

But if the doctor himself, once taking over the care and treatment himself met with misfortune, being captured by the Saracens or falling ill or something else that prevented him from visiting the sick and he died, reason adjudges that in law the doctor is not liable for compensation.

And if a doctor had wrongly treated, as above, a free man or woman who died, reason adjudges that the doctor should be lawfully hung and his property should belong to the lord. But if he had received anything from the dead man, the doctor's property should be handed over to the deceased's relatives, for that is right and reasonable.

Likewise, if a doctor treated a servant, male or female, for a broken arm or leg and said that he would cure it completely, as would be the case if he had acted properly, and he made a solemn covenant but then broke it and acted badly, applying useless plasters which left men forever crippled, reason judges that the doctor is liable to take the servant and pay his master what he cost. If he cannot pay all, reason adjudges further that he must leave the servant with his lord or lady and instead should pay as much as the value of that servant, male or female, has fallen, for he has been left injured by his intervention. If he crippled a Christian man or woman, reason adjudges that he should lose his right thumb and owe no further damages so long as he took nothing for treatment, otherwise he is rightly responsible for giving it back.

CH. 233. THE LAW REGULATING PHYSIC

Here you will have the reason and law of medicines and of the activities of physicians who give the sick a syrup, drug or electuary from which he dies as a result of bad treatment.

If it happens by misadventure that my slave, man or woman, falls ill and a doctor goes to his lord or lady and says that he will cure him and agrees a fee with the lord, and then if the doctor gives laxatives or heating substance by which the seat of the disease is all putrefied and he betakes himself to bed; and if he should have given him astringents and cold substances and did not, with the result that he died, reason judges and commands to judge that the doctor is liable to give me another servant or the amount he was worth on the day he died, and that is the law and judgement of the Assise.

Likewise, if my servant should be ill with fever so that he has great heat within his body, and the doctor bleeds him before the due time and removes too much blood so that, both by the weakness of the fever that he has so disturbed and by the bleeding, the fever climbed into the head of the patient, he relapsed and died, reason commands to judge that the doctor is held liable in law and by the Assise to pay compensation to the value of the servant, male or female, on the day of death, or what he cost when first bought, for this is the right and judgement of the Assise.

Item, if my slave should become cold and have a cold disease and a doctor comes and says to his lord, 'I'll cure him', and contracts with his lord and takes up the cure, and if it happens that he is bled for his coldness and this happens because of his ignorance of urine, and failure to judge, and the patient becomes entirely dry, loses his voice or is dried worse because of his previous chill and by the bleeding which had been done, and he dies, reason adjudges and commands that he should be liable to pay to the lord or lady in law as much as he had cost, for this is the reason and judgement of the Assises.

Likewise, if I had a servant, male or female, with dropsy, possessing an enlarged belly, and a doctor is contracted to cure and this doctor taps the belly where the illness is and then doesn't know how to let out the water that was inside, but lets all the fluid come out at the first or second occasion, and the patient is so weakened that he loses his breath and dies, reason judges and commands to judge that the doctor should replace the servant, male or female, by law and by the Assise.

Likewise, if my slave was ill with a quotidian fever, hot and cold, and a doctor comes to his lord or lady and says he will cure him by the application of a drug and agrees with the lord to do so and takes the servant into his care, and then he gives the drug at prime or at midnight and in this drug there was so much scammony that it was so strong that he died, just as if he had drunk it; or if he went to the toilet before it was day and vomited all he had in him, heart, bowels and lungs, and died; or if the doctor had not diagnosed the illness as he should but gave him medicine and he could not go out, reason adjudges that he died of the aforesaid signs and that the doctor must pay compensation in law and by the Assise.

Likewise, if my servant has a bowel disease and a doctor comes and says he will cure it and agrees with the lord or lady and takes the cure in hand, and if it happens that he gives him a powder or strong herb to drink, and he drinks it and dies, reason judges him liable, in reason and law, to pay compensation.

Likewise, if my servant has a bowel disease and a doctor undertakes the cure, and if he takes a very hot iron and wants to cure the haemorrhoids from which the illness comes, and he does not know how to do it so that he burns and makes the end of the bowel damaged at the rectum so that the bowel constricts itself and closes with the cauterisation so that he can no more open his bowels and dies, reason judges and commands to judge that the doctor is bound to pay compensation for that servant, lawfully, for what the lord paid for him.

Item, if my slave is ill with measles, or a dry ulcer or some other disease and I come to a doctor and contract for his cure so that half of the money for which he is sold will be his and the other is that of the owner, and the doctor undertakes the cure and does what he can, to no avail, and he dies, reason judges that the doctor is not liable to pay compensation for the servant, male or female, since he loses all his work in the first place and all that he was going to have; and that is the right and judgment of the Assise.

Likewise, if a doctor has treated in this way a free man or woman, reason judges and commands the doctor be hung, even when he is the doctor to the lord of the land. But before being hung, he must be beaten through the town, urine flask in hand, for that is right and reasonable, to warn others of his crime, for that is the right and reason of the court.

Know well that in all these crimes there should be witnesses, so that if the doctor is accused, if he denies having acted in the above way, these witnesses will swear by the saints that they saw him before them treat this patient with these drugs or syrups and that this is why the patient who had another disease died, and they heard the patient say that because the doctor had given him such things he felt strongly in his body that he would die. Then the doctor ought to be tried for the murder either of the servant, for which he should pay compensation, or of a Christian, for which he should be hung, as said above, for that is right. For otherwise the doctor ought not to be tried on the unsupported word of people or of the patient.

Besides, no foreign doctor, that is one coming from Outremer or pagan lands, should practise as a urine doctor until he has been examined by other doctors, the best in the land, in the presence of the bishop of the place wherein this is to be done. If it is recognised that he can correctly practise medicine, the bishop will give him a licence to treat in that particular town where he will see, from the bishop's letter which he will have as testimony, that doctors are proven and can rightly treat by means of urine. And that is the right and reason of the Assise of Jerusalem.

Likewise, if it turns out that he is a poor doctor who cannot practise, reason adjudges that the bishop and court should order him to leave the city or if not, that he should remain without practising on anyone. If it happens that a doctor practises in the town without the leave of the court or bishop, the court should arrest him and beat him out of town, according to the law and decision of the Assise of Jerusalem.

Conclusion

The evidence discussed here is illuminating at a number of different levels. On a personal level it can be used to understand the experiences of an individual wounded crusader both on the battlefield and during his convalescence. With a wider view we can assess the role of medical practitioners and health care institutions in the Latin East and how they functioned. From a yet broader perspective the evidence gives an improved understanding of the interaction between Europe, the Byzantine empire, the Islamic world and the fusion of these influences upon health care in the Frankish states. To further understand the topic, these areas have been investigated in a cross-sectional manner with comparisons between different regions, and also using a time dependent approach to highlight how the situation changed over the 200-year history of the states. A broad range of sources, both textual and archaeological, have been consulted in an attempt to obtain as objective and accurate a view as possible. Rather than just relying on one type of evidence, consulting such varied sources in theory reduces the chance that conclusions will be inaccurate and misleading.

Furthermore, I have tried hard to resist becoming inappropriately positivist in my interpretation. There is often a temptation to infer too much when investigating a topic such as this. Unlike some others in the past I have not over-interpreted the proportion of hospitals providing medical care, I have not made unsubstantiated claims over the efficacy of medical treatments, I have not assumed that the range of treatments used was as extensive as in medical texts of the period and I have not assumed that all anecdotes in the texts were actually true. However, the integration here of the information relevant to injuries, surgery and medical treatment in the crusades has demonstrated a fascinating aspect of life in the medieval eastern Mediterranean that has been little understood before now. What is perhaps even more instructive is how accurate, or otherwise, many of the widely held modern views regarding medicine in the crusades appear to be. While some of these views do have evidence to support them, others have few or no facts behind them and have been perpetuated by unquestioning authors. Others still are flatly in contradiction to the available information and must surely now be laid aside for good.

It seems sensible to consider first the established opinions that do appear to be supported by sound evidence. The hospital in the Frankish states does seem to have been a major step forward for medieval Europeans who emigrated to the eastern Mediterranean. The evidence suggests that the Franks initially established European-style *hospitalia* in the Latin East, which did not provide active medical treatment. Over the decades they adopted Eastern ideas on the role of the hospital, and a number of medicomilitary orders were providing medical treatment by the end of the twelfth century. Several decades after these changes in the East, there was an evolution in the role of the hospital in Europe so that from the thirteenth century onwards the medical function began to be adopted there too. The European houses of these medicomilitary orders, along with the positive experiences of Eastern hospitals held by returning crusaders, seem likely routes for this change in medieval Europe. Another opinion which has largely held up to expectation is that of the importance of Frankish medical legislation. It is the earliest surviving detailed legislation on medical negligence in the Latin world and in consequence is of unique value.

As expected, there is considerable evidence for trauma in the crusades and this has come from both written and archaeological sources. Much of the trauma occurred on the battlefield, where the weapons of the time were highly effective in causing disability and death. Some were also inflicted in the torture chamber and this highlights the levels to which those in power would stoop to extract information or punish their enemies. A further expected source of trauma was the court of law, where mutilation and capital punishment were well-accepted sentences. There is also sound evidence for the practice of emergency surgery for the treatment of a wide variety of wounds and other serious injuries. Yet another expected finding is that I have been unable to discover much evidence for Muslim medical practitioners at work within the Frankish states. In a Latin Christian-dominated society it might be expected that those Muslims with a transferable profession such as medicine would have moved across the border to work elsewhere, in an atmosphere where they would not be intimidated or discriminated against. Of course, the absence of such named individuals in the Latin sources may merely reflect the perspective of the sources I have been able to use. It is possible that Muslims did work there but that the evidence for this was only recorded in Arabic texts which are not widely known today. However, the presence of other non-Christian practitioners such as Jews are attested to in these Latin sources, and consequently the silence regarding Muslim practitioners may be suggesting that few worked in the Latin East compared with members of other cultural groups.

However, we are still left with a considerable number of widely held concepts regarding crusader and Frankish medicine which seem to be either unsubstantiated or in some cases frankly incorrect. I have been unable to find any evidence that convinces me that a typical Frankish medical practitioner in the Latin East was technically any better or worse at treating a patient than one of their Jacobite, Jewish or Muslim colleagues. There is fairly limited evidence with which to examine this problem, but in my opinion the evidence which has come to light so far does not support the widely held view that Frankish practitioners from Europe were ignorant and technically inferior to those who learnt their medicine in the East. Another point worth discussing is that of medieval dissection and autopsy. It is commonly thought that autopsy and medical dissection of humans by Latin practitioners first began in Italy in the 1280s. However, at a much earlier date (1103) we have the case of the wounding of King Baldwin in battle, which is followed by an attempt to perform an autopsy on a Muslim prisoner given a similar wound. While the prisoner was spared and a bear used for the same purpose, both events were highly unusual in the Latin world this early and should be of great interest to those studying the history of anatomy and dissection. Incidentally, such ingenuity and innovation appears in stark contrast to the concept of the ignorant and incompetent crusading doctor.

Another concept at odds with the evidence is why hardly any modern authors mention the involvement of European medical practitioners in the crusades, with the consequence that few of the elite are presumed to have gone east. This study has shown how a significant number of master physicians and surgeons went east on expeditions, as well as the less well educated practitioners. It is possible that medieval authors did not bother recording this information in many cases, as it may have been sufficiently common an occurrence to be regarded as unremarkable. Consequently, the effects of the experience on so many of those leading practitioners who subsequently guided the evolution of medicine in Europe have largely gone unnoticed by modern researchers. This thought leads on to the preconceptions regarding the role of the crusades as a portal for the exchange of medical knowledge between cultures. While it is typically implied that the Frankish states come a very poor third after Sicily and Spain in the transfer of such information between Europe and other cultures, the find-ings here suggest otherwise. This preconception, which I believe to be also a misconception, is based on the fact that the major criterion often used for assessing the importance of each of these routes is the translation of medical texts from Arabic into Latin. Little weight is given to the practi-cal skills learnt by European practitioners while on crusade, the changing function of the hospital, the licensing of practitioners and a whole host of other areas where the Europeans in the Latin East adopted new ideas which subsequently became common practice in Europe. I think it is no longer reasonable to perceive the Frankish states as of little importance in the exchange of medical knowledge in the medieval Mediterranean, as it seems clear that they acted as a route for different kinds of knowledge than was the case for the translating centres in Spain and Italy.

A number of accepted views regarding the medieval hospital are also unsupported by the evidence discussed here. There is no evidence to suggest that the Hospital of St John, or any other Frankish institution in the Latin East, was providing medical care in the early years after the conquest. This only happened a number of decades later, and when it did it was in addition to, and not in place of, the core function of providing food and accommodation for pilgrims. The earliest suggestion which I have been able to identify for this evolution is in a text written some time between 1128 and 1237, while the earliest specific mention of actual medical practitioners in these hospitals is from the 1180s. Another point of contention is that several works have stated that the teachings of Salerno were the dominant influence upon medical practice in the hospitals of the Frankish states. However, the investigation of dietary modification for inpatients contradicts this, and suggests that by the late twelfth century it was probably Eastern, rather than European, ideas which dominated. Yet another unsubstantiated belief regarding hospitals in the crusades is that the wounded were left to fend for themselves if they were unable to hire a doctor to treat them. In fact, the mobile field hospital of the Order of St John and the field hospitals spontaneously established during the Third Crusade show how this was by no means the case. A further unsubstantiated view is that planned, elective surgery was used rarely in the medieval period, and that analgesia was not employed because of the risk of killing the patient. A number of elective operations have been described from written Frankish sources and the use of opium by medical practitioners is also highlighted. I do believe that less elective surgery was performed than emergency surgery for trauma, and that elective operations were generally the safer options available. However, it does nevertheless demonstrate that the practice of surgery was by no means limited to the treatment of injuries.

Why should there be so many misconceptions regarding medicine in the crusades? When so many other subspecialisms within the history of medicine have moved on from the attitudes of a century ago, crusader medicine is still in almost the same place in many respects. There are many reasons for this, as we might expect. The complicated nature of the study of the crusades, as outlined in the introduction, means that there has been less scholarly work performed on this topic than for mainland Europe over the same time period. Numerous modern books on medical practice, hospitals and medical training focus on medieval England, France, Italy and Spain but this is the first ever book on crusader medicine. Secondly, the articles written on medicine in the Frankish states can broadly be grouped into two. The first group questions the old ideas and looks for evidence in original sources in the assessment of their hypothesis. The second takes well established ideas as written in stone and states them as fact, when the original evidence upon which they were based is open to differing interpretations or is even never quoted. Unfortunately, far too many articles in the latter group have been written over the years. Despite the fact that the views passed on from one article to the next have no validity, their influence is still felt. A third factor behind these misconceptions, to which we are all vulnerable, is that researchers may not be looking in the right places for the evidence. As time passes new sources of information will always become available, often demonstrating how unbalanced the conclusions of the past actually were. Further research in well-targeted areas may result in our having to rethink some of our ideas once again in the years to come.

There are still many aspects of Frankish medicine of which we have little or no knowledge, and these topics would be ideal targets for further work. Only those conditions associated with warfare, trauma and surgery have been investigated in detail in this book, although certain related topics such as the exchange of knowledge with the crusades and Frankish medical legislation have also been reviewed. In a subsequent book I intend to investigate those diseases and medical conditions which have not been discussed here. This will assess topics such as malnutrition, infectious disease and epidemics, parasites, mental illness and the spread of disease with the crusades. The work will also address the various attitudes to disease held by the educated elite, the less educated general population and the clergy, along with the role of the *physicus* in medical treatment in the Latin East. One significant limitation on the evidence presented here is the preponderance of evidence from European or Latin sources. There is much less evidence from Eastern sources. This is partly because most of the published texts concerning the crusades are those of Latin authors. Another factor is that my linguistic skills do not stretch to Arabic, Armenian, Greek or Syriac, so these sources are not as well covered as I would like. Future work by scholars with the skills to investigate manuscripts in these languages has the potential to demonstrate a completely different perspective on medicine in the crusades, that of the Eastern practitioner. Past compilations of medical practitioners in England and France have highlighted many of the individuals known to have participated in the crusades. However, no such comprehensive study of German or Italian practitioners has yet been published. When this work is undertaken we would expect a significant number of further individuals to be identified as having taken part in a crusade.

Study of manuscripts in library archives continues to identify unexpected texts, either because they are bound together with other material or they have been mislabelled or miscatalogued in the past. Future systematic surveys of such material may well highlight new sources of evidence for those interested in medicine in the time of the crusades. Certainly the medical manuscripts from the Latin East recently highlighted by Emilie Savage-Smith and Charles Burnett show the success of this approach. The publication of editions of sources which are at present only in manuscript form should also be of great potential benefit. Collections of documents which might seem at first glance to be of limited appeal can have a tremendous impact upon a variety of fields of scholarship. The notarial records of Lamberto di Sambuceto have incidentally highlighted a large number of practitioners such as barbers, apothecaries and surgeons in Frankish Cyprus, groups that are rarely mentioned in other types of manuscript. Study of similar documents originating from other parts of the Latin East may well be just as illuminating.

On a different note, it was most surprising to find that so little is known about field hospitals on the medieval battlefield. While there is a small amount of information on them in the Islamic world and now firm evidence for the Latin East, there is a conspicuous absence of information regarding field hospitals in past studies of military medicine in early medieval Europe. This may, of course, imply that there were no field hospitals at that time in Europe, but it may be merely that the sources for them have not come to our attention. An in-depth assessment of this topic might be a fruitful line of investigation in the future. The medical negligence laws from the kingdom of Jerusalem are also in need of more detailed research. There has been little comparison of these with either Arabic legislation and the Islamic *hisba* manuals, or with Byzantine legislation. It would be interesting to see whether the Frankish views on negligence concurred or contrasted with the rulings in other comparable codes, and whether the Franks were more or less rigorous in the standards they set for acceptable medical practice.

Finally, the archaeological excavations must continue to provide that evidence which the written record can never give. Enlarging the range of cemeteries examined in the Latin East will clearly increase the physical number of skeletal remains studied, and so allow statistical analyses not possible with data from small excavations. Larger numbers will also increase the chance of identifying rare diseases or operative procedures on bone that may only have been performed intermittently. Study at sites with differing characteristics, such as cities, villages, castles and battlefields, should allow us to investigate the health implications associated with such environments. As well as increasing the number of sites under study, we can also improve the way we study them. Progressive use of bioarchaeological techniques in partnership with other scientific specialisms allows much greater information to be gleaned from modern excavations. Whereas in the past an archaeologist would be satisfied merely to have recovered a pharmacy jar, now we can also study the contents to determine which medicines were kept in it. Instead of merely cleaning a medieval latrine block to allow its display for tourists, now we can also determine the parasites contained in the intestines of those who originally used the facilities. The use of such bioarchaeological techniques in the study of hospitals and other relevant sites has tremendous potential for the future.

If it is possible to summarise the evolution in medical care that took place during the lifetime of the Frankish states then comparison between military medicine at the start and end of the crusader period might be the simplest way. The practical recommendations for military health care contained in Arnold of Villanova's *Regimen Almarie* of 1310[1] must have evolved out of the harsh lessons learned on almost any medieval expedition, be it a crusade to the Middle East or Spain or alternatively in battles between rival powers in Europe itself. Had these rules been written two hundred years earlier then perhaps many of the worst moments in the history of crusading warfare might have been avoided. The huge death toll from infectious disease in the siege of Antioch on the First Crusade, in part a result of mosquitoes from the nearby marshes[2] and the floating dead in the water supply in the Seventh Crusade at Mansourah in Egypt[3] are perhaps two of the most noteworthy.

---

[1] McVaugh 1992.   [2] Albert of Aachen bk 3, ch. 40.
[3] John of Joinville 1874 pp. 158–60; John of Joinville 1955 p. 96.

Certainly, by the beginning of the fourteenth century there seems to have been a much greater awareness of how to minimise unnecessary deaths in an army on the march than was the case when the crusades began two hundred years before. Medicine in the Mediterranean world changed hugely from the eleventh to fourteenth centuries and the crusades must surely have played an important role in this transformation.

Bibliography

PRIMARY SOURCES

'Abd al-Rahman b. Nasr al-Shayzari. *The Book of the Islamic Market Inspector.* Ed. al-Sayyid al-Baz al-'Arimi, trans. R. P. Buckley. Oxford: Oxford University Press 1999.

Acta Aragonensia. Jaymes II (1291–1327). Ed. H. Finke, 3 vols. Basel: Scientia Verlag Aalen 1908.

Adam of Cremona. *Ärztliche Verhaltungsmassregeln auf dem Heerzug ins Heilige Land für Kaiser Friedrich II, Geschrieben von Adam v. Cremona (ca.1227).* Ed. F. Hönger. Borna-Leipzig: Buchdruckerei Robert Noske 1913.

Aggregationes de Crisi et Creticis Diebus. Medieval Prognosis and Astrology. Ed. C. O'Boyle. Cambridge: Wellcome Unit 1991.

Al-Samarqandī. *The Medical Formulary of Al-Samarqandī.* Ed. and trans. M. Levey and N. Al-Khaledy. Philadelphia: University of Pennsylvania 1967.

Albert of Aachen. *Historia Iherosolimitana.* Ed. and trans. S. Edgington. Oxford: Oxford Medieval Texts (in press).

Albucasis. *On Surgery and Instruments: a Definitive Edition of the Arabic Text of Albucasis, with English Translation.* Ed. and trans. M. S. Spink and G. L. Lewis. London: Wellcome Institute 1973.

Ambroise. *Estoire de la Guerre Sainte. Histoire en Vers de la Troisième Croisade (1190–1192).* Ed. G. Paris. Paris: L'Imprimerie Nationale 1897.

Ambroise. *The History of the Holy War,* in *Three Old French Chronicles of the Crusades,* pp. 1–160. Ed. G. Paris, trans. E. N. Stone. Washington: University of Washington 1939 .

Anatomia Porci Cophonis, in *Anatomical Texts of the Earlier Middle Ages,* pp. 48–53. Ed. G. W. Corner. Washington: Carnegie Institution 1927.

Annali Bolognesi. Ed. L. V. Savioli, 2 vols. Bassano 1784–9.

Archives de L'Hôtel-Dieu de Paris (1157–1300). Ed. L. Brièle. Paris: L'Imprimerie Nationale 1894, pp. 534–5.

Arnold of Villanova. *The Earliest Printed Book on Wine, by Arnold of Villanova [1235–1311].* Ed. and trans. H. E. Sigerist. New York: Schuman 1943.

Assises d'Antioch. Reproduites en Français. Ed. L. M. Alishan. Venice: Société Mekhithariste de Saint-Lazare 1876.

Assises de Jérusalem. Les Livres des Assises et des Usages dou Reaume de Jérusalem. Ed. E. H. Kausler, I. Stuttgart: Adolf Krabbe 1839.

Assises de Jérusalem. Ed. M. Beugnot, 2 vols. Recueil des Historiens des Croisades. Paris: Lois 1841–3.

Assizes of the Lusignan Kingdom of Cyprus. Ed. N. Coureas. Nicosia: Cyprus Research Centre 2002.

Avicenna. *A Treatise on the Canon of Medicine of Avicenna.* Ed. and trans. O. C. Gruner. London: Luzac 1930.

Barhebraeus (Gregorius Abul-Pharajius). *Historia Compendiosa Dynastiarum.* Ed. E. Pococke. Oxford 1663 (for an English translation of this text, see appendix in B. Z. Kedar and E. Kohlberg (1995), *Theodore of Antioch*).

Barhebraeus. *Chronicon Ecclesiasticum.* Ed. J. B. Abbeloos and T. J. Lamy, 3 vols. Louvain and Paris 1872–7.

Barhebraeus. *The Chronography of Gregory Abu'l-Faraj, 1225–1286.* Ed. and trans. E. A. W. Budge. Oxford: Oxford University Press 1932a.

Barhebraeus. *The Abridged Version of the Book of Simple Drugs of Ahmad Ibn Muhammad al-Ghâfiqî by Gregorius abu'l-Farag (Barhebraeus).* Ed. and trans. M. Meyerhof and G. P. Sobhy, 2 vols. Cairo: Al-Eltemad 1932b.

Baudouin d'Avensnes. Extraits de la chronique attribuée à Baudoin d'Avensnes, fils de la Comtesse Marguerite de Flandre. Ed. Guigniaut and de Wailly. In *Recueil de Historiens des Gaules et de la France*, XXI. Paris: L'Imprimerie Impériale 1855.

Beiträge zur Geschichte der Kreuzzüge. Ed. R. Röhricht. Berlin: Weidmannsche Buchhandlung 1874.

Benvenutus Grassus. *Benvenuti Grassi Hierosolimitani Doctoris Celeberrimi ac Expertissimi de Oculis eorumque Egritudinibus & Curis Feliciter Incipit.* Ed. Ferrara. Severinus 1474.

Benvenutus Grassus. *De Oculis Eorumque Egritudinibus et Curis.* Ed. Ferrara, trans. C. A. Wood. Stanford: Stanford University Press 1929.

Benvenutus Grassus. *The Wonderful Art of the Eye. A Critical Edition of the Middle English Translation of his De Probatissima Arte Oculorum.* Ed. and trans. L. M. Eldredge. Michigan: Michigan State Press 1996.

Calendar of Close Rolls Preserved in the Public Record Office. Edward I. AD 1272–1279. London: HMSO 1900, p. 247.

Calendar of the Patent Rolls Preserved in the Public Record Office. Edward I, AD 1272–1281. London: HMSO 1901, p. 200.

Calendar of the Patent Rolls Preserved in the Public Record Office. Henry III, AD 1247–1258. 56 vols. (1901–16). London: HMSO 1908, XLII, p. 623.

Calendar of the Patent Rolls Preserved in the Public Record Office. Henry III, AD 1258–1266. London: HMSO 1910, p. 276.

Calendar of the Patent Rolls Preserved in the Public Record Office. Henry III, AD 1266–1272. London: HMSO 1913.

Cambridge, Corpus Christi College Library, MS 26, fol. 3v–4r, 'the house of Saint Thomas the Martyr.

Canso d'Antioca: an Occitan Epic Chronicle of the First Crusade. Ed. and trans. C. Sweetenham and L. M. Paterson. Aldershot: Ashgate 2003.

Cartulaire de Notre-Dame de Chartres. Ed. E. De Lépinois and L. Merlet, 3 vols. Chartres: Garnier 1862–5.

Cartulaire Général de l'Ordre des Hospitaliers des Saint Jean de Jérusalem, 1100–1310. Ed. J. Delaville le Roulx, 4 vols. Paris: Ernest Leroux, 1894–1906.

Cartulaires du Bas-Poitou. Ed. P. Marchegay. Vendée, France: Les Roches-Baritaud 1877.

Cartulary of Oseney Abbey. Ed. H. E. Salter, 6 vols. Oxford: Oxford Historical Society 1929–36.

Chartularum Universitatis Parisiensis. Ed. H. Denifle, 4 vols. Paris 1889–97.

Chartulary of St John of Pontefract. Ed. R. Holmes, Record Series no. 2, 2 vols. Yorkshire Archaeological Society 1899–1902.

Chronique de Primat. Ed. J. du Vignay in *Recueil des Historiens des Gaules et de la France*, XXIII, pp. 1–106. Paris: L'Imprimerie Royale 1894.

Comte de Marsy (1884) Fragment d'un cartulaire de l'Ordre de Saint-Lazare en Terre Sainte. Documents. *Archives de l'Orient Latin* **2**: 121–57.

Continuation of William of Tyre. *La Continuation de Guillaume de Tyr (1184–1197)*. Ed. M. R. Morgan. Paris: Paul Geuthner 1982.

Continuation of William of Tyre, 1184–97. In *The Conquest of Jerusalem and the Third Crusade: Sources in Translation*, pp. 11–145. Ed. M. R. Morgan, trans. P. W. Edbury. Aldershot: Ashgate 1996.

De Claris Archigymnasii Bononiensis Professoribus. Ed. M. Sarti and M. Fattorini, 2 vols. Bologna 1886–96.

Decrees of the Ecumenical Councils. Ed. and trans. N. P. Tanner, 2 vols. London: Sheed & Ward 1990.

De Vita et Actibus Regis Francorum Ludovici et de Miraculis. Ed. Daunou and Naudet, In *Recueil des Historiens des Gaules et de la France*, XX. Paris: L'Imprimerie Royale 1840.

Die Statuten des Deutschen Ordens nach den altesten Handschriften. Ed. M. Perlbach. Halle: Max Niemeyer 1890.

Disciplinary Decrees of the General Councils: Text, Translation and Commentary. Ed. H. J. Schroeder. St Louis: Herder Brook 1937.

Documents Historiques Relatifs à la Vicomte de Carlat. Ed. G. Saige and Le Comte de Dienne. Monaco: Collection de Documents Historiques Publiés par Ordre de S. A. S. le Prince Albert Ie 1900.

Documents Illustrative of the Social and Economic History of the Danelaw. Ed. and trans. F. M. Stenton. London: Oxford University Press 1920.

Ernoul. *Chronicle d'Ernoul et de Bernard le Trésorier*. Ed. M. L. de Mas Latrie. Paris: Jules Renouard 1871.

Ernoul. *The Chronicle of Ernoul and Bernard the Treasurer*. In *The Conquest of Jerusalem and the Third Crusade: Sources in Translation*. Ed. M. L de Mas Latrie, trans. P. W. Edbury. Aldershot: Ashgate 1996.

Eudes de Champagne. In M. Malewicz (1974) Libellus de efficatia artis astrologice. Traité astrologique d'Eudes de Champagne, XIIe siècle. *Mediaevalia Philosophica Polonorum* **20**: 1–95 (includes discussion as well as the Latin text).

Fonti per la Storia della Medicina e della Chirurgia per il Regno di Napoli nel Periodo Angioino (a. 1273–1410). Ed. R. Calvanico. Naples: l'Arte Tipografica 1962.

Galen. *On Anatomical Procedures*. Ed. and trans. C. Singer. Oxford: Oxford University Press 1956.

Galvano de Levanto. In C. Kohler (1898), Traité du recouvrement de la Terre Sainte addresse, vers l'an 1295, à Philippe le Bel par Galvano de Levanto, médecin genois. *Revue de l'Orient Latin* **6**: 343–69 (discussion and Latin edition of the text).

Geoffrey of Villehardouin. *La Conquête de Constantinople*. Ed. E. Faral. Paris: Louis Halpen 1938.

Geoffrey of Villehardouin. *The Conquest of Constantinople*. In *Joinville and Villehardouin: Chronicles of the Crusades*. Trans. M. R. B. Shaw. Harmondsworth: Penguin 1963.

Gervase of Canterbury. *The chronicle of the reigns of Stephen, Henry II and Richard I*. Ed. W. Stubbs. *Rerum Britannicarum Medii Aevi Scriptores, or Chronicles and Memorials of Great Britain and Ireland During the Middle Ages*, Rolls series 73. London: Longman 1879.

Geschichte der Christlichen Arabischen Literatur. Ed. G. Graf, 5 vols. Vatican: Biblioteca Apostolica Vaticana 1944–53.

Gesta Abbatum Monasterii Sancti Albani. Ed. H. T. Riley. *Rerum Britannicarum Medii Aevi Scriptores, or Chronicles and Memorials of Great Britain and Ireland in the Middle Ages*, Rolls series 28, 3 vols. London: Longman 1867–9.

Gilbertus Anglicus. *Compendium Medicine*. Lyons 1510.

Gilo of Paris. *The Historia Vie Hierosolimitanae of Gilo of Paris and a Second Anonymous Author*. Ed. C. W. Grocock and J. E. Sidberry. Oxford: Clarendon Press 1997.

Glossarium ad Scriptores Mediae et Infimae Latinitatis. Ed. C. D. DuCange, 6 vols. Paris 1733–6.

Great Roll of the Pipe for the First Year of the Reign of King Richard the First, AD 1189–1190. Ed. J. Hunter. London: Eyre and Spottiswoode 1844.

Great Roll of the Pipe for the Eighteenth Year of the Reign of King Henry the Second, AD 1171–2. London: Pipe Roll Society 1894.

Great Roll of the Pipe for the Second Year of the Reign of King Richard the First. Michaelmas 1190. Ed. D. M. Stenton, NS vol. *i*, 2 Richard I. London: Pipe Roll Society, 1925.

Guibert of Nogent. *Dei Gesta Per Francos*. Ed. R. B. C. Huygens. Turnhout: Brepols 1996.

Guibert of Nogent. *The Deeds of God Through the Franks: Gesta Dei Per Francos*. Trans. R. Levine. Woodbridge: Boydell Press 1997.

Guillaume de Nangis. *Gesta Philippi Regis Franciae, Filii Sanctae Memoriae Regis Ludovici*. Ed. Daunou and Naudet. In *Recueil des Historiens des Gaules et de la France*, xx. Paris: L'Imprimerie Royale 1840.

Hayton. *La flor des estoires de le terre d'orient*. In *Recueil des Historiens des Croisades: Historiens Arméniens*, ii, pp. 113–253. Paris: L'Imprimerie Nationale 1906.

Historia Diplomatica Frederici Secundi. Ed. J.-L.-A. Huillard-Bréholles, 6 vols. Paris 1852–61.

Ibn Abi Usaybiʿa. Text as Appendix B in E. Kohlberg and B. Z. Kedar (1988), A Melkite physician in Frankish Jerusalem and Ayyubid Damascus: Muwaffaq al-Din Yaʿqub b. Siqlab. *Asian and African Studies* **22**: 113–26.

Ibn al-Athir. *Kamil at-Tawarikh* [The perfect history]. In *Arab Historians of the Crusades*. Ed. F. Gabrieli and trans. E. J. Costello. London: Routledge and Kegan Paul 1969.

Ibn al-Firkah. *The Book of Arousing Souls to Visit Jerusalem's Holy Walls*. In *Palestine – Mohammedan Holy Land*. Ed. and trans. C. D. Matthews. New Haven: Yale University Press 1949.

Ibn al-Furat. *Ayyubids, Mamlukes and Crusaders. Selections from the Tarikh al-Duwal wa 'l-Muluk of Ibn al-Furat*. Ed. and trans. M. C. Lyons, U. Lyons and J. S. C. Riley-Smith, 2 vols. Cambridge: W. Heffer 1971.

Ibn al-Qifti. Text as appendix A, in E. Kohlberg and B. Z. Kedar (1988). A Melkite physician in Frankish Jerusalem and Ayyubid Damascus: Muwaffaq al-Din Yaʿqub b. Siqlab. *Asian and African Studies* **22**: 113–26.

Ibn Butlan. *Le Taqwim al-Sihha (Tacuini Sanitatis) d'Ibn Butlan: un Traité médical du XIe Siècle. Histoire du Texte, Edition Critique, Traduction, Commentaire*. Ed. H. Elkhadem. Louvain: Aedibus Peeters 1990.

Ibn Jubayr. *The Travels of Ibn Jubayr*. Ed. and trans. R. C. J. Broadhurst. London: Jonathan Cape 1952.

Ibn Jumayrʿ. *Treatise to Salah ad-Din on the Revival of the Art of Medicine*. Ed. and trans. H. Fahndrich. Wiesbaden: Deutsche Morgenländische Gesellschaft 1983.

Ibn Shaddad. *The Rare and Excellent History of Saladin*. Ed. and trans. D. S. Richards. Aldershot: Ashgate 2001.

Index Britanniae Scriptorum. Ed. J. Bale, R. L. Poole and M. Bateson. Oxford: Clarendon Press 1902.

Innocent IV. Quelques lettres d'Innocent IV. Extraits des Manuscrits de la Bibliothèque Nationale. Ed. J. B. Hauvréau. *Notices et Extraits des Manuscrits de la Bibliothèque Nationale et autres Bibliothèques*, 42 vols. (1787–1933), xxiv (ii), pp. 157–246. Paris: Institut National de France 1876.

Jacques of Vitry. *Historia Hierosolimitana*, in *Gesta Dei Per Francos*. Ed. J. Bongars, 2 vols., i, pt 2, pp. 1047–1124, Hanover 1611.

The History of Jerusalem (AD 1180). Trans. A. Stewart. Library of the Palestine Pilgrim Text Society, xi. New York: AMS Press 1971.

Johannis Saraceni. *Tabulae ceratae Johannis Sarraceni, in thesauro cartarum servatae*. Ed. Guigniaut and de Wailly. In *Recueil de Historiens des Gaules et de la France*, xxi. Paris: L'Imprimerie Impériale 1855.

John of Joinville. *Histoire de Saint Louis. Jean Sire de Joinville*. Ed. N. de Wailly. Paris: Librairie de Firmin Didot Frères 1874.

John of Joinville. *The Life of St Louis*. Ed. N. de Wailly, trans. R. Hague. London: Sheed & Ward 1955.

John of Joinville. In *Joinville and Villehardouin. Chronicles of the Crusades*. Ed. N. de Wailly, trans. M. R. B. Shaw. Harmondsworth: Penguin 1963.

John Mandeville. In *Early Travels in Palestine*. Ed. and trans. T. Wright. London: H. G. Bohn 1848.

John Mandeville. *The Travels of Sir John Mandeville*. Ed. and trans. C. W. R. D. Moseley. Harmondsworth (UK): Penguin 1983.

John of Würzburg. In *Jerusalem Pilgrimage 1099–1185*, pp. 244–73. Ed. and trans. J. Wilkinson, J. Hill and W. F. Ryan. London: Hakluyt Society 1988.

John of Würzburg. *Peregrinationes Tres: Saewulf, John of Würzburg, Theodericus*, pp. 78–138. Ed. R. B. C. Huygens. Turnhout: Brepols 1994.

Kedar, B. Z. A twelfth century description of the Jerusalem Hospital. In *The Military Orders*. II: *Welfare and Warfare*, pp. 3–26. Ed. H. Nicholson. Aldershot: Ashgate 1998 (this contains a Latin edition of the text in question).

Kedar, B. Z. (1999) On the origins of the earliest laws of Frankish Jerusalem: the Canons of the Council of Nablus, 1120. *Speculum* **74**: 310–35 (this contains both a critique and also the full Latin text of the canons).

Lamberto de Sambuceto. *Actes Passés à Famagouste de 1299 à 1301*. Ed. C. Desimoni. Gênes: Institut Royal des Sourds-Muets 1883.

Lamberto de Sambuceto. *Gênes et l'Outre-Mer. I. Les Actes de Caffa du Notaire Lamberto di Sambuceto 1289–1290*. Ed. M. Balard. Paris: Mouton 1973.

Lamberto de Sambuceto. *Notai Genovesi in Oltremare Atti Rogati a Cipro da Lamberto di Sambuceto (3 luglio 1300 – 3 agosto 1301)*. Ed. V. Polonio. Genoa: University of Genoa 1982.

Lamberto de Sambuceto. *Notai Genovesi in Oltremare Atti Rogati a Cipro da Lamberto di Sambuceto (6 luglio – 27 ottobre 1301)*. Ed. R. Pavoni. Genoa: University of Genoa 1982.

Lamberto de Sambuceto. *Notai Genovesi in Oltremare Atti Rogati a Cipro da Lamberto di Sambuceto (11 ottobre 1296 – 23 guigno 1299)*. Ed. M. Balard. Genoa: University of Genoa 1983.

Lamberto de Sambuceto. *Notai Genovesi in Oltremare Atti Rogati a Cipro da Lamberto di Sambuceto (gennaio – agosto 1302)*. Ed. R. Pavoni. Genoa: University of Genoa 1987.

Layettes de Trésor des Chartres. Ed. M. J. De Laborde, 5 vols. Paris: E. Plon 1863–1909.

Le Cartulaire du Chapitre du Saint-Sépulchre de Jérusalem. Ed. G. Bresc-Bautier. Paris: Paul Geuthner 1984.

Le Confesseur de Marguerite. Vie de Saint Louis par le Confesseur de la Reine Marguerite. Ed. Daunou and Naudet. In *Recueil des Historiens des Gaules et de la France*, xx. Paris: L'Imprimerie Royale 1840.

L'Estat de la Cité de Iherusalem [v.1231]. In *Itinéraires à Jérusalem et Descriptions de la Terre Sainte Rédigée en Français au XIe, XIIe et XIIIe Siècles*, pp. 31–52. Ed. H. Michelant and G. Raynaud. Geneva: Société de l'Orient Latin 1882.

Le Livre au Roi. Introduction, Notes et Edition Critique. Ed. M. Greilsammer. Paris: L'Académie des Inscriptions et Belles Lettres 1995.

Les Archives, la Bibliothèque et le Trésor de l'Ordre de Saint-Jean de Jérusalem à Malte. Ed. J. Delaville le Roulx. Paris: Ernest Thorin 1883.

Les Régistres de Grégoire IX. Ed. L. Auvray, 4 vols. Paris: Thorin 1896–1955.

Les Registres d'Innocent IV. Ed. E. Berger, 4 vols. Paris: Thorin 1884–1920.

Liber Augustalis. In *Historia Diplomatica Frederici Secundi*, 6 vols., IV (i), pp. 1–178. Ed. J. L. A. Huillard-Bréhols. Paris: H. Plon 1854.

Liber Augustalis, or Constitutions of Melfi Promulgated by the Emperor Frederick II for the Kingdom of Sicily in 1231. Ed. J. L. A. Huillard-Bréhols, trans. J. M. Powell. New York: Syraceuse University Press 1971.

Marsilio Zorzi. *Der Bericht des Marsilio Zorzi Codex Querini-Stampalia IV 3 (1064).* Ed. O. Berggötz. Frankfurt: Peter Lang 1991.

Matthew Paris. *English History from the Years 1235–1273.* Ed. Watts, trans. J. A. Giles. 3 vols. London: Henry G. Bohn 1852–4.

Matthew Paris, Monachi Sancti Albani. *Historia Anglorum, Sive ut Vulgo Dicitur, Historia Minor.* Ed. F. Madden. *Rerum Britannicarum Medii Aevi Scriptores, or Chronicles and Memorials of Great Britain and Ireland During the Middle Ages*, Rolls series 44, 3 vols. London: Longman 1866–9.

Matthew Paris, Monachi Sancti Albani. *Chronica Majora.* Ed. H. R. Luard. *Rerum Britannicarum Medii Aevi Scriptores, or Chronicles and Memorials of Great Britain and Ireland During the Middle Ages*, Rolls series 57, 7 vols. London: Longman 1872–83.

Matthew Paris, *Itinéraire de Londres à Jérusalem.* In *Itinéraires à Jérusalem et descriptions de la Terre Sainte*, pp. 123–39. Ed. H. Michelant and G. Raynaud. Geneva: Société de l'Orient Latin 1882.

Minstrel of Reims. *Récits d'un Ménestrel de Reims au Treizième Siècle.* Ed. N. de Wailly. Paris: Librairie de la Société de l'Histoire de France 1876.

Minstrel of Reims. *Chronicle of Reims.* In *Three Old French Chronicles of the Crusades*, pp. 247–366. Ed. N. de Wailly, trans. E. N. Stone. Washington: University of Washington 1939.

Monasticon Anglicanum: a History of the Abbies and other Monasteries, Hospitals and Friaries and Cathedrals and Collegiate Churches with their Dependencies in England and Wales. Ed. W. Dugdale, 6 vols. London: Longman & Joseph Harding 1821–30 (with regard to Gilbertus Anglicus, a number of manuscripts write 'magistro E. de Aquila' rather than the expected 'G' but they are all thought to be referring to the Gilbert).

Moses Maimonides. *Glossary of Drug Names.* Ed. M. Meyerhof, trans. F. Rosner. Philadelphia: American Philosophical Society 1979.

Naser-e Khosraw. *Book of Travels (Safarnama).* Trans. W. M. Thackston. Albany (USA): Bibliotheca Persica 1986.

Obituaires de la Province de Sens. Ed. A. Molinier, Paris: L'Imprimerie Nationale 1902.

Odo of Deuil. *De Profectione Ludovici VII in Orientem.* Ed. and trans. V. G. Berry. New York: Columbia University Press, 1948.

Oliver of Paderborn. *Historia Damiatina.* In *Die Schriften des Kölner Domscholasters, Spätern Bischofs von Paderborn und Kardinal-Bischofs von Sabina Oliverus.* Ed. H. Hoogeweg. Tübingen: Bibliothek des Literarischen Vereins in Stuttgart, series no. 20, 1894.

Oliver of Paderborn. *The Capture of Damietta*. Ed. H. Hoogeweg, trans. J. J. Gavigan. Philadelphia: University of Pennsylvania 1948.

Orderic Vitalis. *The Ecclesiastical History of Orderic Vitalis*. Ed. and trans. M. Chibnall, 6 vols. Oxford: Clarendon Press 1968–80 (Latin and English text).

Oribasius of Pergamon. *Dieting for an Emperor. Books 1 and 4 of Oribasius' Medical Compilations*. Ed. and trans. M. Grant. Leiden: E. J. Brill 1997.

Paulus Aegineta. *The Seven Books of Paulus Aegineta*. Ed. and trans. F. Adams, 3 vols. London: Sydenham Society 1844–7.

Pelrinages et pardouns de Acre. In *Itinéraires à Jérusalem et Descriptions de la Terre Sainte Rédigée en Français aux XIe, XIIe et XIIIe Siècles*, pp. 227–36. Ed. H. Michelant and G. Raynaud. Geneva: Société de l'Orient Latin 1882.

Petahyah of Regensburg (Petachiae Ratisbonensis). *Itinerarium*. Ed. J. C. Wagenseilia, col. MCLXVI–MCCXII, in *Thesaurus Antiquitatum Sacrarum*. Ed. B. Ugolino. Venice: J. G. Herthz 1746.

Philippe de Navarre. *Récit de Philippe de Navarre (1211–1242)*. In *Les Gestes des Chiprois*. Ed. G. Raynaud. Geneva: Société de l'Orient Latin 1887.

Qusta Ibn Luqua. *Medical Regime for the Pilgrims to Mecca. The Risala fi tadbir safar al hajj*. Ed. G. Bos. Leiden: E. J. Brill 1992.

Ralph de Diceto, Decani Lundonensis. *Opera Historica*. Ed. W. Stubbs. *Rerum Britannicarum Medii Aevi Scriptores, or Chronicles and Memorials of Great Britain and Ireland During the Middle Ages*, Rolls series 68, 2 vols. London: Longman 1876.

Raymond d'Aguilers. *Historia Francorum qui Ceperunt Iherusalem*. Ed. and trans. J. H. Hill and L. L. Hill. Philadelphia: American Philosophical Society 1968.

Raymond d'Aguilers. *Le Liber de Raymond d'Aguilers*. Ed. J. H. Hill and L. L. Hill. Paris: Paul Geuthner 1969.

Regesta Regni Hierosolymitani. Ed. R. Röhrichte, 2 vols. Innsbruck: Libraria Academica Wagneriana 1893–1904.

Regimen Sanitatis Salerni. The School of Salernum. Ed. J. Harington. Salerno: Ente Provinciale Per Il Tourismo 1953.

Richard de Templo. *Itinerarium Peregrinorum et Gesta Regis Ricardi*. Ed. W. Stubbs. *Rerum Britannicarum Medii Aevi Scriptores, or Chronicles and Memorials of Great Britain and Ireland During the Middle Ages*, Rolls series 38(i). London: Longman 1864.

Richard de Templo. *Chronicle of the Third Crusade: A Translation of 'Itinerarium Peregrinorum et Gesta Regis Ricardi'*. Trans. H. Nicholson. Aldershot: Ashgate 1997.

Riolan, J. *Curieuses Recherches sur les Escholes en Médecine de Paris et de Montpellier*, p. 92. Paris: Gaspar Meturas 1651.

Roger of Howden. *The Annals of Roger of Hoveden, Comprising the History of England and of Other Countries of Europe from AD 732 to AD 1201*. Trans. H. T. Riley, 2 vols. London: H. G. Bohn 1853.

Roger of Howden. *Chronica Magistri Rogeri de Hoveden*. Ed. W. Stubbs. *Rerum Britannicarum Medii Aevi Scriptores, or Chronicles and Memorials of Great*

Britain and Ireland During the Middle Ages, Rolls series 51, 4 vols. London: Longmans, 1868–71.

Roger of Wendover. *Flowers of History (1066–1215 AD)*. Trans J. A. Giles, 2 vols. Felinbach: Llanerch 1994 (reprint of 1849 edition).

Roger of Wendover. *Flores Historiarum*. Ed. H. G. Hewlett. *Rerum Britannicarum Medii Aevi Scriptores, or Chronicles and Memorials of Great Britain and Ireland During the Middle Ages*, Rolls series 84, 3 vols. London: Longman, 1886–9.

Röhricht, R. (1881) Etudes sur les derniers temps du royaume Jérusalem. A. La croisade du Prince Edouard d'Angleterre (1270–1274). Appendice. *Archives de l'Orient Latin* **1**: 630–2.

Rotuli Chartarum. Ed. T. D. Hardy, London: Commissioners on the Public Records 1837.

Rule of the Templars. La Règle du Temple. Ed. H. de Curzon, Paris: Librairie Renouard 1886.

Rule of the Templars. Ed. H. de Curzon, trans. J. M. Upton-Ward, Woodbridge: Boydell Press 1992.

Sacrorum Conciliorum Nova et Amplissima Collectio. Ed. J. D. Mansi, new edition. Florence and Venice, 1759–98.

Saewulf. *A reliable account of the situation of Jerusalem, 1101–3*, in *Jerusalem Pilgrimage 1099–1185*, pp. 94–116. Ed. and trans. J. Wilkinson, J. Hill and W. F. Ryan. London: Hakluyt Society 1988.

Saewulf. *Peregrinationes Tres: Saewulf, John of Würzburg, Theodericus*, pp. 58–77. Ed. R. B. C. Huygens. Turnhout: Brepols 1994.

Studien zur Geschichte des Fünften Kreuzzuges. Ed. R. Röhricht, Innsbruck: Wagnerschen Universitäts 1891.

Synodicum Nicosiense and other Documents of the Latin Church of Cyprus, 1196–1373. Ed. C. Schabel. Nicosia: Cyprus Research Centre 2001.

Tabulae Ordinis Theutonici. Ed. E. G. W. Strehlke. Berlin: Weidmann 1869.

Tacuinum Sanitatis. The Medieval Health Handbook. Ed. L. G. Arano, trans. O. Ratti and A. Westbrook. London: Barrie & Jenkins 1976.

Templar of Tyre. *Cronaca de Templare de Tiro (1243–1314)*. Ed. L. Minervini. Naples: Liguori 2000.

Testimonia Minora de Quinto Bello Sacro. Ed. R. Röhricht, 5 vols. Geneva: Société de l'Orient Latin (série historique), 1877–87.

The City of Jerusalem. Ed. H. Michelant and G. Raynaud, trans. C. R. Conder. PPTS series VI, pp. 1–49. London: Library of the Palestine Pilgrims Texts Society 1897.

Theodericus. *Peregrinationes Tres: Saewulf, John of Würzburg, Theodericus*, pp. 142–97. Ed. R. B. C. Huygens. Turnhout: Brepols 1994.

Theodorich. In *Jerusalem Pilgrimage 1099–1185*, pp. 274–314. Ed. and trans. J. Wilkinson, J. Hill and W. F. Ryan. London: Hakluyt Society 1988.

Theodorich Borgognoni. *Cyrurgia*. In *Cyrurgia Guidonis de Chauliaco, et Cyrurgia Bruni, Theoderici, Rogerii, Rolandi, Bertapali, Lanfranci*, pp. 106–146. Ed. B. Locatellus, Venice 1498.

Theodorich Borgognoni. *The Surgery of Theodorich, ca.* AD *1267.* Ed. B. Locatellus, trans. E. Campbell and J. Colton, 2 vols. New York: Appleton-Century-Crofts 1955–60.

Tritton, A. S. and Gibb, H. A. R. (1933) The first and second crusades from an anonymous Syriac chronicle. *Journal of the Royal Asiatic Society* (no vol.): 69–101 and 274–305.

Usama ibn Munqidh. *An Arab-Syrian Gentleman and Warrior in the Period of the Crusades. Memoirs of Usamah ibn-Munqidh.* Ed. and trans. P. K. Hitti. New York: Columbia University Press 1929.

Viage Literario á las Inglesias de España. Ed. J. L. Villanueva, 22 vols. Madrid 1803–52.

Walter the Chancellor. *Galterii Cancellarii, Bella Antiochena.* Ed. H. Hagenmeyer. Innsbruck: Wagnerschen Universitäts-Buchhandlung 1896.

Walter the Chancellor. *The Antiochene Wars.* Ed. H. Hagenmeyer, trans. T. S. Asbridge and S. B. Edgington. Aldershot: Ashgate 1999.

William of Tyre. *A History of Deeds Done Beyond the Sea.* Trans. E. A. Babcock and A. C. Krey, 2 vols. New York: Columbia University 1943.

William of Tyre. *Guillaume de Tyr: Chronique.* Ed. R. B. C. Huygens, 2 vols. Brepols: Turnhout 1986.

Work on Geography, Descriptio Locorum Circa Hierusalem Adjacentum. In *Les Églises de la Terre Sainte*, pp. 414–33. Ed. M. de Vogüé. Paris: Victor Didron 1860.

Work on Geography. Ed. M. de Vogüé. In *Jerusalem Pilgrimage 1099–1185*, pp. 181–211. Trans. J. Wilkinson, J. Hill and W. F. Ryan. London: Hakluyt Society 1988.

SECONDARY WORKS

Adamson, P. B. (1976) Schistosomiasis in antiquity. *Medical History* **20**: 176–88.

(1982) The military surgeon: his place in history. *Journal of the Royal Army Medical Corps* **128**: 43–50.

(1988) Dracontiasis in antiquity. *Medical History* **32**: 204–9.

Agrimi, J. and Crisciani, C. (1994) The science and practice of medicine in the thirteenth century according to Guglielmo da Saliceto, Italian surgeon. In L. Garcia-Ballester, R. French, J. Arrizabalaga and A. Cunningham (eds.), *Practical Medicine from Salerno to the Black Death* (Cambridge: Cambridge University Press), pp. 60–87.

(1998) Charity and aid in mediaeval Christian civilization. In M. D. Grmek, B. Fantini, A. Shugaar (eds.), *Western Medical Thought from Antiquity to the Middle Ages* (Cambridge (Mass.): Harvard University Press), pp. 170–96.

Allan, N. (1990) Hospice to hospital in the Near East: an instance of continuity and change in late antiquity. *Bulletin of the History of Medicine* **64**: 446–62.

Alston, M. N. (1944) The attitude of the church towards dissection before 1500. *Bulletin of the History of Medicine* **16**: 221–38.

Alvarez-Milan, C. (2000) Practice versus theory: tenth century case histories from the Islamic Middle East. *Social History of Medicine* **13**: 293–306.

Amiran, D. H. K., Arieh, E. and Turcotte, T. (1994) Earthquakes in Israel and adjacent areas: macroseismic observations since 100 BCE. *Israel Exploration Journal* **44**: 260–305.

Amouroux, M. (1999) Colonization and the creation of hospitals: the eastern extension of western hospitality in the eleventh and twelfth centuries. *Mediterranean Historical Review* **14**: 31–43.

Amundsen, D. W. (1971) Visigothic medical legislation. *Bulletin of the History of Medicine* **45**: 553–69.

(1973) The liability of the physician in Roman law. In H. Karplus (ed.), *International Symposium on Society, Medicine and Law. Jerusalem, March 1972* (Amsterdam: Elsevier), pp. 17–30.

(1974) The medical legislation of the Assizes of Jerusalem. In F. N. L. Poynter (ed.), *Proceedings of the XXIII International Congress of the History of Medicine, London 2–9 September 1972* (London: Wellcome Institute of the History of Medicine), I, pp. 517–22.

(1977) The liability of the physician in classical Greek legal theory and practice. *Journal of the History of Medicine and Allied Sciences* **32**: 172–203.

Amundsen, D. W. and Ferngren, G. B. (1979) The forensic role of physicians in Roman law. *Bulletin of the History of Medicine* **53**: 39–56.

Anon. (1750) Douzième siècle. Etat des lettres en France dans le cours de ce siècle. *Histoire Littéraire de la France* **9**: 1–225 (pp. 191–6 cover medical practitioners).

(1885) Raimond Lulle, Ermite. *Histoire Littéraire de la France* **29**: 1–386.

Atiya, A. S. (1962) *The Crusade: Historiography and Bibliography* (Bloomington: Indiana University Press).

Auchterlonie, P. (1987) *Arabic Biographical Dictionaries: a Summary Guide and Bibliography* (Durham: Middle East Libraries Committee).

Azmi, H. A. A. (1984) Contribution of Muslim physicians to the development of surgery during the Middle Ages. *Studies in History of Medicine* **8**: 49–59.

Bachrach, B. S. (1999) The siege of Antioch: a study in military demography. *War in History* **6**: 127–46.

Baer, W. S. (1931) The treatment of chronic osteomyelitis with the maggot (larva of the blow fly). *Journal of Bone and Joint Surgery* **13**: 438–75.

Bahat, D. (2002) Hospices and hospitals in Mamluk Jerusalem. In Y. Lev (ed.), *Towns and Material Culture in the Medieval Middle East* (Leiden: E. J. Brill), pp. 73–88.

Baker, C. F. (1996) Islamic and Jewish medicine in the medieval Mediterranean world: the Genizah evidence. *Journal of the Royal Society of Medicine* **89**: 577–80.

Barber, M. (1994) *The New Knighthood: a History of the Order of the Temple* (Cambridge: Cambridge University Press).

(2001) The charitable and medical activities of the Hospitallers and Templars. In G. R. Evans (ed.), *A History of Pastoral Care* (London: Cassell), pp. 148–68.

Barnes, E. (2003) The dead do tell tales. In C. K. Williams and N. Bookidis (eds.), *Corinth: the Centenary, 1896–1996* (Princeton: American School of Classical Studies at Athens), pp. 435–43.

Barnes, E. and Ortner, D. J. (1997) Multifocal eosinophilic granuloma with a possible trepanation in a fourteenth century Greek young skeleton. *International Journal of Osteoarchaeology* 7: 542–47.

Bar-Sela, A. and Hoff, H. E. (1962) Isaac Israeli's fifty admonitions to the physicians. *Journal of the History of Medicine* 17: 245–57.

Bar-Sela, A., Hoff, H. E. and Faris, E. (1964) Moses Maimonides' two treatises on the Regimen of Health. *Transactions of the American Philosophical Society* 54: 3–50.

Bartlett, R. (1986) *Trial by Fire and Water: The Medieval Judicial Ordeal* (Oxford: Clarendon Press).

Baur, M. L. (1927) Recherches sur l'histoire de l'anesthésie avant 1846. *Janus* 31: 213–25.

Bayon, H. P. (1953) The masters of Salerno and the origins of professional medical practice. In E. A. Underwood (ed.), *Science, Medicine and History* (London: Oxford University Press), 1, pp. 203–19.

Beddie, J. S. (1933) Some notices of books in the east in the period of the crusades. *Speculum* 8: 240–2.

Bellamy, J. (1973) *Crime and Public Order in England in the Later Middle Ages* (London: Routledge and Kegan Paul).

Ben Dov, M. (1993) The restoration of St Mary's Church of the German knights in Jerusalem. In Y. Tasfrir (ed.), *Ancient Churches Revealed* (Jerusalem: Israel Exploration Society), pp. 140–2.

Bennett, D. (1999) Three xenon texts. *Medicina Nei Secoli Arte E Scienza* 11: 507–19.

Bennett, M. (1992) *La Règle du Temple* as a military manual, or how to deliver a cavalry charge. Appendix in J. M. Upton-Ward, *The Rule of the Templars* (Woodbridge: Boydell Press), pp. 175–88.

Berryman, H. E. and Haun, S. J. (1996) Applying forensic techniques to interpret cranial fracture patterns in an archaeological specimen. *International Journal of Osteoarchaeology* 6: 2–9.

Berthaud, H. (1907) Les médecins et chirurgiens des rois capétiens du XIe au XIIIe siècle. *Bulletin de la Société Française d'Histoire de la Médecine* 6: 39–89.

Biesterfeldt, H. H. (1984) Some opinions on the physician's renumeration in mediaeval Islam. *Bulletin of the History of Medicine* 58: 16–27.

Billard, M. (1991) Violent traumatic injuries on human skeletal remains buried with horses in a Gallo-Roman collective grave (Lyon-Vaise, France, AD 200–300). *International Journal of Osteoarchaeology* 1: 259–64.

Bird, J. (2001) Medicine for body and soul: Jacques de Vitry's sermons to hospitallers and their charges. In P. Biller and J. Zeigler (eds.), *Religion and Medicine in the Middle Ages* (York: York Medieval Press), pp. 91–134.

Bisset, N. G. (1989) Arrow and dart poisons. *Journal of Ethnopharmacology* 25: 1–41.

Bliquez, L. J. (1984) Two lists of Greek surgical instruments and the state of surgery in Byzantine times. *Dumbarton Oaks Papers* **38**: 187–204.

(1993) The role of instruments in the study of Greco-Roman surgery. *Caduceus* **9**: 77–86.

(1996) Prosthetics in classical antiquity: Greek, Etruscan and Roman prosthetics. *Aufstieg und Niedergang der Römischen Welt* **37**: 2640–76.

(1999) The surgical instrumentarium of Leon Iatrosophistes. *Medicina Nei Secoli Arte E Scienza* **11**: 291–322.

Bliquez, L. J. and Kazhdan A. (1984) Four testimonia to human dissection in Byzantine times. *Bulletin of the History of Medicine* **58**: 554–7.

Boas, A. J. (2001) *Jerusalem in the Time of the Crusades: Society, Landscape and Art in the Holy City Under Frankish Rule* (London: Routledge).

Bourman, W. C. and Sanghvi, I. S. (1963) Pharmacological actions of hemlock (*Conium maculatum*) alkaloids. *Journal of Pharmacy and Pharmacology* **15**: 1–25.

Boylston, A. (2000) Evidence for weapon-related trauma in British archaeological samples. In M. Cox and S. Mays (eds.), *Human Osteology in Archaeology and Forensic Science* (London: Greenwich Medical Media), pp. 357–80.

Boylston, A., Novak, S., Sutherland, T., Holst, M. and Coughlan, J. (1997) Burials from the battle of Towton. *Royal Armouries Yearbook* **2**: 36–9.

Brachet, A. (1903) *Pathologie Mentale des Rois de France. Louis XI et ses Ascendants* (Paris: Hachette).

Bradbury, J. (1979) Greek fire in the west. *History Today* **29**: 326–31.

(1985) *The Medieval Archer* (Woodbridge: Boydell Press).

(1994) *The Medieval Siege* (Woodbridge: Boydell Press).

Bragman, L. J. (1927) Maimonides' treatise on Hemorrhoids. *New York State Journal of Medicine* **27**: 598–601.

Brain, P. (1979) In defence of ancient bloodletting. *South African Medical Journal* **56**: 149–54.

(1986) *Galen on Bloodletting: a Study of the Origins, Development and Validity of his Opinions, with a Translation of the Three Works* (Cambridge: Cambridge University Press).

Brefold, J. (1994) *A Guidebook for the Jerusalem Pilgrimage in the Later Middle Ages: a Case for Computer-Aided Textual Criticism* (Hilversum: Veloren).

Brittain, R. P. (1966) The history of legal medicine: the Assises of Jerusalem. *Medico-Legal Medicine* **34**: 72–3.

Brocard, H. (1877) Inventaire des reliques et autres curiosités de l'église cathédrale de Langres. *Bulletin de la Société Historique et Archéologique de Langres* **1**: 152–78.

Brodman, J. W. (1998) *Charity and Welfare: Hospitals and the Poor in Medieval Catalonia* (Philadelphia: University of Philadelphia Press).

Brooks, E. St. J. (1956–7) Irish possessions of St. Thomas of Acre. *Proceedings of the Royal Irish Academy* **58c**: 21–44.

Brothwell, D. R. (1994) Ancient trephining: multifocal evolution or trans-world diffusion? *Journal of Paleopathology* **6**: 129–38.

Brothwell, D. R. and Møller-Christensen, V. (1963) Medico-historical aspects of a very early case of mutilation. *Danish Medical Bulletin* **10**: 21–5.

Brown, E. A. R. (1981) Death and the human body in the later Middle Ages: the legislation of Boniface VIII on the division of the corpse. *Viator* **12**: 221–70.

Browning, R. (1985) A further testimony to human dissection in the Byzantine world. *Bulletin of the History of Medicine* **59**: 518–20.

Bruce, G. M. (1941) A note on penal blinding in the Middle Ages. *Annals of Medical History* **3**: 369–71.

Brundage, J. A. (1993) Latin jurists in the Levant: the legal elite of the crusader states. In M. Shatzmiller (ed.), *Crusaders and Muslims in Twelfth Century Syria* (Leiden: E. J. Brill), pp. 18–42.

Bruneton, J. (1999) *Pharmacognosy, Phytochemistry, Medicine Plants.* Trans. C. K. Hatton (2nd edn., London: Intercept).

Brunius, U., Zederfeldt, B. and Ahren, C. (1967) Healing of skin incisions closed by non-suture technique. *Acta Chirurgica Scandinavica* **133**: 509–16.

Bull, R. J. (ed.) (1987) *The Joint Expedition to Caesarea Maritima. Preliminary Reports* (Madison: Drew University Institute for Archeological Research).

Bullen, J., Griffiths, F., Rogers, H. and Ward, G. (2000) Sepsis: the critical role of iron. *Microbes and Infection* **2**: 409–15.

Bullough, V. L. (1958) The development of the medical guilds at Paris. *Medievalia et Humanistica* **12**: 33–40.

   (1960) The teaching of surgery at the University of Montpellier in the thirteenth century. *Journal of the History of Medicine and Allied Sciences* **15**: 202–4.

   (1961) Medical study at mediaeval Oxford. *Speculum* **36**: 600–12.

   (1962a) Population and the study and practice of mediaeval medicine. *Bulletin of the History of Medicine* **36**: 62–9.

   (1962b) The mediaeval medical school at Cambridge. *Mediaeval Studies* **24**: 161–8.

Bullough, V. L. and Campbell, C. (1980) Female longevity and diet in the Middle Ages. *Speculum* **55**: 317–25.

Burkitt, H. G., Quick, C. R. G. and Gatt, D. (1996) *Essential Surgery: Problems, Diagnosis and Management* (2nd edn., Edinburgh: Churchill Livingstone).

Burnett, C. (1994) Michael Scot and the transmission of scientific culture from Toledo to Bologna via the court of Frederick II Hohenstaufen. *Micrologus* **2**: 101–26.

   (1997) Translating from Arabic into Latin in the Middle Ages: theory, practice and criticism. In S. G. Lofts and P. W. Rosemann (eds.), *Editer, Traduire, Interpréter. Essais de Méthodologie Philosophique* (Louvain: Peeters), pp. 55–78.

   (1998–9) The Sortes Regis Amalrici: an Arabic divinatory work in the Latin Kingdom of Jerusalem? *Scripta Mediterranea* **19–20**: 229–37.

   (2000) Antioch as a link between Arabic and Latin culture in the twelfth and thirteenth centuries. In I. Draelants, A. Tihon, B. van den Abeele (eds.), *Occident et Proche-Orient: Contacts Scientifiques au Temps des Croisades* (Louvain: Brepols), pp. 1–78.

Burnett, C. and Jacquart, D. (eds.) (1994) *Constantine the African and 'Ali Ibn Al-'Abbas Al-Majusi: The Pantegni and Related Texts* (Leiden: E. J. Brill).

Burns, R. I. (1972) The medieval crossbow as surgical instrument: an illustrated case history. *Bulletin of the New York Academy of Medicine* **48**: 983–9.

Bylebyl, J. J. (1990) The medical meaning of physica. *Osiris* **6**: 16–41.

Cahen, C. (1934) Indigènes et croisés. Quelques mots à propos d'un médecin d'Amaury et de Saladin. *Syria* **15**: 351–60.

Cameron, M. L. (1993) *Anglo-Saxon Medicine* (Cambridge: Cambridge University Press).

Capasso, L. and Di Tota, G. (1996) Possible therapy for headaches in ancient times. *International Journal of Osteoarchaeology* **6**: 316–19.

Capparoni, P. (1923) *Magistri Salernitani Nondum Cogniti: A Contribution to the History of the Medical School of Salerno* (London: John Bale).

Carlin, M. (1989) Medieval English hospitals. In L. Granshaw and R. Porter (eds.), *The Hospital in History* (London: Routledge), pp. 21–39.

Carlino, A. (1999) *Books of the Body: Anatomical Ritual and Renaissance Learning*. Trans. J. Tedeschi and A. C. Tedeschi (Chicago: University of Chicago Press).

Carter, A. J. (1996) Narcosis and nightshade. *British Medical Journal* **313**: 1630–2.
  (1999) Dwale: an anaesthetic from old England. *British Medical Journal* **319**: 1623–6.

Chandra, R. K. (1986) Nutritional regulation of immunity and infection. *Journal of Pediatric Gastroenterology and Nutrition* **5**: 844–52.

Chereau, A. (1862) Les médecins et les chirurgiens de Saint Louis, roi de France. *L'Union Médicale* n.s. **14**: 209–15.

Cochrane, L. (1994) *Adelard of Bath: the First English Scientist* (London: British Museum).

Codellas, P. S. (1942) The Pantokrator, the imperial Byzantine medical center of xiith century AD in Constantinople. *Bulletin of the History of Medicine* **12**: 392–410.

Committee on Trauma (1994) *Advanced Trauma Life Support (ATLS)* (Chicago: American College of Surgeons).

Conrad, L. I. (1994) Did al-Walid I found the first Islamic hospital? *ARAM* **6**: 225–44.
  (1999) Usama ibn Munqidh and other witnesses to Frankish and Islamic medicine in the era of the crusades. In Z. Amar, E. Lev and J. Schwartz (eds.), *Medicine in Jerusalem Throughout the Ages* (Tel Aviv: Bar Ilan University), pp. XXVII–LII.
  (2001) Book review. *Social History of Medicine* **14**: 133–5.

Cope, Z. (1958) The treatment of wounds through the ages. *Medical History* **2**: 163–74.

Cornand, G. (1979) Trachome et armées. *Revue Internationale du Trachome et de Pathologie Oculaire Tropicale et Subtropicale* **56**: 99–110.

Corner, G. W. (1927) *Anatomical Texts of the Earlier Middle Ages* (Washington: Carnegie Institution).

(1937) On early Salernitan surgery and especially the 'Bamberg Surgery'. *Bulletin of the History of Medicine* **5**: 1–32.

Cosman, M. P. (1972) Medieval medical malpractice and Chaucer's physician. *New York State Journal of Medicine* **72**: 2439–44.

(1973) Medieval medical malpractice: the dicta and the dockets. *Bulletin of the New York Academy of Medicine* **49**: 22–47.

(1982) The medieval medical third party: compulsory consultation and malpractice insurance. *Annals of Plastic Surgery* **8**: 152–62.

Coureas, N. (2001) The provision of charity and hospital care on Latin Cyprus. *Epeteris: Annual Journal of the Cyprus Research Centre* **27**: 33–50.

(2002) *The Assizes of the Lusignan Kingdom of Cyprus* (Nicosia: Cyprus Research Centre).

Courville, C. B. (1965) War wounds of the cranium in the Middle Ages, as disclosed in the skeletal material from the battle of Visby (1361 AD). *Bulletin of the Los Angeles Neurological Society* **30**: 27–33.

Croft, P. (2000) The faunal remains. In R. P. Harper and D. Pringle (eds.), *Belmont Castle: the Excavation of a Crusader Stronghold in the Kingdom of Jerusalem* (Oxford: Oxford University Press), pp. 173–94.

Cunha, E. and Silva, A. M. (1997) War lesions from the famous Portuguese medieval battle of Aljubarrota. *International Journal of Osteoarchaeology* **7**: 595–9.

D'Alverny, M.-T. (1967) Astrologues et théologiens au XIIe siècle. In *Mélanges Offerts à M.-D. Chenu* (Paris), pp. 40–50.

(1982) Translations and translators. In R. L. Benson, G. Constable and C. D. Lanham (eds.), *Renaissance and Renewal in the Twelfth Century* (Oxford: Clarendon Press), pp. 421–62.

Daugherty, C. G. (1995) The death of Socrates and the toxicology of hemlock. *Journal of Medical Biography* **3**: 178–82.

Daumet, G. (1918) Une femme-médecin au XIIIe siècle. *Revue des Etudes Historiques* **84**: 69–71.

Dauriol, M. (1847) A substitute for the vapour of ether to annul sensation during operations. *The Lancet* **1**: 540.

Deffarge, A. (1928) *Histoire Critique des Anesthétiques Anciens, et en Particulier des Eponges Somnifères à Base de Drogues Végétales* (Bordeaux: Biere).

Delaville le Roulx, J. (1904) *Les Hospitaliers en Terre Sainte et à Chypre (1100–1310)* (Paris).

Delisle, L. (1890) *Littérature Latine et Histoire du Moyen Age* (Paris).

(1896) Testaments d'Arnaud de Villeneuve et de Raimond Lulle, 20 juillet 1305 et 26 avril 1313. *Journal des Savants*, 342–55.

Del Gaizo, M. (1894) *Il Magistero Chirurgico di Teodorico dei Borgognoni* (Naples: Tocco).

Demaitre, L. (1975) Theory and practice in medical education at the University of Montpellier in the thirteenth and fourteenth centuries. *Journal of the History of Medicine* **30**: 103–23.

Demel, B. (1998) Welfare and warfare in the Teutonic Order: a survey. In H. Nicholson (ed.), *The Military Orders. II: Welfare and Warfare* (Aldershot: Ashgate), pp. 61–73.

Demirhan, A. (1980) The evolution of opium in the Islamic world and Anatolian Turks. *Studies in History of Medicine* **4**: 73–97.

De Moulin, D. (1971) Cutting for stone in the early Middle Ages. *Bulletin of the History of Medicine* **45**: 76–9.

Denny, N. and Filmer-Sankey, J. (eds.) (1973) *The Travels of Sir John Mandeville* (London: Collins).

Derenne, J.-Ph., Debru, A., Grassin, A. E. and Whitelaw, W. A. (1994) The earliest history of diaphragm physiology. *European Respiratory Journal* **7**: 2234–40.

Dichter, B. (1979) *The Orders and Churches of Crusader Acre* (Acre: Municipality of Acre).

Dickson, G. (2000) Medieval Christian crowds and the origins of crowd psychology. *Revue d'Histoire Ecclésiastique* **95**: 54–75.

D'Irsay, S. (1925) The life and works of Gilles de Corbeil. *Annals of Medical History* **7**: 362–78.

Dolev, E. (1996) Medicine in the crusaders' kingdom of Jerusalem. In M. Waserman and S. S. Kottek (eds.), *Health and Disease in the Holy Land* (Lewiston: Edwin Mellen), pp. 157–72.

Dolev, E. and Knoller, N. (2001) Military medicine in the crusaders' kingdom of Jerusalem. *Israel Medical Association Journal* **3**: 389–92.

Dols, M. W. (1987) The origins of the Islamic hospital: myth and reality. *Bulletin of the History of Medicine* **61**: 367–90.

(1992) *Majnun: the Madman in Medieval Islamic Society* (Oxford: Clarendon Press).

DuBois, P. (1991) *Torture and Truth* (New York: Routledge).

Dunlop, D. M. (1960) Bimaristan. i. Early period and Muslim east. In *Encyclopedia of Islam*, I(ii). Ed. H. A. R. Gibb, J. H. Kramers, E. Levi-Provencal, J. Schacht, B. Lewis and Ch. Pellat (2nd edn., Leiden: E. J. Brill), pp. 1223–4.

Edbury, P. W. (1996) *The Conquest of Jerusalem and the Third Crusade* (Aldershot: Scolar Press).

(1997) *John of Ibelin and the Kingdom of Jerusalem* (Woodbridge: Boydell).

Edge, D. and Paddock, J. M. (1996) *Arms and Armour of the Medieval Knight* (London: Saturn).

Edgington, S. (1994) Medical knowledge of the crusading armies: the evidence of Albert of Aachen and others. In M. Barber (ed.), *The Military Orders. I: Fighting for the Faith and Caring for the Sick* (Aldershot: Ashgate), pp. 320–6.

(1998a) Albert of Aachen and the Chansons de Geste. In J. France and W. G. Zajac (eds.), *The Crusades and their Sources* (Aldershot: Ashgate), pp. 23–37.

(1998b) Medical care in the Hospital of St John in Jerusalem. In H. Nicholson (ed.), *The Military Orders. II: Welfare and Warfare* (Aldershot: Ashgate), pp. 27–33.

(1999) The Hospital of St John in Jerusalem. In Z. Amar, E. Lev and J. Schwartz (eds.), *Medicine in Jerusalem Throughout the Ages* (Tel Aviv: Bar Ilan University), pp. ix–xxv.

Edgington, S. (ed.) (in press) *Albert of Aachen. Historia Iherosolimitana* (Oxford: Oxford Medieval Texts).

Edwards, H. (1976) Theodorich of Cervia, a mediaeval antiseptic surgeon. *Proceedings of the Royal Society of Medicine* **69**: 553–5.

Eknoyan, G. (1994) Arabic medicine and nephrology. *American Journal of Nephrology* **14**: 270–8.

Elad, A. (1995) *Medieval Jerusalem and Islamic Worship: Holy Places, Ceremonies, Pilgrimage* (Leiden: E. J. Brill).

Eldredge, L. M. (ed.) (1996) *The Wonderful Art of the Eye by Benvenutus Grassus. A Critical Edition of the Middle English Translation of his De Probatissima Arte Oculorum* (Michigan: Michigan State Press).

Elgood, C. (1951) *A Medical History of Persia and the Eastern Caliphate* (Cambridge: Cambridge University Press).

Elkhadem, H. (1990) Le Taqwim al-Sihha (Tacuini Sanitatis) d'Ibn Butlan: Histoire du Texte. *Acta Belgica Historiae Medicinae* **3**: 139–46.

Ell, S. R. (1984) Blood and sexuality in medieval leprosy. *Janus* **71**: 153–64.
  (1996) Pilgrims, crusades and plagues. In M. Waserman and S. S. Kottek (eds.), *Health and Disease in the Holy Land* (Lewiston: Edwin Mellen), pp. 173–87.

Ellenblum, R. (2003) Frontier activities: the transformation of a Muslim sacred site into the Frankish castle of Vadum Jacob. *Crusades* **2**: 83–97.

Ellenblum, R., Marco, S., Agnon, A., Rockwell, T. and Boas, A. (1998) Crusader castle torn apart by earthquake at dawn, 20 May 1202. *Geology* **26**: 303–6.

Ellis, E. S. (1946) *Ancient Anodynes: Primitive Anaesthesia and Allied Conditions* (London: Heinemann).

Emden, A. B. (1957–9) *A Biographical Register of the University of Oxford to AD 1500*, 3 vols. (Oxford: Clarendon Press).

Epstein, S. (1984) *Wills and Wealth in Medieval Genoa, 1150–1250* (Cambridge, Mass.: Harvard University Press).

Evans, W. C. (1996) *Trease and Evans' Pharmacognosy* (14th edn., London: W. B. Saunders).

Favreau, M.-L. (1975) *Studien zur Frühgeschichte des Deutschen Ordens*. Kieler Historische Studien XXI (Stuttgart: Ernst Klett).

Feigenbaum, A. (1955a) On the use of embryonic tissue for therapeutic purposes, enhancing wound healing, by an eye practitioner of the 12th century – Benvenutus Grapheus Hierosolymitanus. *Acta Medica Orientalia* **14**: 26–9.
  (1955b) Notes on ocular diseases and their treatment, including surgical procedures, contained in the work of Benvenutus Grapheus Hierosolymitanus, an eye practitioner of the 12th century. *Acta Medica Orientalia* **14**: 75–82.
  (1957) Archeological evidence of the occurrence of regular seasonal ophthalmias in ancient Egypt. *Janus* **46**: 165–72.

Ficarra, B. J. (1996) Disease to death during the crusades. In M. Waserman and S. S. Kottek (eds.), *Health and Disease in the Holy Land* (Lewiston: Edwin Mellen), pp. 135–55.

Fiorato, V., Boylston, A. and Knüsel, C. (eds.) (2000) *Blood Red Roses: The Archaeology of a Mass Grave from the Battle of Towton, AD 1461* (Oxford: Oxbow).

Fisher, G. J. (1996) Historical and bibliographical notes. xx. Haly Abbas. In F. Sezgin, M. Amawi, C. Ehrig-Eggert and E. Neubauer (eds.), *'Ali Ibn Al-'Abbas Al-Majusi (4th/10th cent.)* (Frankfurt: Johann Wolfgang Goethe University), pp. 11–19.

Fitzgerald, M. J. T. (1985) *Neuroanatomy: Basic and Applied* (London: Bailliere Tindall).

Forey, A. (1973) *The Templars in the Corona de Aragon* (London: Oxford University Press).

(1977) The military order of St Thomas of Acre. *English Historical Review* **92**: 481–503.

(1984) The militarisation of the hospital of St John. *Studia Monastica* **26**: 75–89.

(1992) *The Military Orders from the Twelfth to the Early Fourteenth Centuries* (Basingstoke: Macmillan).

(1998) Literacy and learning in the military orders during the twelfth and thirteenth centuries. In H. Nicholson (ed.), *The Military Orders.* II: *Welfare and Warfare* (Ashgate: Aldershot), pp. 185–206.

France, J. (1998) The anonymous Gesta Francorum and the Historia Francorum qui Ceperunt Iherusalem of Raymond of Aguilers and the Historia de Hierosolymitano Itinere of Peter Tudebode: an analysis of the textual relationship between primary sources for the First Crusade. In J. France and W. G. Zajac (eds.), *The Crusades and their Sources* (Aldershot: Ashgate), pp. 39–69.

(2001) Recent writing on medieval warfare: from the fall of Rome to c.1300. *The Journal of Military History* **65**: 441–73.

France, J. and Zajac, W. G. (eds.) (1998) *The Crusades and their Sources* (Aldershot: Ashgate).

Freeman, P. W. M. and Pollard, A. (eds.) (2001) *Fields of Conflict: Progress and Prospect in Battlefield Archaeology*. BAR International Series no. 958 (Oxford: Archaeopress).

French, R. K. (1978) The thorax in history. III: Beginning of the Middle Ages. *Thorax* **33**: 295–306.

(1994) Astrology in medical practice. In L. Garcia-Ballester, R. French, J. Arrizabalaga and A. Cunningham, *Practical Medicine from Salerno to the Black Death* (Cambridge: Cambridge University Press), pp. 30–59.

(1999) *Dissection and Vivisection in the European Renaissance* (Aldershot: Ashgate).

Friedman, Y. (2000) See Jerusalem and die: Jerusalem as a last stop in crusader times. In J. Schwartz, Z. Amar and I. Ziffer (eds.), *Jerusalem and Eretz Israel* (Tel Aviv: Eretz Israel Museum), pp. 89–99.

(2002) *Encounters Between Enemies: Captivity and Ransom in the Latin Kingdom of Jerusalem* (Leiden: E. J. Brill).

Frohberg, U. (1989) Oral and maxillofacial surgery: the state of the art in early medieval Europe. *Bulletin of the History of Dentistry* **37**: 105–7.

Gabriel, R. A. and Metz, K. S. (1992) *A History of Military Medicine* I (New York: Greenwood Press).

Garcia-Ballester, L. (1987) Medical science in thirteenth century Castille: problems and prospects. *Bulletin of the History of Medicine* **61**: 183–202.

(1994) A marginal learned medical world: Jewish, Muslim and Christian medical practitioners and the use of Arabic medical sources in late medieval Spain. In L. Garcia-Ballester, R. French, J. Arrizabalaga and A. Cunningham (eds.), *Practical Medicine from Salerno to the Black Death* (Cambridge: Cambridge University Press), pp. 353–94.

Garcia-Ballester, L., McVaugh, M. R. and Rubio-Vela, A. (1989) Medical licensing and learning in fourteenth century Valencia. *Transactions of the American Philosophical Society* **79**: 1–128.

Gautier, P. (1974) Le typikon du Christ Saveur Pantocrator. *Revue des Études Byzantines* **32**: 1–145.

Getz, F. (1991) *Healing and Society in Medieval England: A Middle English Translation of the Pharmaceutical Writings of Gilbertus Anglicus* (Madison: University of Wisconsin).

(1995) Medical education in later medieval England. In V. Nutton and R. Porter (eds.), *The History of Medical Education in Britain* (Amsterdam: Rodopi), pp. 76–93.

(1998) *Medicine in the English Middle Ages* (Princeton: Princeton University Press).

Gil-Sotres, P. (1994) Derivation and revulsion: the theory and practice of medieval phlebotomy. In L. Garcia-Ballester, R. French, J. Arrizabalaga and A. Cunningham (eds.), *Practical Medicine from Salerno to the Black Death* (Cambridge: Cambridge University Press), pp. 110–55.

Gilchrist, R. (1995) *Contemplation and Action: the Other Monasticism* (London: Leicester University Press).

Giles, J. A. (ed.) (1852–4) *Matthew Paris: English History from the Years 1235–1273*, 3 vols. (London: Henry G. Bohn).

Girdler, R. W. (1990) The Dead Sea transform fault system. *Tectonophysics* **180**: 1–13.

Glick, T. F. (1971) Muhtasib and mustasaf: a case study of institutional diffusion. *Viator* **2**: 59–81.

Goldmann, Z. (1966) The hospice of the Knights of St John in Akko. *Archaeology* **19**: 182–9.

(1994) *Akko in the Time of the Crusaders: the Convent of the Order of Saint John* (Akko (Israel): Government Tourist Office).

Goldstein, H. I. (1931) Maggots in the treatment of wound and bone infections. *Journal of Bone and Joint Surgery* **13**: 476–8.

Gordon, E. C. (1991) Accidents among medieval children as seen from the miracles of six English saints and martyrs. *Medical History* **35**: 145–63.

Goss, V. P. and Bornstein, C. V. (eds.) (1986) *The Meeting of Two Worlds: Cultural Exchange Between East and West During the Period of the Crusades* (Kalamazoo: Western Michigan University).

Gougaud, L. (1924) La pratique de la phlébotomie dans les cloîtres. *Revue Mabillon* **14**: 1–13.

Grandclaude, M. (1923) *Etude Critique sur les Livres des Assises de Jérusalem* (Paris: Jouve).

(1926) Classement summaire des manuscripts des principaux Livres des Assises de Jérusalem. *Revue Historique de Droit Français et Etranger* **5**: 418–75.

Grauer, A. L. and Roberts, C. A. (1996) Paleoepidemiology, healing and possible treatment of trauma in the medieval cemetery population of St Helen-on-the-Walls, York, England. *American Journal of Physical Anthropology* **100**: 531–44.

Green, M. H. (1994) Documenting medieval women's medical practice. In L. Garcia-Ballester, R. French, J. Arrizabalaga and A. Cunningham (eds.), *Practical Medicine from Salerno to the Black Death* (Cambridge: Cambridge University Press), pp. 322–52.

Gross, R. L. and Newberne, P. M. (1980) Role of nutrition and immunologic function. *Physiological Reviews* **60**: 188–251.

Habib Khan, A. and Riaz Ali Perwaz, S. (1980) Zahrawi's contribution to dentistry. *Studies in History of Medicine* **7**: 115–29.

Haddad, F. S. (1986–7) Surgical firsts in Arabic medical literature. *Studies in History of Medicine and Science* **10–11**: 95–103.

Hallback, D. (1976–7) A medieval (?) bone with a copper plate support, indicating an open surgical treatment. *OSSA* **3–4**: 63–82.

Hamarneh, S. K. (1993) Health sciences in al-Andalus, Tunisia and Egypt during 10–12th centuries. *Studies in History of Medicine and Science* **12**: 1–42.

Hamarneh, S. K. and Awad, H. A. (1977) Early surgical instruments excavated in Old Cairo, Egypt. *International Surgery* **62**: 520–4.

Hamilton, B. (1999) The way to Rome and Jerusalem: pilgrim routes from France and Germany at the time of the crusades. In M. A. Anton-Villasanchez (ed.), *Santiago, Roma, Jerusalem. Actas del III Congreso Internacional de Estudios Jacobeos* (Santiago de Compostela: Xunta de Galicia), pp. 135–44.

Hamilton, R. W. (1949) *The Structural History of the Aqsa Mosque: A Record of Archaeological Gleanings from the Repairs of 1938–1942* (London: Oxford University Press).

Hammond, E. A. (1960) Incomes of medieval English doctors. *Journal of the History of Medicine and Allied Sciences* **15**: 154–69.

Handerson, H. E. (1918) *Gilbertus Anglicus: Medicine of the Thirteenth Century* (Cleveland: Cleveland Medical Library Association).

Hartung, E. F. (1934) Medical regulations of Frederick the Second of Hohenstaufen. *Medical Life* **41**: 587–601.

Harvey, B. (1993) *Living and Dying in England, 1100–1540: the Monastic Experience* (Oxford: Clarendon).

Haskins, C. H. (1960) *Studies in the History of Mediaeval Science* (New York: Frederick Ungar).

Hauben, D. J. and Sonneveld, G. J. (1983) The influence of war on the development of plastic surgery. *Annals of Plastic Surgery* **10**: 65–9.

Henderson, J. (1989) The hospitals of late mediaeval and renaissance Florence: a preliminary survey. In L. Granshaw and R. Porter (eds.), *The Hospital in History* (London: Routledge), pp. 63–92.

Hiestand, R. (1988) König Balduin und sein Tanzbär. *Archiv für Kulturgeschichte* **70**: 343–380.

(1989) Skandinavische Kreuzfahrer, griechischer Wein und eine leichenöffnung im Jahre 1110. *Würzburger Medizinhistorische Mitteilungen* **7**: 143–53.

Hill, D. R. (1998) Trebuchets. In D. A. King (ed.), *Studies in Medieval Islamic Technology* (Aldershot: Ashgate), ch. XIX.

Hillenbrand, C. (1999) *The Crusades: Islamic Perspectives* (Edinburgh: Edinburgh University Press).

Hillgarth, J. N. (1971) *Ramon Lull and Lullism in Fourteenth Century France* (Oxford: Clarendon Press).

Holck, P. (2002) Two 'medical' cases from medieval Oslo. *International Journal of Osteoarchaeology* **12**: 166–72.

Horden, P. (1988) A discipline of relevance: the historiography of the later mediaeval hospital. *Social History of Medicine* **1**: 359–74.

Horwitz, L. K. and Dahan, E. (1996) Animal husbandry practices during the historic periods. In A. Ben-Tor, M. Avissar and Y. Portugali (eds.), *Yoqne'am I: the Late Periods*. Qedem Reports no. 3 (Jerusalem: Hebrew University), pp. 246–55.

Hubbard, R. N. L. B. and McKay, J. (1986) Medieval plant remains. In D. Pringle (ed.), *The Red Tower* (London: British School of Archaeology in Jerusalem), pp. 187–91.

Hume, E. E. (1940) *Medical Work of the Knights Hospitallers of St John of Jerusalem* (Baltimore: Johns Hopkins).

Hunt, L.-A. (1997–8) Manuscript production by Christians in 13th–14th century Greater Syria and Mesopotamia and related areas. *ARAM* **9–10**: 289–336 (also reprinted in L.-A. Hunt, *Byzantium, Eastern Christendom and Islam: Art at the Crossroads of the Medieval Mediterranean* (London: Pindar Press 2000), II, pp. 153–97).

Hunt, R. W. (1950) Stephen of Antioch. *Mediaeval and Renaissance Studies* **2**: 172–3.

Hunt, T. (1990) *Popular Medicine in Thirteenth-Century England* (Cambridge: D. S. Brewer).

(1992) *The Medieval Surgery* (Woodbridge: Boydell Press).

Hurnand, N. D. (1969) *The King's Pardon for Homicide before AD 1307* (Oxford: Clarendon Press).

Infusino, M., O'Neill, Y. V. and Calmes, S. (1989) Hog beans, poppies and mandrake leaves – a test of the efficacy of the medieval 'soporific sponge'. In R. S. Atkinson and T. B. Boulton (eds.), *The History of Anaesthesia* (London: Royal Society of Medicine – Parthenon Publishing), pp. 29–33.

Ingelmark, B. E. (1939–40) The skeletons. In Thordman, B., Norlund, O. and Ingelmark, B. E. *Armour from the Battle of Visby, 1361*, 2 vols. (Stockholm: Kungl. Vitterhets Historie Och Atikvitets Akademien), I, pp. 149–209.

Irwin, R. (1998) Usamah ibn Munqidh: an Arab-Syrian gentleman at the time of the crusades reconsidered. In J. France and W. G. Zajac (eds.), *The Crusades and their Sources* (Aldershot: Ashgate), pp. 71–87.

Iskandar, A. Z. (1962) Galen and Rhazes on examining physicians. *Bulletin of the History of Medicine* **36**: 362–5.

Jackson, R. (1988) *Doctors and Diseases in the Roman Empire* (London: British Museum).

Jackson, S. W. (1972) Unusual mental states in Medieval Europe. 1. Medical syndromes of mental disorder: 400–1100 AD. *Journal of the History of Medicine* **27**: 262–97.

Jacoby, D. (1979) Crusader Acre in the thirteenth century: urban layout and topography. *Studi Medievali* **20**: 1–46.

Jacquart, D. (1979) *Dictionnaire Biographique des Médecins en France au Moyen Age. Supplément* (Geneva: Droz).

(1981) *Le Milieu Médical en France du XIIe au XVe Siècle* (Geneva: Droz).

(1994) Medical practice in Paris in the first half of the fourteenth century. In L. Garcia Ballester, R. French, J. Arrizabalaga and A. Cunningham (eds.), *Practical Medicine from Salerno to the Black Death* (Cambridge: Cambridge University Press), pp. 186–210.

Jadon, S. (1970a) A comparison of the wealth, prestige and medical works of the physicians of Salah al-Din in Egypt and Syria. *Bulletin of the History of Medicine* **44**: 64–75.

(1970b) The physicians of Syria during the reign of Salah al-Din 570–589 AH, 1174–1193 AD. *Journal of the History of Medicine and Allied Sciences* **25**: 323–40.

James, R. and Nasmyth-Jones, R. (1992) The occurrence of cervical fractures in victims of judicial hanging. *Forensic Science International* **54**: 81–91.

James, T. (1983) A history of bloodletting. *Adler Museum Bulletin* **9**: 21–8.

Janssens, P. A. (1987) A copper plate on the upper arm in a burial at the church in Vrasene (Belgium). *Journal of Paleopathology* **1**: 15–18.

Jarcho, S. (1944) Guide for physicians (Musar Harofim) by Isaac Judaeus (880?–932?). *Bulletin of the History of Medicine* **15**: 180–8.

(1987) A history of semitertian fever. *Bulletin of the History of Medicine* **61**: 411–30.

Jaspert, N. (1997) Heresy and holiness in a Mediterranean dynasty: the house of Barcelona in the thirteenth and fourteenth centuries. In D. A. Agius and I. R. Netton (eds.), *Across the Mediterranean Frontiers: Trade, Politics and Religion, 650–1450* (Turnhout: Brepols), pp. 105–35.

Johansen, K. and Watson, J. (1998) Compartment syndrome: new insights. *Seminars in Vascular Surgery* **11**: 294–301.

Jones, W. R. (1983) The clinic in three mediaeval societies. *Diogenes* **122**: 86–101.

Judd, M. A. and Roberts, C. A. (1998) Fracture patterns at the medieval leper hospital in Chichester. *American Journal of Physical Anthropology* **105**: 43–55.

(1999) Fracture trauma in a medieval British farming village. *American Journal of Physical Anthropology* **109**: 229–43.

Juvin, P. and Desmonts, J.-M. (2000) The ancestors of inhalational anesthesia: the soporific sponges (xith–xviith centuries): how a universally recommended technique was abruptly discarded. *Anesthesiology* **93**: 265–9.

Karger, B., Sudhues, H., Kneubuehl, B. P. and Brinkmann, B. (1998) Experimental arrow wounds: ballistics and traumatology. *The Journal of Trauma: Injury, Infection and Critical Care* **45**: 495–501.

Karmi, G. (1979) State control of the physicians in the Middle Ages: an Islamic model. In A. W. Russell (ed.), *The Town and State Physician in Europe from the Middle Ages to the Enlightenment* (Wolfenbuttel: Herzog August Bibliothek), pp. 63–84.

Kass, E. H. and Sossen, H. S. (1959) Prevention of infection of the urinary tract in the presence of indwelling catheters. *Journal of the American Medical Association* **169**: 1181–3.

Kedar, B. Z. (1995) Benvenutus Grapheus of Jerusalem, an oculist in the era of the crusades. *Korot* **11**: 14–41.

(1998) A twelfth century description of the Jerusalem Hospital. In H. Nicholson (ed.), *The Military Orders.* II: *Welfare and Warfare* (Aldershot: Ashgate), pp. 3–26.

(1999) On the origins of the earliest laws of Frankish Jerusalem: the Canons of the Council of Nablus, 1120. *Speculum* **74**: 310–35.

(2001) Convergences of oriental Christian, Muslim and Frankish worshipers: the case of Saydnaya and the Knights Templar. In Z. Hunyadi and J. Laszlovszky (eds.), *The Crusades and the Military Orders* (Budapest: Central European University), pp. 89–100.

Kedar, B. Z. and Pringle, D. (1985) La Feve: a crusader castle in the Jezreel Valley. *Israel Exploration Journal* **35**: 164–79, plates 20–1.

Kedar, B. Z. and Kohlberg, E. (1995) The intercultural career of Theodore of Antioch. *Mediterranean Historical Review* **10**: 164–76.

Kerridge, I. H. and Lowe, M. (1995) Bloodletting: the story of a therapeutic technique. *The Medical Journal of Australia* **163**: 631–3.

Kettenes-Van Den Bosch, J. J., Salemink, C. A. and Khan, I. (1981) Biological activity of the alkaloids of *Papaver bracteatum* Lindl. *Journal of Ethnopharmacology* **3**: 21–38.

Keys, T. E. (1963) *The History of Surgical Anesthesia* (New York: Dover).

King, E. J. (1932) *The Seals of the Order of St John of Jerusalem* (London: Methuen).

(1934) *The Rules, Statutes and Customs of the Hospitallers: 1099–1310* (London: Methuen).

Kirkup, J. R. (1981) The history and evolution of surgical instruments. *Annals of the Royal College of Surgeons of England* **63**: 279–85.

Kirsch, P. E. (1969) Some aspects of law and medicine in the Latin Kingdom of Jerusalem. In C. H. Wechte and H. Karplus (eds.), *Proceedings of the Fifth International Medical-Legal Seminar, Israel, March 15–25, 1969* (Jaffa: Hebrew University), pp. 9–16.

Klein-Franke, F. (1986) What was the fatal disease of al-Malik al-Salih Najm al-Din Ayyub? In M. Sharon (ed.), *Studies in Islamic History and Civilization* (Leiden: E.J. Brill), pp. 153–7.

Knight, I. and Eldridge, J. (1984) *The Heights and Weights of Adults in Great Britain* (London: HMSO).

Knüsel, C. J. (2000) Activity-related skeletal change. In Fiorato, V., Boylston, A. and Knüsel, C. (eds.), *Blood Red Roses: the Archaeology of a Mass Grave from the Battle of Towton AD 1461* (Oxford: Oxbow Books), pp. 103–18.

Knüsel, C. J. and Goggel, S. (1993) A cripple from the medieval hospital of Ss. James and Mary Magdalen, Chichester. *International Journal of Osteoarchaeology* 3: 155–65.

Knüsel, C. J., Kemp, R. L. and Budd, P. (1995) Evidence for remedial medical treatment of a severe knee injury from Fishergate Gilbertine Monastery in the City of York. *Journal of Archaeological Science* 22: 369–84.

Kohanski, T. (ed.) (2001) *The Book of John Mandeville* (Arizona: Arizona State University).

Kohlberg, E. and Kedar, B. Z. (1988) A Melkite physician in Frankish Jerusalem and Ayyubid Damascus: Muwaffaq al-Din Ya'qub b. Siqlab. *Asian and African Studies* 22: 113–26.

Kohler, C. (1898) Traité du recouvrement de la Terre Sainte addresse, vers l'an 1295, à Philippe le Bel par Galvano de Levanto, médecin genois. *Revue de l'Orient Latin* 6: 343–69 (discussion and Latin edition of the text).

Kristeller, P. O. (1945) The school of Salerno: its development and its contribution to the history of learning. *Bulletin of the History of Medicine* 17: 138–94.

Kritikos, P. G. and Papadaki, S. P. (1967) The history of the poppy and of opium in antiquity in the eastern Mediterranean area. *Bulletin on Narcotics* 19: 5–10.

Kroll, J. and Bachrach, B. (1984) Sin and mental illness in the Middle Ages. *Psychological Medicine* 14: 507–14.

Kunitz, S. J. (1987) Making a long story short: a note on men's height and mortality in England from the first through the nineteenth centuries. *Medical History* 31: 269–80.

Kunzl, E. (1996) Forschungsberichte zu den antiken medizinischen Instrumenten. *Aufstieg und Niedergang der Römischen Welt* 37: 2433–639.

(1999) Roman medical tools according to archaeological sources. *Michmanim* 13: 60–9.

Kuriyama, S. (1995) Interpreting the history of bloodletting. *Journal of the History of Medicine and Allied Sciences* 50: 11–46.

Lang, S. J. (1992) John Bradmore and his book Philomena. *Social History of Medicine* 5: 121–30.

Langbein, J. H. (1977) *Torture and the Law of Proof* (Chicago: University of Chicago).

Langlois, Ch.-V. (1887) *Le Règne de Philippe III Le Hardi* (Paris: Hachette).

Lanhers, M.-C., Fleurentin, J., Cabalion, P., Rolland, A., Dorfman, P., Misslin, R. and Pelt, J.-M. (1990) Behavioral effects of *Euphorbia hirta* L.: sedative and anxiolytic properties. *Journal of Ethnopharmacology* 29: 189–98.

Lascaratos, J. (1992) The penalty of blinding during Byzantine times: medical remarks. *Documenta Ophthalmologica* 81: 133–44.

Lascaratos, J. and Marketos, S. (1996) A little known emperor physician: Manuel I Comnenus of Byzantium (1143–1180). *Journal of Medical Biography* 4: 187–90.

(1998) The cause of death of the Byzantine Emperor John 1 Tzimisces (969–976): poisoning or typhoid fever? *Journal of Medical Biography* **6**: 171–4.

Lascaratos, L. and Voros, D. (1998) The fatal wounding of Emperor John II Comnenus. *Journal of Wound Care* **7**: 195–6.

Latham, R. E. (1994) *Revised Medieval Latin Word List, From British and Irish Sources* (London: British Academy/Oxford University Press).

Leclerq, J. (1965) Traités contemporains de Dante sur les sujets qu'il a traités. *Studi Medievali*, series 3, **6**: 491–535.

Leiser, G. (1983) Medical education in Islamic lands from the seventh to the fourteenth century. *Journal of the History of Medicine and Allied Sciences* **38**: 48–75.

Leopold, A. (2000) *How to Recover the Holy Land: the Crusade Proposals of the Late Thirteenth and Early Fourteenth Centuries* (Aldershot: Ashgate).

Leven, K.-H. (1991) Byzantinische Kaiser und ihre Leibärzte zur Darstellung der Medizin der Komnenenzeit durch Niketas Choniates. *Würzburger Medizin-historische Mitteilungen* **9**: 73–104.

Levey, M. (1963) Fourteenth century Muslim medicine and the hisba. *Medical History* **7**: 176–82.

(1970) Embalming procedures of al-Razi. *Pharmacy in History* **12**: 169.

Levy, R. (1929) *Baghdad Chronicle* (Cambridge: Cambridge University Press).

Lewis, B. (1964) Maimonides, Lionheart and Saladin. *Eretz-Israel* **7**: 70–5.

Lieber, E. (1979) Galen: physician as philosopher. Maimonides: philosopher as physician. *Bulletin of the History of Medicine* **53**: 268–85.

Lilley, J. M., Stroud, G., Brothwell, D. R. and Williamson, M. H. (1994) *The Jewish Burial Ground at Jewbury* (York Archaeological Trust: York).

Lloyd, S. (1988) *English Society and the Crusade, 1216–1307* (Oxford: Clarendon).

Lokhorst, G.-J. (1982) An ancient Greek theory of hemispheric specialisation. *Clio Medica* **17**: 33–8.

Lorentzon, M. (1992) Mediaeval London: care of the sick. *History of Nursing Society Journal* **4**: 100–10.

Lunardini, A., Caramella, D., Mallegni, F. and Fornaciari, G. (2000) Frontal fracture with therapeutic trepanation in an early medieval skull from northern Italy. *Journal of Paleopathology* **12**: 21–5.

Luttrell, A. (1994) The Hospitallers' medical tradition: 1291–1530. In Barber, M. (ed.), *The Military Orders: Fighting for the Faith and Caring for the Sick* (Variorum: Aldershot), pp. 64–81.

(1996) The earliest Templars. In M. Balard (ed.), *Autour de la Première Crusade*, Série Byzantina Sorbonensia 14 (Paris: Publications de la Sorbonne), pp. 193–202.

(1997) The earliest Hospitallers. In B. Z. Kedar, J. Riley-Smith and R. Hiestand (eds.), *Montjoie* (Variorum: Aldershot), pp. 37–54

(1998) Margarida d'Erill, hospitaller of Alguaire 1415–1456. *Anuario de Estudios Medievales* **28**: 219–49.

Maalouf, A. (1984) *The Crusades Through Arab Eyes*. Trans. J. Rothschild (London: Al Saqi).

MacCallan, A. F. (1913) *Trachoma and its Complications in Egypt* (Cambridge: Cambridge University Press).

MacFarlane, R. G. (1962) The reactions of the blood to injury. In H. Florey (ed.), *General Pathology* (London: Lloyd-Luke Medical Books) pp. 216–33.

MacKinney, L. C. (1960) A thirteenth century medical case history in miniatures. *Speculum* **35**: 251–9.

(1962) The beginnings of western scientific anatomy: new evidence and a revision in interpretation of Mandeville's role. *Medical History* **6**: 233–9.

Malewicz, M. (1974) Libellus de efficatia artis astrologice. Traité astrologique d'Eudes de Champagne, xiie siècle. *Mediaevalia Philosophica Polonorum* **20**: 1–95. (includes discussion as well as the Latin text).

Manchester, K. and Elmhirst, O. E. C. (1980) Forensic aspects of an Anglosaxon injury. *OSSA* **7**: 179–88.

Martin, R. (1959) *Lehrbuch der Anthropologie*, 2 vols. (3rd edn., Stuttgart: Gustav Fischer), ii, p. 787.

Matthews, L. G. (1967) The City of York's first spicers, grocers and apothecaries. *Pharmaceutical Historian* **1**: 2–3.

Mauron, J. (1986) Food, mood and health: the mediaeval outlook. *International Journal for Vitamin and Nutrition Research* **29** suppl.: 9–26.

Mayer, H. E. (1988) *The Crusades*. Trans J. Gillingham (2nd edn., Oxford: Oxford University Press).

Mays, S. A. (1996) Healed limb amputations in human osteoarchaeology and their causes: a case study from Ipswich, UK. *International Journal of Osteoarchaeology* **6**: 101–13.

McMinn, R. M. H. (ed.) (1994) *Last's Anatomy. Regional and Applied* (9th edn., Edinburgh: Churchill Livingstone).

McVaugh, M. R. (1992) Arnold of Villanova's Regimen Almarie (Regimen Castra Sequentium) and medieval military medicine. *Viator* **23**: 201–13.

(1993) *Medicine Before the Plague. Practitioners and their Patients in the Crown of Aragon, 1285–1345* (Cambridge: Cambridge University Press).

(1994) Royal surgeons and the value of medical learning: the Crown of Aragon, 1300–1350. In L. Garcia-Ballester, R. French, J. Arrizabalaga and A. Cunningham (eds.), *Practical Medicine from Salerno to the Black Death* (Cambridge: Cambridge University Press), pp. 211–36.

(1997) Bedside manners in the Middle Ages. *Bulletin of the History of Medicine* **71**: 201–23.

(1998a) Treatment of hernia in the later Middle Ages: surgical correction and social construction. In R. French, J. Arrizabalaga, A. Cunningham and L. Garcia-Ballester (eds.), *Medicine from the Black Death to the French Disease* (Ashgate: Aldershot), pp. 131–55.

(1998b) Therapeutic strategies: surgery. In M. D. Grmek and B. Fantini (eds.), *Western Medical Thought from Antiquity to the Middle Ages*. Trans A. Shugaar (Cambridge, Mass.: Harvard University Press), pp. 273–90.

(2000) Surgical education in the Middle Ages. *Dynamis* **20**: 283–304.

(2001) Cataracts and hernias: aspects of surgical practice in the fourteenth century. *Medical History* **45**: 319–40.

Meagher, D. J. (2001) Delirium: optimising management. *British Medical Journal* **322**: 144–9.

Meaney, A. L. (1981) *Anglo-Saxon Amulets and Curing Stones*, series no. 96 (Oxford: British Archaeological Reports).

Mencacci, L. (1996) L'assistenza sanitaria nello spedale di Altopascio. In A. Cenci (ed.), *L'Ospitalità in Altopascio. Storia e Funzioni di un Grande centro Ospitaliero* (Lucca: Comune di Altopascio), pp. 130–48.

Merrillees, R. S. (1962) Opium trade in the Bronze Age Levant. *Antiquity* **36**: 287–92.

Metcalf, D. M. (1995) *Coinage of the Crusades and the Latin East* (2nd edn., London: Royal Numismatic Society).

Meyerhof, M. (1936) The history of trachoma treatment in antiquity and during the Arabic Middle Ages. *Bulletin of the Ophthalmological Society of Egypt* **29**: 26–87.

Militzer, K. (1998) The role of hospitals in the Teutonic Order. In H. Nicholson (ed.), *The Military Orders.* II: *Welfare and Warfare* (Aldershot: Ashgate), pp. 51–9.

Miller, J. E. (1960) Javelin thrower's elbow. *Journal of Bone and Joint Surgery* **42B**: 788–91.

Miller, R. L., Ikram, S., Armelagos, G. J., Walker, R., Harer, W. B., Shiff, C. J., Baggett, D., Carrrigan, M. and Maret, S. M. (1994) Diagnosis of Plasmodium falciparum infections in mummies using the rapid manual ParaSight^{TM}-F test. *Transactions of the Royal Society of Tropical Medicine and Hygiene* **88**: 31–2.

Miller, T. S. (1978) The knights of Saint John and the Hospitallers of the Latin west. *Speculum* **53**: 709–33.

(1984) Byzantine hospitals. *Dumbarton Oaks Papers* **38**: 53–63.

(1990) The Sampson Hospital of Constantinople. *Byzantinische Forschungen* **15**: 101–35.

(1997) *The Birth of the Hospital in the Byzantine Empire* (2nd edn., Baltimore: Johns Hopkins University Press).

(1999) Byzantine physicians and their hospitals. *Medicina Nei Secoli Arte E Scienza* **11**: 323–35.

Milne, J. S. (1907) *Surgical Instruments in Greek and Roman Times* (Oxford: Clarendon Press).

Mitchell, P. D. (1994) Pathology in the crusader period: human skeletal remains from Tel Jezreel. *Levant* **26**: 67–71.

(1997) Further evidence of disease in the crusader period population of Le Petit Gérin (Tel Jezreel). *Tel Aviv* **24**: 169–79.

(1998) The archaeological approach to the study of disease in the Crusader States, as employed at *Le Petit Gérin*. In H. Nicholson (ed.), *The Military Orders.* II: *Welfare and Warfare* (Aldershot: Ashgate), pp. 43–50.

(1999a) The integration of the palaeopathology and medical history of the crusades. *International Journal of Osteoarchaeology* **9**: 333–43.

(1999b) Tuberculosis in the Crusades. In G. Palfi, O. Dutour, J. Deak and I. Hutas (eds.), *Tuberculosis: Past and Present*. (Golden Book-TB Foundation: Budapest-Szeged, Hungary), pp. 43–9.

(2000a) An evaluation of the leprosy of King Baldwin IV of Jerusalem in the context of the mediaeval world. Appendix in B. Hamilton, *The Leper King and his Heirs. Baldwin IV and the Crusader Kingdom of Jerusalem* (Cambridge: Cambridge University Press), pp. 245–58.

(2000b) The evolution of social attitudes to the medical care of those with leprosy within the Crusader States. *Cahiers du GRHIS (Rouen)* **11**: 21–30.

(2002) The myth of the spread of leprosy with the crusades. In: C. A. Roberts, M. E. Lewis and K. Manchester (eds.), *The Past and Present of Leprosy* (Oxford: Archaeopress), pp. 171–7.

(2003) Pre-Columbian treponemal disease from 14th century AD Safed, Israel and the implications for the medieval eastern Mediterranean. *American Journal of Physical Anthropology* **121**: 117–24.

(2004a) Evidence for elective surgery in the Frankish states of the near east in the crusader period (12th–13th centuries). In K. P. Jankrift and F. Steger (eds.), *Gesundheit-Krankheit: Kulturtransfer medizinischen Wissens von der Spätantike bis in die Frühe Neuzeit*. (Cologne: Böhlau-Verlag), pp. 121–38.

(2004b) The palaeopathology of skulls recovered from a medieval cave cemetery near Safed, Israel. *Levant* **36**: 243–50.

(in press) (a) The infirmaries of the Order of the Temple in the Frankish states of the medieval eastern Mediterranean. In B. Bowers (ed.), *The Medieval Hospital and Medical Practice: Bridging the Evidence*. (Aldershot: Ashgate) (in press).

(in press) (b) Disease. In A. V. Murray (ed.), *Encyclopedia of the Crusades* (ABC-Clio: Santa Barbara).

(in press) (c) War Injuries. In A. V. Murray (ed.), *Encyclopedia of the Crusades* (ABC-Clio: Santa Barbara).

(in press) (d) The torture of military captives in the crusades to the medieval Middle East. In M. Yazigi and N. Christie (eds.), *Noble Ideals and Bloody Realities: Warfare in the Middle Ages, 1378–1492* (Leiden: E. J. Brill).

Mitchell, P. D. and Stern E. (2000) Parasitic intestinal helminth ova from the latrines of the 13th century crusader Hospital of St John in Acre, Israel. In M. La Verghetta and L. Capasso (eds.), *Proceedings of the XIIIth European Meeting of the Paleopathology Association, Chieti, Italy 2000* (Teramo: Edirafital SpA), pp. 207–13.

Mitchell, P. D., Huntley, J. and Stern, E. (in press) Bioarchaeological analysis of the 13th century latrines of the crusader Hospital of St John at Acre, Israel. In W. Zajac (ed.), *The Military Orders. III: Their History and Heritage* (Aldershot: Ashgate).

Moffat, B. and Fulton, J. (1988) *SHARP Practice 2. The Second Report on Researches into the Medieval Hospital at Soutra, Lothian Region, Scotland* (Edinburgh: SHARP).

Moffat, B., Thomson, B. S. and Fulton, J. (1989) *The Third Report on the Researches into the Medieval Hospital at Soutra* (Edinburgh: SHARP).

Mogle, P. and Zias, J. (1995) Trephination as a possible treatment for scurvy in a Middle Bronze Age (c.2200 BC) skeleton. *International Journal of Osteoarchaeology* **5**: 77–81.

Møller-Christensen, V. (1938) *The History of Forceps*. Trans. W. E. Calvert (London: Oxford University Press).

Molleson, T. and Blondiaux, J. (1994) Riders' bones from Kish, Iraq. *Cambridge Archaeological Journal* **4**: 312–16.

Morris, C. (1992) The eleventh century school of Salerno. *Sydsvenska Medicinhistoriska Sallskapets Arsskrift* **29**: 77–84.

Munro, D. C. and Haagensen, C. D. (1933) Arabian medicine as represented in the memoirs of Usamah ibn Munqidh. *Annals of Medical History* **5**: 226–35.

Munter, A. H. (1936) A study of the lengths of the long bones of the arms and legs in man, with special reference to Anglosaxon skeletons. *Biometrika* **28**: 258–94.

Murray-Jones, P. (1994) John of Aderne and the Mediterranean tradition of scholastic surgery. In L. Garcia-Ballester, R. French, J. Arrizabalaga and A. Cunningham (eds.), *Practical Medicine from Salerno to the Black Death* (Cambridge: Cambridge University Press), pp. 289–321.

Nabri, I. A. (1983) El Zahrawi (936–1013 AD), the father of operative surgery. *Annals of the Royal College of Surgeons of England* **65**: 132–4.

Neugebauer, R. (1979) Medieval and early modern theories of mental illness. *Archives of General Psychiatry* **36**: 477–83.

Nicolle, D. (1979) An introduction to arms and warfare in classical Islam. In R. Elgood (ed.), *Islamic Arms and Armour* (London: Scolar Press), pp. 162–86.

(1980) The Monreale capitals and the military equipment of later Norman Sicily. *Gladius* **15**: 87–103.

(1983) The Cappella Palatina ceiling and the Muslim military inheritance of Norman Sicily. *Gladius* **16**: 45–145.

(1988) *Arms and armour in the Crusading era: 1050–1350*. (New York: Kraus), I, pp. 318–35 and II, pp. 804–11.

(1993) Wounds, military surgery and the reality of crusading warfare; the evidence of Usamah's memoirs. *Journal of Oriental and African Studies* **5**: 33–46.

(1994) The reality of Mamluk warfare: weapons, armour and tactics. *Al-Masaq* **7**: 77–110.

(1999) Medieval warfare: the unfriendly interface. *The Journal of Military History* **63**: 579–600.

Niermeyer, J. F. and van de Kieft, C. (2002) *Mediae Latinitatis Lexicon Minus* (Leiden: E. J. Brill).

Norris, J. (1983) The 'scurvy disposition': heavy exertion as an exacerbating influence on scurvy in modern times. *Bulletin of the History of Medicine* **57**: 325–38.

Novak, S. A. (2000) Battle-related trauma. In V. Fiorato, A. Boylston and C. Knüsel (eds.), *Blood Red Roses: the Archaeology of a Mass Grave from the Battle of Towton AD 1461* (Oxford: Oxbow Books), pp. 90–102.

Nutton, V. (1969) Medicine and the Roman army: a further consideration. *Medical History* **13**: 260–70.

(1979) Continuity or rediscovery? The city physician in classical antiquity and mediaeval Italy. In A. W. Russell (ed.), *The Town and State Physician in Europe from the Middle Ages to the Enlightenment* (Wolfenbüttel: Herzog August Bibliothek), pp. 9–46.

(1986) Essay review. *Medical History* **30**: 218–21.

Oakshott, E. (1994) *The Sword in the Age of Chivalry* (2nd edn., Woodbridge: Boydell Press).

O'Boyle, C. (1994) Surgical texts and social contexts: physicians and surgeons in Paris, c.1270–1430. In L. Garcia-Ballester, R. French, J. Arrizabalaga and A. Cunningham (eds.), *Practical Medicine from Salerno to the Black Death* (Cambridge: Cambridge University Press), pp. 156–85.

(1998) *The Art of Medicine: Medical Teaching at the University of Paris, 1250–1400* (Leiden: E. J. Brill).

Olivieri, B. (1968) The 'Spongia Soporifera'. *Salerno* **2**: 45–55.

Olry, R. (1997) Medieval neuroanatomy: the text of Mondino dei Luzzi and the plates of Guido da Vigevano. *Journal of the History of the Neurosciences* **6**: 113–23.

O'Neill, Y. V. (1970) Another look at the 'Anatomia Porci'. *Viator* **1**: 117–24.

(1976) Innocent III and the evolution of anatomy. *Medical History* **20**: 429–33.

Oppenheimer, S. J. (2001) Iron and its relation to immunity and infectious disease. *The Journal of Nutrition* **131**(2S-II): 616–35.

Orme, N. and Webster, M. (1995) *The English Hospital, 1070–1570* (New Haven: Yale University Press).

Ortiz, J. A. and Berger, R. A. (1998) Compartment syndrome in the hand and wrist. *Hand Clinics* **14**: 405–18.

Ortner, D. J. and Ribas, C. (1997) Bone changes in a human skull from the early Bronze Age site of Bab Edh-Dhra', Jordan, probably resulting from scalping. *Journal of Paleopathology* **9**: 137–42.

Ovadiah, A. (1993) A crusader church in the Jewish quarter of the old city of Jerusalem. In Y. Tasfrir (ed.), *Ancient Churches Revealed*. (Jerusalem: Israel Exploration Society), pp. 136–9.

Page, W. (ed.) (1905–28) *The Victoria History of the County of Buckingham*, 5 vols. (London: St Catherine Press).

Pahlitzsch, J. (2001). *Graeci und Suriani im Palästina der Kreuzfahrerzeit* (Berlin: Duncker and Humblot).

Park, K. (1994). The criminal and the saintly body: autopsy and dissection in renaissance Italy. *Renaissance Quarterly* **47**: 1–33.

(1995) The life of the corpse: division and dissection in late medieval Europe. *Journal of the History of Medicine and Allied Sciences* **50**: 111–32.

(1998) Stones, bones and hernias: surgical specialists in fourteenth- and fifteenth-century Italy. In R. French, J. Arrizabalaga, A. Cunningham and L. Garcia-Ballester (eds.), *Medicine from the Black Death to the French Disease* (Ashgate: Aldershot), pp. 110–30.

Parker, S., Roberts, C. and Manchester, K. (1985–6) A review of British trepanations with reports on two new cases. *OSSA* **12**: 141–57.

Parker, T. W. (1963) *The Knights Templar in England* (Tucson: University of Arizona).

Partner, N. F. (1977) *Serious Entertainments: the Writing of History in Twelfth-Century England* (Chicago: University of Chicago).

Partner, P. (1987) *The Knights Templar and their Myth* (Rochester (USA): Destiny Books).

Passmore, R. and Eastwood, M. A. (eds.) (1986) *Human Nutrition and Dietetics* (8th edn., Edinburgh: Churchill Livingstone).

Paterson, L. M. (1988) Military surgery: knights, sergeants and Raimon of Avignon's version of the *Chirurgia* of Roger of Salerno (1180–1209). In C. Harper-Bill and R. Harvey (eds.), *The Ideals and Practice of Medieval Knighthood* II (Woodbridge: Boydell Press), pp. 117–46.

Peers, E. A. (1929) *Ramon Lull, a Biography* (London: Society for Promoting Christian Knowledge).

Pereira, M. (1989) *The Alchemical Corpus Attributed to Raymond Lull* (London: Warburg Institute).

Perrot, R. (1988) The materia medicalis in the therapy of medieval injuries. *Journal of Paleopathology* **1**: 147–56.

Persaud, T. V. (1984) *Early History of Human Anatomy* (Springfield: Charles C. Thomas).

Peters, E. (1985) *Torture* (Oxford: Blackwell).

Phillips, I., Fernandez, R. and Gundara, N. S. (1968) Acetic acid in the treatment of superficial wounds infected by Pseudomonas aeruginosa. *Lancet* **1**: 11–13.

Poirier, P. P. and Taher, M. A. (1980) Historical seismicity in the Near and Middle East, North Africa and Spain from Arabic documents (VIIth–XVIIIth century). *Bulletin of the Seismological Society of America* **70**: 2185–201.

Pollard, T. and Oliver, T. (2002) *Two Men in a Trench: Battlefield Archaeology – the Key to Unlocking the Past* (London: Penguin).

Post, J. B. (1972) Doctor versus patient: two fourteenth-century law suits. *Medical History* **26**: 296–300.

Pounds, N. J. G. (1994) *An Economic History of Medieval Europe* (2nd edn., London: Longman).

Powell, J. M. (1986) *Anatomy of a Crusade, 1213–1221* (Philadelphia: University of Pennsylvania).

Prawer, J. (1951) L'établissement des coutumes du marché à Saint-Jean d'Acre et la date de composition du Livre des Assises des Bourgeois. *Revue Historique de Droit Français et Etranger* **29**: 329–51.

(1953) Historical maps of 'Akko. *Eretz Israel* **2**: 175–84 (in Hebrew).

(1972a) *The World of the Crusades* (London: Weidenfeld and Nicolson).

(1972b) *The Latin Kingdom of Jerusalem: European Colonialism in the Middle Ages* (London: Weidenfeld and Nicolson).

(1976) The Armenians in Jerusalem under the crusaders. In M. E. Stone (ed.), *Armenian and Biblical Studies* (Jerusalem: St James Press), pp. 222–36.

(1980) *Crusader Institutions* (Oxford: Clarendon Press).

Prescott, E. (1992) *The English Medieval Hospital, c.1050–1640* (London: Seaby).

Pringle, D. (1985) Reconstructing the castle of Safad. *Palestine Exploration Quarterly* **117**: 139–49.

(1990–1) Crusader Jerusalem, *Bulletin of the Anglo-Israel Archaeological Society* **10**: 105–13.

(1992) Aqua Bella: the interpretation of a crusader courtyard building. In B. Z. Kedar (ed.), *The Horns of Hattin* (London: Variorum), pp. 147–67.

(1993–) *The Churches of the Crusader Kingdom of Jerusalem*, 3 vols. (Cambridge: Cambridge University Press) (last volume in press).

Pryor, J. H. (1988) In Subsidium Terrae Sanctae: export of foodstuffs and raw materials from the Kingdom of Sicily to the Kingdom of Jerusalem, 1265–1284. *Asian and African Studies* **22**: 127–46.

Rang, H. P. and Dale, M. M. (1987) *Pharmacology* (Edinburgh: Churchill Livingstone).

Raphael, K. (1999) Crusader arms and armour. In S. Rozenberg (ed.), *Knights of the Holy Land: the Crusader Kingdom of Jerusalem* (Jerusalem: The Israel Museum), pp. 149–59.

Rath, G. (1964) Gilles de Corbeil as critic of his age. *Bulletin of the History of Medicine* **38**: 133–8.

Rawcliffe, C. (1988) The profits of practice: the wealth and status of medical men in later medieval England. *Social History of Medicine* **1**: 61–78.

(1998) Hospital nurses and their work. In R. Britnell (ed.), *Daily Life in the Late Middle Ages* (Stroud: Sutton Publishing), pp. 43–64.

(1999) Medicine for the soul: the mediaeval English hospital and the quest for spiritual health. In J. R. Hinnels and R. Porter (eds.), *Religion, Health and Suffering* (London: Kegan Paul International), pp. 316–38.

(2000) God, mammon and the physician: medicine in England before the College. *Journal of the Royal College of Physicians of London* **34**: 266–72.

Reverte, J. M. (1980) Trephined skulls in medieval Spain. *Paleopathology Newsletter* **32**: 5–6.

Rey, E. (1895) Les seigneurs de Giblet. *Revue de l'Orient Latin* **3**: 398–422.

Reynolds, D. F. (2001) *Interpreting the Self: Autobiography in the Arabic Literary Tradition* (Berkeley: University of California Press).

Richard, J. (1982) Hospitals and hospital congregations in the Latin kingdom during the first period of the Frankish conquest. In B. Z. Kedar, H. E. Mayer and R. C. Smail (eds.), *Outremer: Studies in the History of the Crusading Kingdom of Jerusalem* (Jerusalem: Yad Izhak Ben-Zvi Institute), pp. 89–100.

(1992) *Saint Louis: Crusader King of France*. Trans. J. Birrell (Cambridge: Cambridge University Press), p. 325.

Richards, D. S. (1992) A doctor's petition for a salaried post in Saladin's hospital. *Social History of Medicine* **5**: 297–306.

(1994) Saladin's hospital in Jerusalem: its foundation and some later archival material. In K. Athamina and R. Heacock (eds.), *The Frankish Wars and their Influence on Palestine* (Jerusalem: Birzeit University), pp. 70–83.

Riley-Smith, J. (1967) *The Knights of St John in Jerusalem and Cyprus, 1050–1310* (London: Macmillan Press).
(1999) *Hospitallers: the History of the Order of St John* (London: Hambledon Press).
(2002) Casualties and the number of knights on the First Crusade. *Crusades* 1: 13–28.
Riley-Smith, J. S. C. (ed.) (1991) *The Atlas of the Crusades* (London: Times Books).
(1999) *The Oxford History of the Crusades* (Oxford: Oxford University Press).
Rimon, O. (1996) Medical instruments from the Roman Period. In O. Rimon (ed.), *Illness and Healing in Ancient Times* (Haifa: University of Haifa) pp. 62*–71*.
Robinson, C. F. (2003) *Islamic Historiography* (Cambridge: Cambridge University Press).
Robinson, V. (1947) *Victory Over Pain: a History of Anesthesia* (London: Sigma).
Romm, S. (1989) Arms by design: from antiquity to the renaissance. *Plastic and Reconstructive Surgery* **84**: 158–63.
Rose, F. C. (1997) The history of head injuries: an overview. *Journal of the History of the Neurosciences* **6**: 154–80.
Rose, J. C., Taani, F., al-Hourani, S. and Vannini, G. (1998) Crusader period disease in Jordan. In E. Strouhal (ed.), *Abstracts of the xiith European Meeting of the Paleopathology Association, Prague-Pilsen, Czech Republic, August 26–29, 1998* (Prague: Charles University), p. 77.
Rosenthal, F. (1978) The physician in medieval Muslim society. *Bulletin of the History of Medicine* **52**: 475–91.
Rosner, F. (1981) The medical writings of Moses Maimonides. *Clio Medica* **16**: 1–11.
(1996) Moses Maimonides and preventative medicine. *Journal of the History of Medicine and Allied Sciences* **51**: 313–24.
Rosser, J. (1986) Crusader castles of Cyprus. *Archaeology* **39**: 40–7.
Rowsome, P. and Yule, B. (1999) The Arab and Crusader sequence (area 1.14). In K. G. Holum, A. Raban and J. Patrich (eds.), *Caesarea Papers 2. Herod's Temple, the Provincial Governor's Praetorium and Granaries, the Later Harbor, a Gold Coin Hoard, and Other Studies* (Portsmouth (Rhode Island): *Journal of Roman Archaeology*), pp. 285–94.
Rubin, M. (1989) Development and change in English hospitals, 1100–1500. In L. Granshaw and R. Porter (eds.), *The Hospital in History* (London: Routledge), pp. 41–59.
Russel, J. C. (1936) Dictionary of writers of thirteenth century England. *Bulletin of the Institute of Historical Research*, Special Supplement no. 3: 1–209.
Saffron, M. H. (1975) Salernitan anatomists. In C. C. Gillispie (ed.), *Dictionary of Scientific Biography* (New York: Charles Scribner's Sons), xii, pp. 80–3.
Salame-Sarkis, H. (1980) *Contribution à l'Histoire de Tripoli et de sa Région à l'Epoque des Croisades* (Paris: Paul Geuthner).
Salazar, C. F. (1998) Getting the point: Paul of Aegina on arrow wounds. *Sudhoffs Archiv* **82**: 170–87.
(2000) *The Treatment of War Wounds in Graeco-Roman Antiquity* (Leiden: E. J. Brill).

Samaran, C. (1981) Projets Français de croisades de Philippe le Bel à Philippe de Valois. *Histoire Littéraire de la France* **41**: 33–74.

Santos, A. L., Umbelino, C., Goncalves, A. and Pereira, F. D. (1998) Mortal combat during the medieval Christian reconquest in Evora, Portugal. *International Journal of Osteoarchaeology* **8**: 454–6.

Sarton, G. (1927–48) *Introduction to the History of Science*, 3 vols. (Baltimore: Williams and Wilkins).

Savage-Smith, E. (1971a) Galen's account of the cranial nerves and the autonomic system. Part 1. *Clio Medica* **6**: 77–98.

(1971b) Galen's account of the cranial nerves and the autonomic system. Part 2. *Clio Medica* **6**: 173–94.

(1995) Attitudes toward dissection in medieval Islam. *Journal of the History of Medicine and Allied Sciences* **50**: 67–110.

(2000) The practice of surgery in Islamic lands: myth and reality. *Social History of Medicine* **13**: 307–21.

(in press) Between, reader and text: some medieval Arabic marginalia. In C. Burnett and D. Jacquart (eds.), *Writing in the Margin: a Context for the Development of Scientific Ideas, from Late Antiquity to the Rennaissance*. (Paris: L'Ecole Pratique des Hautes Etudes).

Scarborough, J. (1976a) Celsus on human vivisection at Ptolemaic Alexandria. *Clio Medica* **11**: 25–38.

(1976b) Galen's investigations of the kidney. *Clio Medica* **11**: 171–7.

Scarry, E. (1985) *The Body in Pain: the Making and Unmaking of the World* (Oxford: Oxford University Press).

Schacht, J. and Meyerhof, M. (1937) *The Medico-Philosophical Controversy Between Ibn Butlan of Baghdad and Ibn Ridwan of Cairo* (Cairo: Egyptian University).

Schick, C. Aceldama (1892) *Palestine Exploration Fund Quarterly Statement*: 283–9.

(1902) The Muristan or the site of the Hospital of St John of Jerusalem. *Quarterly Statements of the Palestine Exploration Fund*: 42–56.

Scott, G. R. (1940) *A History of Torture* (London: Werner Laurie) (reprinted 1995, London: Studio Editions).

Segal, J. B. (1971) Ibn al-'Ibri. In B. Lewis, V. L. Menage, Ch. Pellat and J. Schacht (eds.), *Encyclopedia of Islam* (new (2nd) edn, Leiden: E. J. Brill), III(ii) pp. 804–5.

Seigworth, G. R. (1980) Bloodletting over the centuries. *New York State Journal of Medicine* **80**: 2022–8.

Selwood, D. (1999) *Knights of the Cloister: Templars and Hospitallers in Central-Southern Occitania c.1100–c.1300* (Woodbridge: Boydell Press).

Setton, K. M. (ed.) (1955–89) *A History of the Crusades*, 6 vols. (1955–89) (Philadelphia: University of Pennsylvania Press, I, and Madison: University of Wisconsin, II–VI).

Shahar, S. (1993) Who were old in the Middle Ages? *Social History of Medicine* **6**: 313–41.

Shatzmiller, J. (ed.) (1989) *Médecine et Justice en Provence Médiévale: Documents de Manosque, 1262–1348* (Aix-en-Provence: University of Provence).

Sigerist, H. E. (1935) The history of medical licensing. *Journal of the American Medical Association* **104**: 1057–60.

(1942) The sphere of life and death in early medieval manuscripts. *Bulletin of the History of Medicine* **11**: 293–303.

(1943) A Salernitan student's surgical notebook. *Bulletin of the History of Medicine* **14**: 505–12.

Simili, A. (1973) The beginnings of forensic medicine in Bologna. In H. Karplus (ed.), *International Symposium on Society, Medicine and Law* (Amsterdam: Elsevier), pp. 91–100.

Sinclair, K. V. (1978) The French prayer for the sick in the hospital of the knights of Saint John of Jerusalem at Acre. *Mediaeval Studies* **40**: 484–8.

Singer, D. W. (1928) The alchemical testament attributed to Raymund Lull. *Archeion* **9**: 43–52.

Singh, G. B., Kaur, S., Satti, N. K., Atal, C. K. and Maheshweri, J. K. (1984) Anti-inflammatory activity of *Euphorbia acaulis* roxb. *Journal of Ethnopharmacology* **10**: 225–33.

Sinha, D. N. (1982) Status of anatomy in the University of Bologna (13th to 18th centuries). *Studies in History of Medicine* **6**: 141–6.

Siraisi, N. G. (1973) *Arts and Sciences at Padua: the Studium of Padua Before 1350* (Toronto: Pontifical Institute).

(1981) *Taddeo Alderotti and his Pupils: Two Generations of Italian Medical Learning* (Princeton: Princeton University Press).

(1990) *Medieval and Early Renaissance Medicine* (Chicago: University of Chicago Press).

(1994a) The faculty of medicine. In H. Ridder-Symoens (ed.), *A History of the University in Europe. 1: Universities in the Middle Ages* (Cambridge: Cambridge University Press), pp. 360–87.

(1994b) How to write a Latin book on surgery: organizing principles and authorial devices in Guglielmo da Saliceto and Dino del Garbo. In L. Garcia-Ballester, R. French, J. Arrizabalaga and A. Cunningham (eds.), *Practical Medicine from Salerno to the Black Death* (Cambridge: Cambridge University Press), pp. 88–109.

Sistrunk, T. G. (1993) The function of praise in the contract of a medieval public physician. *Journal of the History of Medicine and Allied Sciences* **48**: 320–34.

Skinner, P. (1997) *Health and Medicine in Early Medieval Southern Italy* (Leiden: E. J. Brill).

Smith, P. and Zegerson, T. (1999) Morbidity and mortality of post-Byzantine populations from Caesarea. In K. G. Holum, A. Raban and J. Patrich (eds.), *Caesarea Papers 2: Herod's Temple, the Provincial Governor's Praetorium and Granaries, the Later Harbor, a Gold Coin Hoard and Other Studies* (Portsmouth (Rhode Island): *Journal of Roman Archaeology*), pp. 433–40.

Sotres, P. G. (1998) The regimens of health. In M. D. Grmek, B. Fantini and A. Shugaar (eds.), *Western Medical Thought from Antiquity to the Middle Ages* (Cambridge, Mass.: Harvard University Press) pp. 291–318.

Spier, J. (1993) Medieval Byzantine magical amulets and their tradition. *Journal of the Warburg and Courtauld Institutes* **56**: 25–62.

Spufford, P. (1986) *Handbook of Medieval Exchange* (London: Royal Historical Society).

(1988) *Money and its Use in Medieval Europe* (Cambridge: Cambridge University Press).

Stephan, H.-G. (1993) Der Chirurg von der Weser (ca.1200–1265) – ein Glücksfall der Archäologie und Medizingeschichte. *Sudhoffs Archiv* **77**: 174–91.

Stern, E. J. (1999) Ceramic ware from the Crusader Period in the Holy Land. In S. Rozenberg (ed.), *Knights of the Holy Land: the Crusader Kingdom of Jerusalem* (Jerusalem: The Israel Museum), pp. 259–65.

Sterns, I. (1983) Care of the sick brothers by the crusader orders in the Holy Land. *Bulletin of the History of Medicine* **57**: 43–69.

Stirland, A. J. (1984) A possible correlation between os acromiale and occupation in the burials from the Mary Rose. In *Vth European Meeting of the Paleopathology Association, Siena* (Siena: University of Siena), pp. 327–33.

(1993) Asymmetry and activity related change in the male humerus. *International Journal of Osteoarchaeology* **3**: 105–13.

(1996) Patterns of trauma in a unique medieval parish cemetery. *International Journal of Osteoarchaeology* **6**: 92–100.

(2000) *Raising the Dead: the Skeleton Crew of Henry VIII's Great Ship the Mary Rose* (Chichester: John Wiley).

Stirland, A. J. and Waldron, T. (1997) Evidence for activity related markers in the vertebrae of the crew of the Mary Rose. *Journal of Archaeological Science* **24**: 329–35.

Sudhoff, K. (1915) Ein diätetischer Brief an Kaiser Friedrich II. von seinem Hofphilosophen Magister Theodorus. *Archiv für Geschichte der Medizin* **9**: 1–9.

Tabbaa, Y. (1997) *Constructions of Power and Piety in Medieval Aleppo* (Pennsylvania: Pennsylvania State University Press).

Talbot, C. H. (1967) *Medicine in Medieval England* (London: Oldbourne).

Talbot, C. H. and Hammond, E. A. (1965) *The Medical Practitioners in Medieval England. A Biographical Register* (London: Wellcome Historical Medical Library).

Thomas, C., Sloane, B. and Phillpotts, C. (1997) *Excavations at the Priory and Hospital of St Mary Spital, London* (London: Museum of London), p. 111.

Thompson, C. J. S. (1942) *The History and Evolution of Surgical Instruments* (New York: Schuman).

Thurzo, M., Lietava, J. and Vondrakova, M. (1991) A case of an unusually large survived neurocranial trauma with marks of partial trephination from West Slovakia (10th century AD). *Journal of Paleopathology* **4**: 37–45.

Toll, C. (1998) Arabic medicine and hospitals in the Middle Ages: a probable model for the military orders' care of the sick. In H. Nicholson (ed.), *The Military Orders. II: Welfare and Warfare* (Aldershot: Ashgate), pp. 35–41.

Trease, G. E. (1959) The spicers and apothecaries of the royal household in the reigns of Henry III, Edward I and Edward II. *Nottingham Medieval Studies* **3**: 19–52.

Tritton, A. S. and Gibb, H. A. R. (1933) The first and second crusades from an anonymous Syriac chronicle. *Journal of the Royal Asiatic Society*, 69–101 and 274–305.

Trotter, D. A. (1999) Arabic surgery in eastern France and in the Midi: the old French and Occitan versions of the Chirurgie d'Albucasis. *Forum for Modern Language Studies* **35**: 358–71.

Trotter, M. and Gleser, G. C. (1958) A re-evaluation of estimation of stature based on measurements taken during life and of long bones after death. *American Journal of Physical Anthropology* **16**: 79–123.

Tsukayama, D. T. and Gustilo, R. B. (1996) Microbiology of open fractures. In C. M. Court-Brown, M. M. McQueen, A. A. Quaba and A. Sarmiento (eds.), *Management of Open Fractures* (London: Martin Dunitz), pp. 37–42.

Urban, W. (2003) *The Teutonic Knights: a Military History* (London: Greenhill).

van Eikels, K. (1998) Knightly hospitallers or crusading knights? Decisive factors for the spread of the Teutonic Knights in the Rhineland and the Low Countries, 1216–1300. In H. Nicholson (ed.), *The Military Orders. II: Welfare and Warfare* (Aldershot: Ashgate), pp. 75–80.

Vedrani, A. (1921) Ugo Borgognoni e Teodorico Borgognoni. In A. Mieli (ed.), *Gli Scienziati Italiano* (Rome: Dott. Attilio Nardeccheia), 1 (2), pp. 312–20.

Vernia, P. (1988) The muhtasib of Valencia and pharmacy in Aragon. *Pharmacy in History* **30**: 89–93.

Vetch, J. (1807) *An Account of the Ophthalmia which has Appeared in England Since the Return of the British Army from Egypt* (London: Longman, Hurst, Rees & Orme).

Vincent, N. (1996) *Peter des Roches: an Alien in English Politics, 1205–1238* (Cambridge: Cambridge University Press).

Voigts, L. E. and Hudson, R. P. (1992) A drynke that men callen dwale to make a man slepe whyle men kerven him: a surgical anesthetic from late medieval England. In S. Campbell, B. Hall and D. Klausner (eds.), *Health, Disease and Healing in Medieval Culture* (London: Macmillan), pp. 34–56.

Voigts, L. E. and McVaugh, M. (1984) A Latin technical phlebotomy and its middle English translation. *Transactions of the American Philosophical Society* **74**: 1–69.

von Staden, H. (1992) The discovery of the body: human dissection and its cultural contexts in ancient Greece. *The Yale Journal of Biology and Medicine* **65**: 223–41.

Wallis, F. (2000) Inventing diagnosis: Theophilus' *De Urinis* in the classroom. *Dynamis* **20**: 31–73.

Walsh, J. J. (1919) The medical history of two crusades. In *Contributions to Medical and Biological Research, Dedicated to Sir William Osler*, 2 vols. (New York: Paul B. Hoeber,), II, pp. 796–805.

Wangensteen, O. H., Smith, J. and Wangensteen, S. D. (1967) Some highlights in the history of amputation reflecting lessons in wound healing. *Bulletin of the History of Medicine* **41**: 97–131.

Ward, B. (1982) *Miracles and the Medieval Mind. Theory, Record and Event, 1000–1215* (London: Scolar Press).

Warren, C. and Conder, C. R. (1884) *The Survey of Western Palestine: Jerusalem* (London: Palestine Exploration Fund).

Watson, R. R. (ed.) (1984) *Nutrition, Disease Resistance and Immune Function* (New York: Dekker).

Watt, W. M. (1991) *Muslim-Christian Encounters: Perceptions and Misperceptions* (London: Routledge).

Weber, J. and Czarnetzki, A. (2001) Neurotraumatological aspects of head injuries resulting from sharp and blunt force in the early Medieval Period of southwestern Germany. *American Journal of Physical Anthropology* **114**: 352–6.

Weinberg, E. D. (1974) Iron and susceptibility to infectious disease. *Science* **184**: 952–6.

Wells, C. (1964) The human skeleton. In S. E. West, Excavations at Cox Lane [1958] and at the town defences, Shire Hall Yard, Ipswich [1959]. *Proceedings of the Suffolk Institute of Archaeology* **29**: 233–335 (see pp. 329–33).

(1974) The results of 'bone setting' in Anglo-Saxon times. *Medical and Biological Illustration* **24**: 215–20.

Wenham, S. J. (1989) Anatomical interpretations of Anglo-Saxon weapon injuries. In S. C. Hawkes (ed.), *Weapons and Warfare in Anglo-Saxon England*, Monograph no. 21 (Oxford: Oxford University Committee for Archaeology), pp. 123–39.

Wickersheimer, E. (1929) *Recueil des Plus Célèbres Astrologues et Quelques Hommes Doctes Faict par Symon de Phares du Temps de Charles VIIIe* (Paris: Champion).

(1936) *Dictionnaire Biographique des Médecins en France au Moyen Age* (Paris: Droz).

(1951) Organisation et législation sanitaires au Royaume franc de Jerusalem (1099–1291). *Archeion. Archives Internationales d'Histoire des Sciences* **30**: 689–705.

Wilkinson, J., Hill, J. and Ryan, W. F. (eds.) (1988) *Jerusalem Pilgrimage 1099–1185* (London: Hakluyt Society).

Williams, A. (1978) *The Metallurgy of Muslim Armour*, Monograph no. 3, Seminars on Early Islamic Science (Manchester: University of Manchester).

Williams, C. K., Barnes, E. and Snyder, L. M. (1997) Frankish Corinth: 1996. *Hesperia* **66**: 7–47.

Woodings, A. F. (1971) The medical resources and practice of the Crusader States in Syria and Palestine, 1096–1193. *Medical History* **15**: 268–77.

Zias, J. and Pomeranz, S. (1992) Serial craniectomies for intracranial infection 5.5 millennia ago. *International Journal of Osteoarchaeology* **2**: 183–6.

Index